Temporal Bone Imaging

Harshavardhan Mahalingam
Editor

Temporal Bone Imaging

A Case-Based Approach

Springer

Editor
Harshavardhan Mahalingam
Department of Radiology
and Imaging Sciences
Sri Ramachandra Institute
of Higher Education and Research (SRIHER)
Chennai, Tamil Nadu, India

ISBN 978-981-95-6131-5 ISBN 978-981-95-6132-2 (eBook)
https://doi.org/10.1007/978-981-95-6132-2

This Springer imprint is published by the registered company Springer Nature Singapore Pte Ltd.
The registered company address is: 152 Beach Road, #21-01/04 Gateway East, Singapore 189721, Singapore

Contents

About the Book

This book covers the basics of temporal bone imaging essential for beginners, including multiplanar and three-dimensional imaging anatomy, the latest imaging techniques and must-know pathologies presented through image-intensive chapters. A case-based learning method has been employed enabling better knowledge retention and easier application of the concepts to daily practice. Chapters are divided according to pathologies rather than anatomical regions helping readers develop a holistic approach to evaluating computed tomography and magnetic resonance imaging scans. Imaging techniques with relevant imaging anatomy, congenital anomalies of the temporal bone, infections, neoplasia, trauma, cochlear implantation imaging and post-operative imaging are covered, all with an emphasis on image-based learning. This book will be a valuable tool for beginners and post-graduate trainees in radiology and otorhinolaryngology by providing essential information on this complex topic in a lucid and interactive manner. Online supplementary DICOM data are provided in many chapters in Parts 1 and 2. Readers are encouraged to download the DICOM files and view them with a DICOM viewer software. Multiplanar reconstruction of the DICOM data will further aid in developing a deeper understanding of imaging anatomy and pathology.

About the Editor

Harshavardhan Mahalingam completed his MBBS at Madras Medical College, Chennai, India, and post-graduation in radiology at Postgraduate Institute of Medical Education and Research (PGIMER), Chandigarh, India; senior residency and fellowship in cross-sectional imaging at Christian Medical College (CMC), Vellore, India. He is working as a consultant radiologist at Sri Ramachandra Institute of Higher Education and Research (SRIHER), Chennai, India. He has published many papers in peer-reviewed national and international journals and delivered numerous lectures at various national and international conferences.

Part I
Temporal Bone Anatomy and Imaging Techniques

Chapter 1
Gross Anatomy and Development of the Temporal Bone Relevant to Imaging

Harshavardhan Mahalingam

1.1 Anatomy of Temporal Bone

The temporal bones are paired structures that form a part of the lateral aspect and base of the skull. Each temporal bone can be divided into five distinct parts—squamous, petrous, mastoid, tympanic, and styloid. Gross anatomy of the temporal bone is represented in Figs. 1.1, 1.2, and 1.3.

The *squamous* part of the temporal bone forms its superior and lateral component. It is shaped like a shell. Its outer surface is convex and lies beneath the subcutaneous tissue of the scalp. It gives rise to the temporalis muscle. Its inner surface is concave and grooved by meningeal vessels. Superiorly, it articulates with parietal bone and anteriorly with greater wing of sphenoid. The zygomatic process of the temporal bone arises from lateral surface of the temporal bone and articulates with the temporal process of zygomatic bone forming the zygomatic arch. The glenoid or mandibular fossa is located along the inferior aspect of the zygomatic process between the articular eminence anteriorly and the tympanic part of temporal bone posteriorly.

The *mastoid* part of the temporal bone forms its posterior component. It is continuous superiorly with the squamous part. It shows an inferior projection called mastoid process. A groove for digastric muscle is seen on medial aspect of the mastoid process. The occipital, posterior auricular, digastric, sternocleidomastoid, and longissimus capitis muscles are attached to the mastoid. The *sigmoid sulcus* is seen on intracranial aspect of the mastoid for the transverse venous sinus. The mastoid has a number of hollow air-filled spaces within called mastoid air cells and an irregular-shaped larger cavity called *mastoid antrum*. This communicates with the epitympanum via the *aditus ad antrum.*

H. Mahalingam (✉)
Department of Radiology, SRIHER, Chennai, India

H. Mahalingam (ed.), *Temporal Bone Imaging*,
https://doi.org/10.1007/978-981-95-6132-2_1

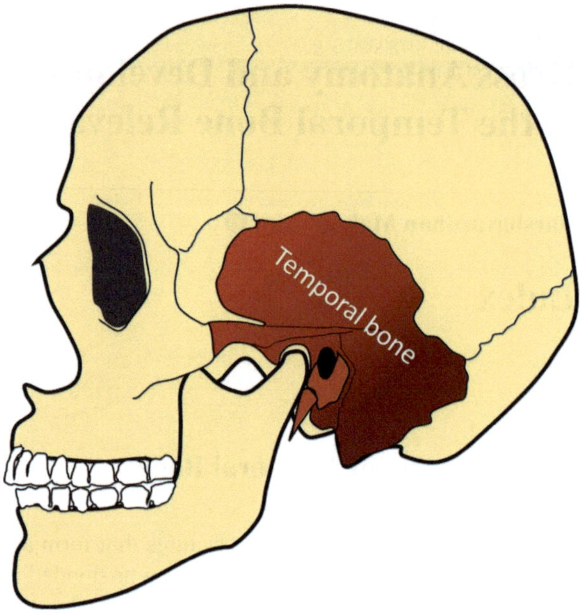

Fig. 1.1 Schematic representation of the skull from lateral view showing the position of the temporal bone

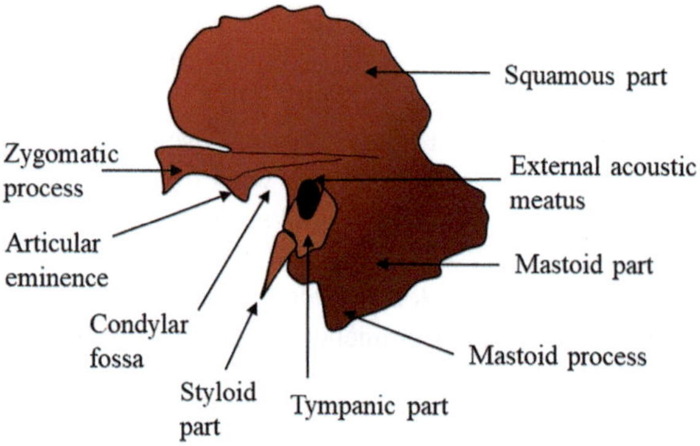

Fig. 1.2 Parts of the temporal bone as viewed from external aspect

The *petrous* part of the temporal bone is a pyramid-shaped structure with base situated laterally and apex pointing medially and anteriorly. It is situated in the skull base between the sphenoid anteriorly and basi-occiput posteriorly. The significant landmarks on anterior face of the pyramid are the depression from the *Meckel's cave* near the apex, the *arcuate eminence* near its midportion, and the tegmen tympani just lateral to the arcuate eminence. The *internal acoustic meatus* is situated in center of the posterior face. Posteroinferior to the internal acoustic meatus is a small slit connecting to *vestibular aqueduct* which transmits the endolymphatic sac. The inferior surface of the petrous temporal bone is irregular and marked anteriorly by the aperture of *carotid canal* and posteriorly by *jugular foramen.* The jugular

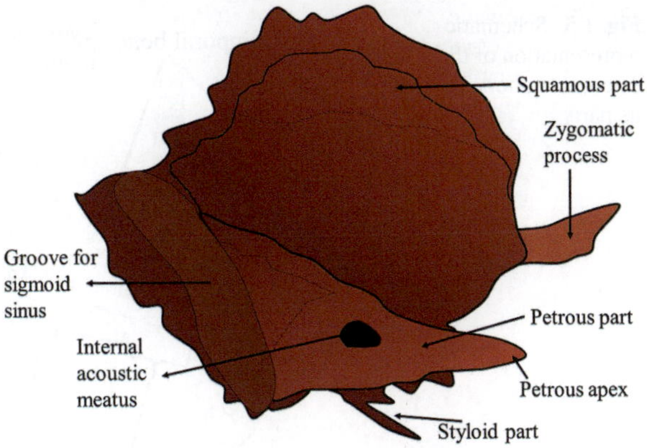

Fig. 1.3 Parts of the temporal bone as viewed from internal aspect

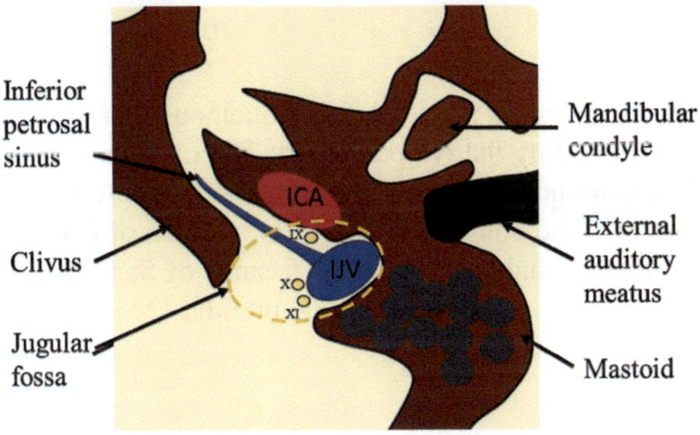

Fig. 1.4 Anatomy of the jugular fossa. ICA, internal carotid artery. IJV, internal jugular vein. IX, glossopharyngeal nerve. X, vagus nerve. XI, spinal accessory nerve

foramen transmits the IX, X, and XI cranial nerves, inferior petrosal sinus, and the sigmoid sinus. Anatomy of the jugular fossa is represented in Fig. 1.4.

The *styloid* process arises from the inferior surface of petrous temporal bone and projects anteriorly and medially. It is around 2.5 cm in length. The stylomastoid foramen is located between the styloid process and mastoid process and transmits the facial nerve.

The *tympanic* part of the temporal bone is located inferior to squamous portion and anterior to the mastoid. It forms the anterior wall, floor, and posterior wall of the bony external auditory canal [1].

1.1.1 The External Auditory Canal (EAC)

It is an S-shaped canal measuring around 2.5 cm to 3 cm in length and extends from the pinna to the tympanic membrane. The canal is directed antero-infero-medially. Its lateral third is fibrocartilaginous while the medial two-third is bony. Anatomy of the external auditory canal is represented in Fig. 1.5. The roof and superior part of

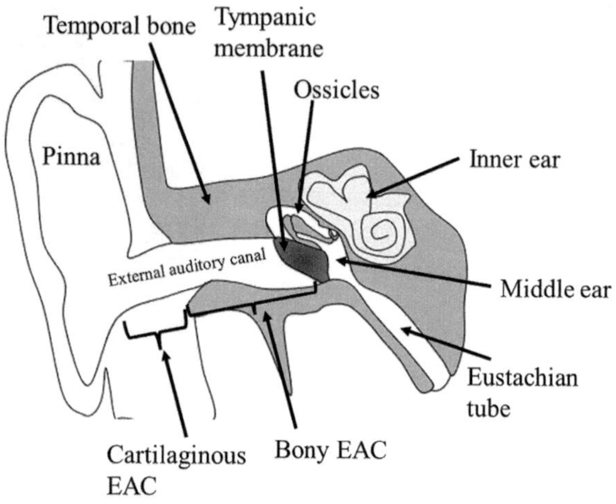

Fig. 1.5 Schematic representation of the external auditory canal and its parts

posterior wall is formed by the squamous part of the temporal bone while the rest are formed by the tympanic part. The canal is narrowest at the osteocartilaginous junction known as isthmus. Sometimes, a defect is observed in the anteroinferior aspect of the bony canal known as foramen of Huschke. The cartilaginous part can also have small defects called fissures of Santorini. These can serve as routes for spread of disease from the canal into the TM joint and infratemporal fossa [2].

1.1.2 Tympanic Membrane

It lies at the medial end of the external auditory canal and separates it from the middle ear cavity. It is oval shaped and measures around 10 mm in maximum diameter. The periphery of the TM is a fibrocartilaginous ring attached to the tympanic sulcus at the medial end of the EAC. There is a defect in the anterosuperior part of the ring at the site of notch of Rivinus in the tympanic sulcus. The anterior and posterior malleolar folds extend from the margins of the defect to the handle of malleus. This part of the TM between the malleolar folds is called *pars flaccida* and the rest of the TM is called *pars tensa*. The *umbo* is the point in the TM at the location of the most inferior part of the handle of malleus which is pulled medially toward the middle ear cavity. The anatomy of the tympanic membrane is represented in Fig. 1.6.

1.1.3 The Middle Ear

The middle ear is an air-filled cleft within the petrous temporal bone lying between the TM laterally and inner ear structures medially. It can be divided into three parts—from superior to inferior, these are epitympanum or attic above level of TM,

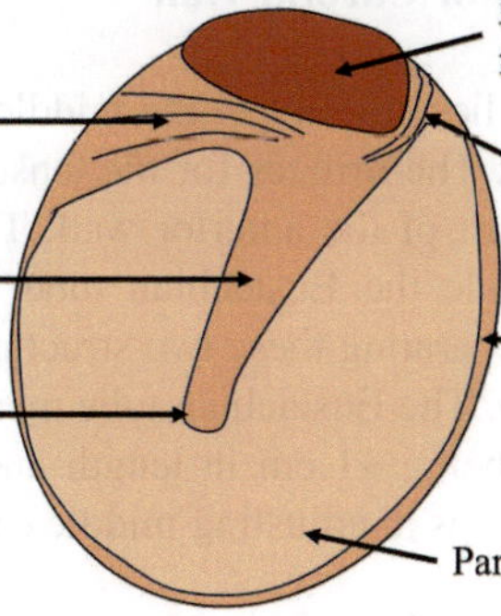

Fig. 1.6 Diagram showing the parts of the tympanic membrane

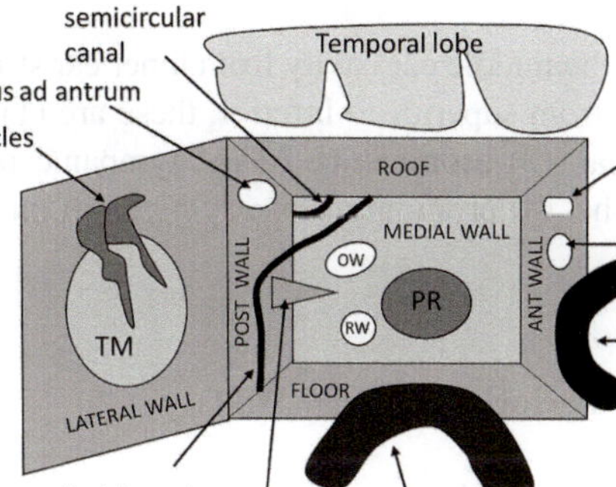

Fig. 1.7 Schematic representation of the walls of the middle ear and the landmarks on each of the wall. OW, oval window; RW, round window

the mesotympanum at level of TM, and hypotympanum below level of TM. The middle ear cavity is much shorter mediolaterally measuring 2 to 6 mm in width, with height and anteroposterior dimension of around 15 mm. For the purpose of description, the middle ear cavity can be considered as cuboid with six walls (Fig. 1.7).

1.1.3.1 Lateral or Membranous Wall

The lateral wall is formed by the tympanic membrane and the squamous temporal bone superior to it. The most medial part of the roof of EAC is called the scutum (located at the superior margin of TM). The tympanic membrane is directed obliquely downward and inward with respect to the EAC forming angle of 55 degrees with the EAC. Three apertures are seen close to the superior aspect of the TM—the petrotympanic fissure (transmits anterior tympanic branch of maxillary artery and anterior ligament of malleus) and the anterior and posterior tympanic apertures (which transmit the chorda tympani branch of facial nerve).

1.1.3.2 Anterior or Carotid Wall

The carotid canal lies anterior to the middle ear cavity and is separated from it by thin cortical bone. The orifices for the tensor tympani and Eustachian tube canals mark the upper part of the anterior wall. The semicanal of the tensor tympani is more superior while the Eustachian tube lies more inferior with the processus cochleariformis separating these two structures. Both the canals are directed anteriorly and inferiorly. The Eustachian tube measures ~3.5 cm in length—the posterolateral bony part being ~1 cm in length and rest being fibrous/cartilaginous. The Eustachian tube helps in adjusting middle ear pressure.

1.1.3.3 Medial or Labyrinthine Wall

It separates the middle ear cavity from inner ear structures and is marked by various structures—from superior to inferior, these are (1) prominence of the lateral semicircular canal, (2) prominence of the tympanic part of the facial canal, (3) oval window niche, (4) promontory overlying basal turn of cochlea, and (5) round window niche.

1.1.3.4 Posterior or Mastoid Wall

The superior part of the posterior wall presents the aditus ad antrum which connects the epitympanum to the mastoid antrum. The pyramidal eminence is seen posterolateral to the oval window. It gives rise to the stapedius muscle, the tendon of which pierces its apex to attach to the stapes. The vertical or mastoid part of facial canal lies near the posterior wall just lateral to the pyramidal eminence. The space medial to the pyramidal eminence is called the sinus tympani while the space lateral to it is called the facial recess (Fig. 1.8).

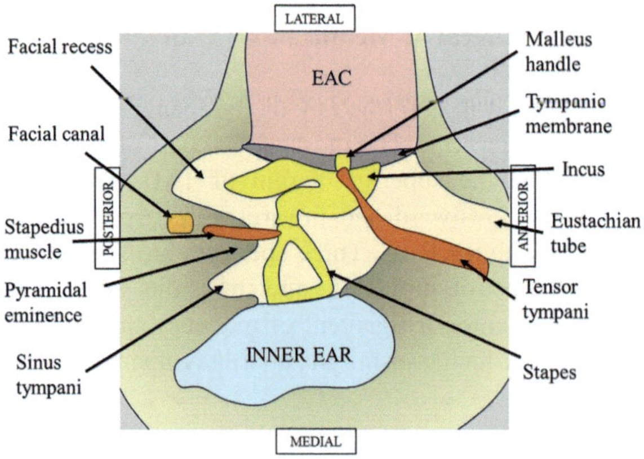

Fig. 1.8 A view of the middle ear cavity from superior aspect showing the anterior and posterior wall structures

1.1.3.5 Roof or Tegmental Wall

The tegmen is a thin plate of bone separating the middle ear and mastoid antrum from the intracranial compartment. The tegmen meets the squamous temporal bone laterally at the petrosquamous sutures which is potential route of spread of infection from the middle ear into the intracranial compartment.

1.1.3.6 Floor or Jugular Wall

The floor is a thin plate of bone separating the middle ear from the internal jugular vein. The thickness of bone is related to size of the jugular bulb. In case of large jugular bulb, the wall may be very thin or dehiscent.

1.1.3.7 Contents of Middle Ear Cavity—The Ossicles and Related Structures

The three ossicles—malleus, incus, and stapes—connect the TM to the oval window. The *malleus* consists of head, neck, and handle/manubrium. The head lies within the epitympanum while the handle attached to the TM. The malleus is attached to the walls of middle ear via three ligaments—anterior, superior, and lateral. The tendon of tensor tympani muscle entering the middle ear cavity from the anterior wall bends laterally to insert into the neck of malleus. The *incus* consists of a body and long and short processes. The anterior surface of the body forms a diarthrodial joint with head of malleus. The short process projects posteriorly while the long process projects inferiorly parallel to the handle of malleus. The posterior incus ligament connects the short process to the posterior wall of middle ear. The long process turns medially at right angles at its lower end to form the lenticular process which forms a diarthrodial joint with head of stapes. The *stapes* consists of head, neck, two crura, and footplate. The footplate is attached to oval window in the medial wall via a syndesmosis and an annular ligament. The stapedial tendon arising from posterior wall inserts into neck of stapes. Ossicular anatomy is depicted in Fig. 1.9.

A nerve plexus is located along the medial wall of middle ear overlying the cochlear promontory. The tympanic branch (Jacobson nerve) of IX nerve and the parasympathetic plexus around internal carotid artery are the major contributors to this plexus [1].

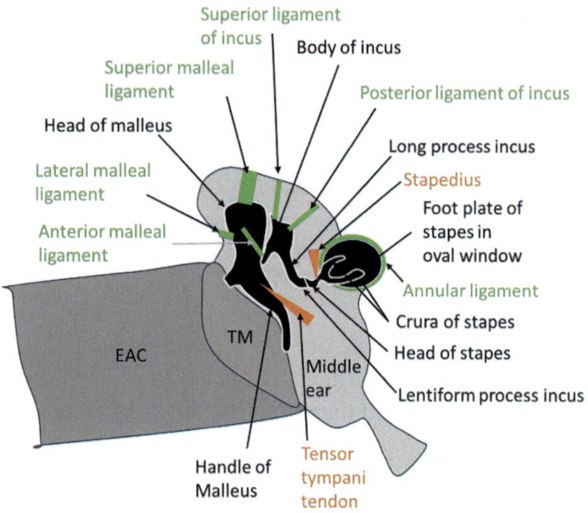

Fig. 1.9 Schematic representation of ossicular anatomy with associated ligaments (in green) and tendons (in orange)

1.1.4 The Facial Nerve in Temporal Bone

The facial nerve has an intricate relationship and complex course within the temporal bone. Its course can be divided into cisternal, IAC, labyrinthine, tympanic, and mastoid segments. The *cisternal segment* is around 24 mm in length and enters the internal acoustic meatus superior to the cochlear nerve. The course within the internal auditory canal is around 7 to 8 mm in length. The *labyrinthine* segment then courses anteriorly within the fallopian or facial nerve canal to end in the first genu. The *first genu* is the site of the *geniculate ganglion*. Distal to this ganglion, the *tympanic part* of nerve takes a hairpin bend to course posteriorly. This segment is around 12 mm in length coursing along the medial wall of middle ear superior to oval window and inferior to lateral semicircular canal. The nerve then changes course near the sinus tympani which marks the *second genu*. The *mastoid segment* then descends vertically close to the posterior wall of the middle ear and exiting the skull through the *stylomastoid foramen*. Three branches arise from the nerve within the temporal bone – the greater superficial petrosal nerve arising from first genu, nerve to stapedius arising from the mastoid part of nerve, and the chorda tympani arising just proximal to the stylomastoid foramen. The tympanic part of the facial canal can often be dehiscent though assessing dehiscence on HRCT sections might often prove difficult [3].

1.1.5 Inner Ear—Bony Labyrinth

The inner ear consists of a membranous labyrinth located within a bony labyrinth. The bony labyrinth consists of cochlea, vestibule, and semicircular canals. The bony labyrinth is filled with *perilymph*. The central part of bony labyrinth is the *vestibule*.

It is continuous anteriorly with the cochlea and posteriorly with the semicircular canal. It has two openings—the oval window and vestibular aqueduct. The *vestibular aqueduct* extends posteriorly from the vestibule to open on posterior surface of the petrous temporal bone. Fissula ante fenestram and fossula post fenestram are two connective tissue-filled extensions from the vestibule toward the middle ear cavity near the oval window. There are *three semicircular canals* connected to the vestibule—superior, posterior, and lateral. The anterior part of each canal is enlarged to form the ampulla. The non-ampullary ends of posterior and superior canal are joined to form a common crus. The *cochlea* is situated anterior to the vestibule. The cochlea is a conical structure with base toward the internal auditory canal and apex pointing infero-antero-laterally. It consists of a bony canal wound around a central bony structure called the *modiolus*, making around two- and three-quarters turns. The modiolus transmits the branches of the cochlear nerve. *Osseous spiral lamina* projects from the modiolus into the cochlear turns which along with the cochlear duct divides the cochlea into scala tympani and scala vestibuli. The *scala tympani* and *scala vestibuli* are intercommunicating at the *helicotrema* at cochlear apex. The bone separating one turn of cochlea from the next is called *interscalar septum.* The projection of the basal turn of cochlea on the medial wall of middle ear is called the *promontory*. The round window opens into the basal turn of cochlea. The *cochlear aqueduct/perilymphatic duct* is a thin canal extending medially from basal turn of the cochlea to inferior surface of the petrous temporal bone running parallel and inferior to internal auditory canal. The perilymph fluid of the semicircular canals, vestibule, and cochlea are intercommunicating.

1.1.6 Inner Ear—Membranous Labyrinth

The membranous labyrinth consists of the cochlear duct, utricle, saccule, and the endolymphatic duct and sac. Membranous labyrinth is filled with *endolymph*. The *cochlear duct* (*aka scala media*) is a blind pouch lying within the bony cochlear canal and divides it into *scala tympani and scala vestibuli*. The cochlear duct is triangular in cross section. It houses the organ of Corti with hair cells. The *utricle* and *saccule* are the endolymphatic structures located within the bony vestibule with the saccule being the more anterior structure. The utricular cavity communicates with the *three semicircular ducts* via five orifices. The saccule communicates with cochlear duct via the ductus reuniens while both the saccule and utricle communicate with endolymphatic sac via the *endolymphatic duct*. The *endolymphatic sac* resides partly within the vestibular aqueduct and partly under the dura of the posterior surface of petrous temporal bone [1]. Figure 1.10 demonstrates the bony and membranous labyrinthine structures. In Fig. 1.10, gray represents perilymph while blue represents endolymph. Figure 1.11 demonstrates the microscopic cross-sectional anatomy of cochlea.

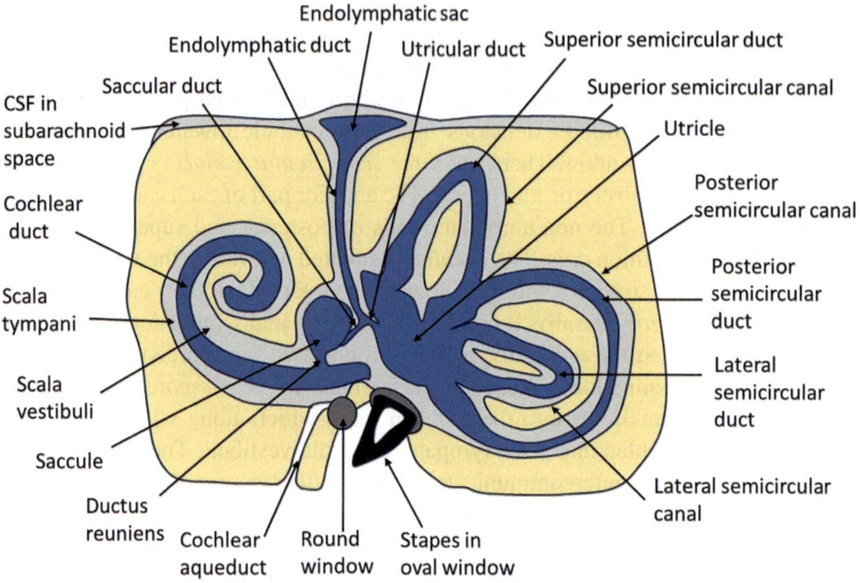

Fig. 1.10 Schematic representation of bony and membranous labyrinth. Perilymph is represented in gray color while endolymph is depicted in blue color. The perilymph is continuous with the CSF via the endolymphatic canal

Fig. 1.11 Cross-sectional anatomy of the cochlea with the cochlear duct depicted in blue color. The scala vestibuli and scala tympani contain perilymph and are continuous with each other at the helicotrema

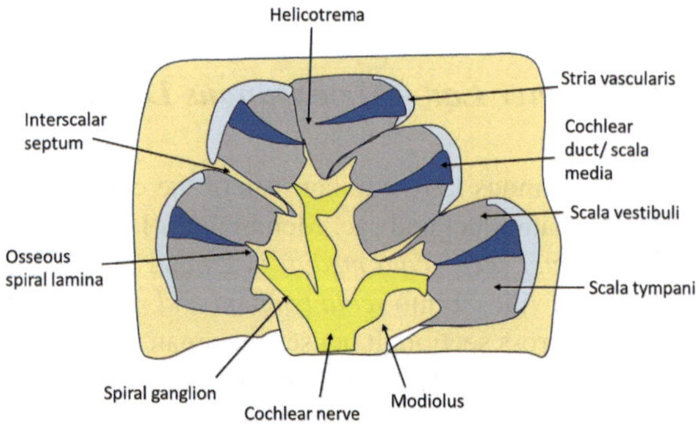

1.1.7 Internal Auditory Canal and Cerebellopontine Angle

The internal auditory canal (IAC) is a bony canal within the petrous temporal bone lined by dura. It runs in medial to lateral direction—from an opening in posterior face of the petrous pyramid (called the porus acusticus internus) to a thin plate of bone (called the fundus or lamina cribrosa) adjacent to inner ear structures. It transmits the facial nerve (VII), vestibulocochlear nerve (VIII), and labyrinthine artery. It is about 9 mm in length and 4 mm in diameter. The fundus of the internal auditory canal is divided into superior and inferior parts by a transverse bony septum, the

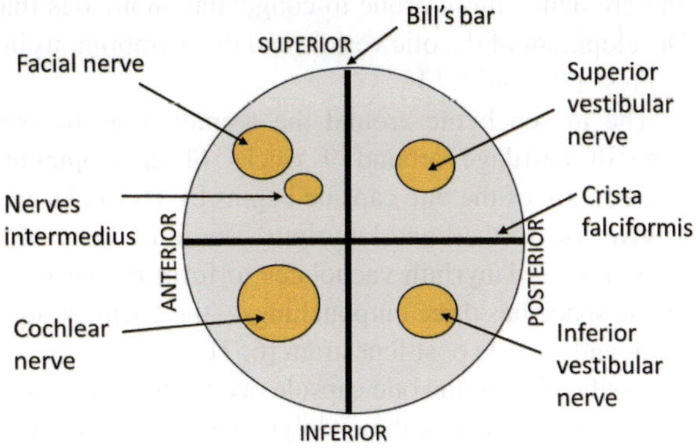

Fig. 1.12 Schematic representation of structures in the fundus of the internal auditory canal

crista falciformis. In the upper compartment, the facial nerve lies anterior and the superior vestibular nerve lies posterior separated by a vertical crest called Bill's bar. In the lower compartment, the cochlear nerve lies anterior while the inferior vestibular nerve lies posterior. Structures at the fundus of the IAC are shown in Fig. 1.12. The singular nerve passes from the posterior semicircular canal to the inferior vestibular nerve at lateral end of IAC through its own separate bony canal. The nervus intermedius is a branch of facial nerve which lies between the facial nerve and superior vestibular nerve in the internal auditory canal and travels through the facial canal to unite with the main motor root at the geniculate ganglion [4, 5].

1.2 Development of the External, Middle, and Inner Ear

1.2.1 The Inner Ear

The membranous labyrinth develops from the neuroectoderm on either side of the head adjacent to the hindbrain from a region called the otic placode around 4th week of development. The otic placode invaginates to form the otic pit and subsequently the otocyst by end of 4th week. The otocyst is fluid filled and lined by ectoderm. This cyst and neural cells from precursors of 7th and 8th cranial nerves migrate to the developing skull base. The otocyst then divides into two parts by around 5th week of development—anteromedial giving rise to cochlear duct and saccule and posterolateral giving rise to utricle and semicircular canals (SCC). The primordial cochlea begins to form by 6th week, forms one turn by 8th week, two and half turns by 10th week, and continues to develop until 24th week of fetal life by which time it reaches its adult form. The lumen of the semicircular ducts is formed by week 8. Complete maturation of the semicircular ducts happens in 2nd trimester with the superior one formed first by week 19 and the lateral one formed last by week 22. The membranous labyrinth, with exception of the endolymphatic sac and duct, reaches adult form by around 6 months of development. The endolymphatic sac and duct enlarge until puberty. The cochlear end organs are last to develop and are hence more prone to congenital anomalies than the vestibular end organs. Development of the otic vesicle and the membranous inner ear structures is depicted in Figs. 1.13 and 1.14.

The mesenchyme around the membranous labyrinth differentiates into outer zone of cartilage around 9 weeks of development (called the otic capsule). Ossification of the otic capsule begins by 16 weeks and is completed by 24th week to give rise to the bony labyrinth. The inner zone of the mesenchyme around the membranous labyrinth vacuolates to form the perilymphatic cavity. The perilymphatic space has three outpouchings—the cochlear aqueduct, the fissula ante fenestram, and fossula post fenestram [6, 7].

Ossification of the otic capsule occurs around 16th to 24th week of development. It completely encases the endolymphatic structures with exception of small rim of cartilage around oval window and around the fissula ante fenestram. The otic capsule

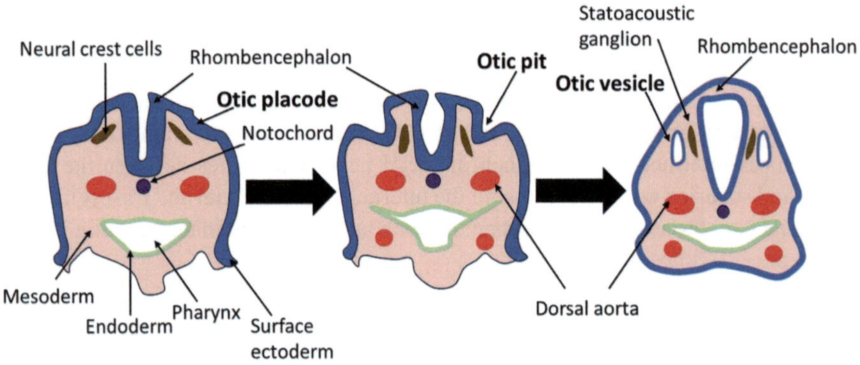

Fig. 1.13 Development of the otic vesicle from the surface ectoderm of the embryo. These stages are seen in 4th to 5th week of embryonic development. The cochlear nerve develops from the neural crest cells

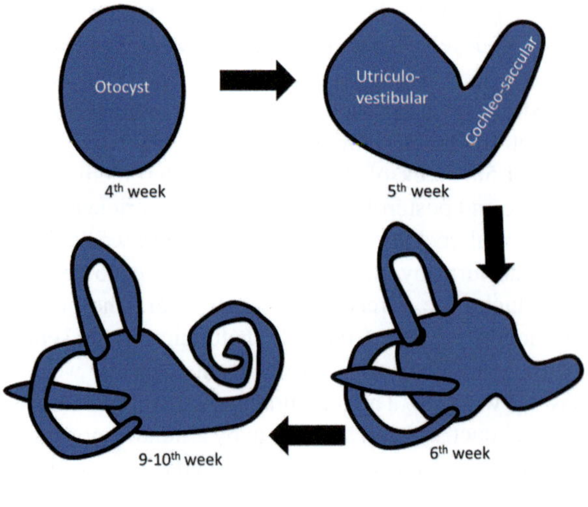

Fig. 1.14 Development of the membranous labyrinth from otocyst/vesicle. Note that the cochlear duct is last to form among the structures of membranous labyrinth

consists of multiple layers of enchondral bone with endosteal bone lining the labyrinth. The endosteal bone when disturbed by pathology may proliferate obliterating the labyrinth. The enchondral bone forming the otic capsule is unique in the human body in that it undergoes little to no remodelling after birth and has poor osteogenic response. Hence, fractures of otic caspule do not heal completely. Periosteal new bone formation however continues into adulthood and later undergoes pneumatization [8].

1.2.2 The External and Middle Ear

Around 4 weeks of development, branchial arches separated by grooves appear on both sides of the head. The first branchial groove deepens to form the external auditory canal. Similarly, pouches develop from the endoderm of the pharynx and the first pouch extends superolaterally to form the Eustachian tube and middle ear cavity. The external auditory meatus reaches adult configuration by around 6 months of development. Development of the external and middle ear is depicted in Fig. 1.15.

The auricle of the external ear develops from six hillocks arising from the first and second branchial arches around 6 weeks of development and fuse by third month. Cartilages from the 1st and 2nd arches form the ear ossicles. The malleus and incus assume adult form by midterm of fetal life. The stapes however undergoes some remodelling after birth. The ossicles become engulfed by the first pharyngeal pouch by 22nd week of development. The middle ear becomes pneumatized by 30 weeks of development with the mastoid antrum undergoing similar changes by 35 weeks. These spaces are filled with fluid during fetal life and become air filled after birth [9].

The tympanic membrane is formed by all three germ layers—surface ectoderm of the 1st branchial cleft, mesoderm, and endoderm of 1st pharyngeal pouch.

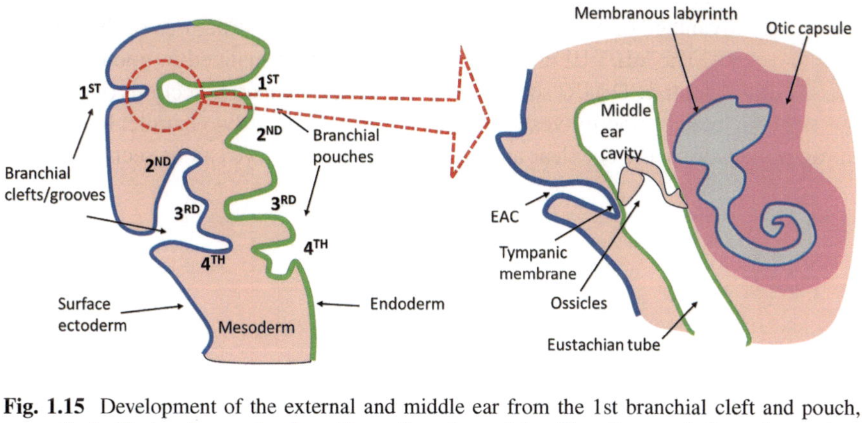

Fig. 1.15 Development of the external and middle ear from the 1st branchial cleft and pouch, respectively. First and second arch cartilages form the ossicles. The otic capsule forms by condensation of the mesenchyme around the membranous labyrinth

Air cells of temporal bone develop after birth for many years. Epithelium-lined projections arise from the middle ear and project into space created by conversion of marrow into loose connective tissue. This process is dynamic and can be arrested by repeated episodes of otitis media in childhood. The mastoid part of the temporal bone is virtually absent at birth and develops beginning around 2nd year of life as extensions from the petrous and squamous parts of the temporal bone. Air cells pneumatize from the antrum in two directions—down to the mastoid tip and laterally into squamous part; the bone dividing these two sets of cells is called the Korner's septum.

References

1. Som PM, Curtin HD. Head and neck imaging. Mosby Elsevier; 2011. p. 2994.
2. Juliano AF, Ginat DT, Moonis G. Imaging review of the temporal bone: Part I. Anatomy and inflammatory and neoplastic processes. Radiology. 2013;269(1):17–33.
3. Gupta S, Mends F, Hagiwara M, Fatterpekar G, Roehm PC. Imaging the facial nerve: a contemporary review. Radiol Res Pract. 2013;2013:248039.
4. Kozerska M, Skrzat J. Anatomy of the fundus of the internal acoustic meatus – micro-computed tomography study. Folia Morphol. 2015;74(3):352–8.
5. Rubinstein D, Sandberg EJ, Cajade-Law AG. Anatomy of the facial and vestibulocochlear nerves in the internal auditory canal. AJNR Am J Neuroradiol. 1996;17(6):1099–105.
6. Whitfield TT. Development of the inner ear. Curr Opin Genet Dev. 2015;32:112–8.
7. Feraco P, Piccinini S, Gagliardo C. Imaging of inner ear malformations: a primer for radiologists. Radiol Med (Torino). 2021;126(10):1282–95.
8. Som PM, Curtin HD. Head and neck imaging E-book: expert consult- online and print. Elsevier Health Sciences; 2011. p. 3079.
9. Anthwal N, Thompson H. The development of the mammalian outer and middle ear. J Anat. 2016;228(2):217–32.

Chapter 2
Temporal Bone Imaging Techniques

Kiran Gopinathan

Cross-sectional imaging is the current investigation of choice for a noninvasive detailed assessment of both anatomy and pathology in the temporal bone. Computed tomography (CT) and magnetic resonance imaging (MRI) are both complimentary in this aspect, each having its own merits and demerits.

2.1 CT Technique

High-resolution computed tomography (HRCT) provides better spatial resolution compared to MRI and is the modality of choice to assess bony anatomy, fractures, calcifications, cortical erosions, air, and fat.

Indications:

- Trauma
- Congenital ear anomalies
- Infections
- Inflammatory diseases
- Neoplasms
- Pre- and postoperative evaluation (e.g., cochlear implantation, tympanoplasty, mastoidectomy)

Our institutional protocol for HRCT imaging of the temporal bone (using 128-slice helical GE scanner) has the following parameters:

- 140 kV
- 150 mAs

K. Gopinathan (✉)
Department of Radiology, SRIHER, Chennai, India
e-mail: g.kiran@sriramachandra.edu.in

H. Mahalingam (ed.), *Temporal Bone Imaging*,
https://doi.org/10.1007/978-981-95-6132-2_2

- 0.6 mm slice thickness
- 1024 × 1024 high-resolution matrix
- 15–20 cm field of view (FOV)

Images are acquired from above the superior-most mastoid air cells above the bony portion of the external auditory canal (EAC) through the mastoid tip inferiorly with the baseline parallel to the infraorbitomeatal line [1] (Fig. 2.1). Helical scanning of the temporal bone is usually done without gantry angulation and has been reported to result in lower effective dose as well as organ dose to the lens of the eye than sequential direct axial and coronal scanning with gantry tilt [2].

Image acquisition is followed by 0.6 mm thickness reconstructions in the coronal and axial planes using a high-resolution algorithm (also called bone algorithm) for each ear separately (10 cm FOV) with window level of 1000 HU and window width of 4000 HU [3].

Axial reconstruction is done in a plane parallel to the lateral semicircular canal (LSC). Example of an axial image is represented in Fig. 2.2. Cranial extent is up to the superior margin of the petrous apex and caudally up to the inferior tip of the mastoid process.

The coronal images are reconstructed perpendicular to the axial plane from the anterior margin of the petrous apex to the posterior margin of the mastoid bone (Fig. 2.3). Example of a coronal image is represented in Fig. 2.4.

Axial 2 mm thickness reconstructions are also done in soft tissue window.

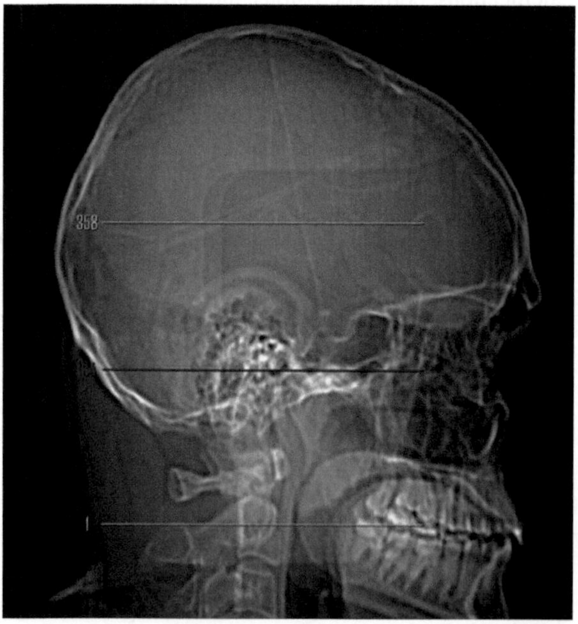

Fig. 2.1 CT scanogram of the skull depicting the craniocaudal extent of coverage for acquisition of HRCT temporal bone and the axis of acquisition

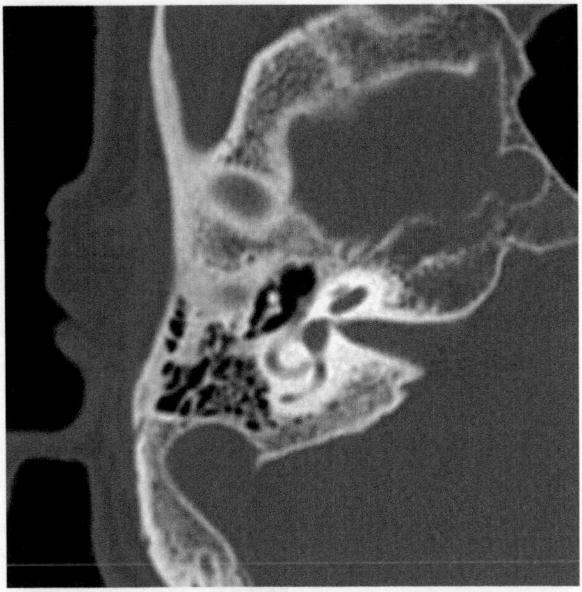

Fig. 2.2 Example of an axial HRCT image reconstructed parallel to the lateral semicircular canal

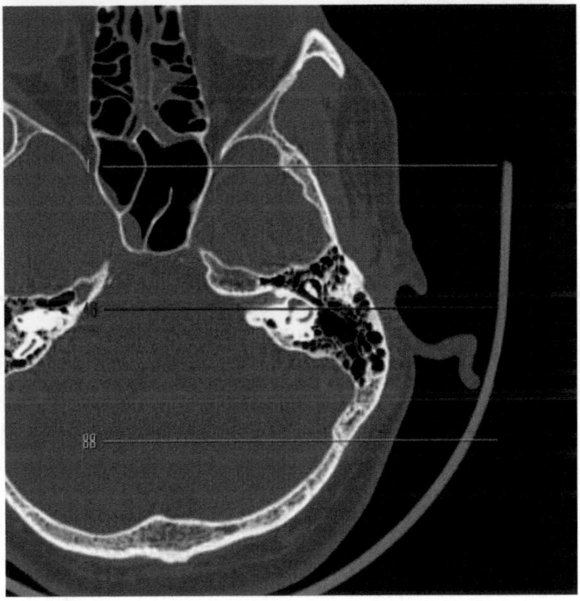

Fig. 2.3 Axial HRCT image depicting the anteroposterior extent of the coronal reconstruction

Post-contrast imaging is not routinely done except in suspected cases of neoplasms and to assess intracranial extension of infection such as meningitis, epidural abscess, and dural venous thrombosis.

Special planes of reconstruction [1]:

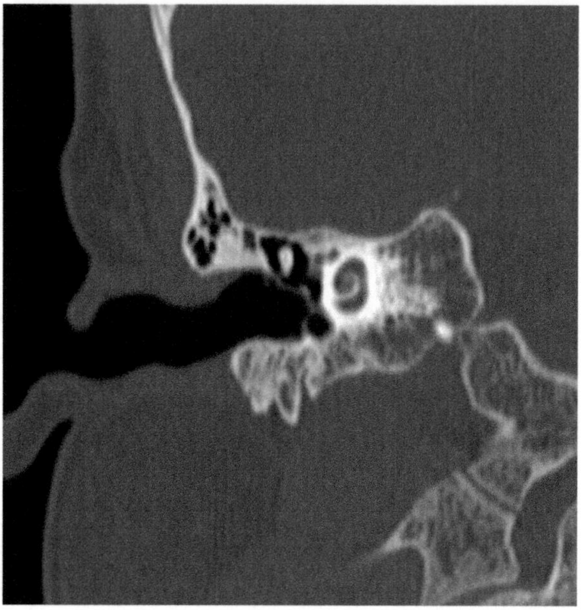

Fig. 2.4 Example of a coronal HRCT image reconstructed perpendicular to the lateral semicircular canal

- Stenvers plane
- It is an oblique coronal projection where the images are reconstructed parallel to the long axis of the petrous temporal bone and perpendicular to the superior semicircular canal (SSC). The cochlea is seen en face in this plane.
- Pöschl plane
- Images are reconstructed perpendicular to the long axis of the petrous temporal bone and parallel to the SSC. Dehiscence of roof of SCC is clearly depicted in this plane.

Cone-beam computed tomography (CBCT) systems, conventionally used in dental imaging, operate using an X-ray beam with a conical geometry between the source and the detector in contrast to the fan-beam geometry of conventional CT. With the use of a 2D flat panel detector, a volumetric data set can be acquired with a single rotation of the gantry enabling a high spatial resolution (≤0.1 mm) and low radiation dose (up to 10–100 μSv using low-dose protocols) [4]. This has made CBCT a compelling alternative to helical CT in imaging the temporal bone.

But CBCT is not without its limitations. The long acquisition time (up to 40 s), which makes it prone to motion artifacts, is a major deterrent in pediatric/elderly population. Added to this is the poor soft tissue contrast resolution, which makes it unsuitable for general diagnostic imaging and thereby reluctance to invest in such a system solely for this purpose.

2.2 MRI Technique

MR imaging offers better characterization of soft tissue lesions, cranial nerve involvement, membranous labyrinth, and bone marrow signal changes. There is no single specific protocol for MR imaging of the temporal bone, and the MRI sequences performed are tailored to the indication of the study.

A 3 mm thickness axial fast spin echo (FSE) T2-weighted images with fat saturation (FS) of the entire brain is generally done to screen for other pathologies.

Axial and coronal 2 mm thickness FSE T2-weighted images with FS provide good anatomic detail with fluid in the bony/membranous labyrinth acting as natural contrast and abnormal fluid signal intensities within the tympanic and mastoid air spaces appearing hyperintense on T2.

Heavily T2-weighted 3D sequence such as FIESTA, CISS, DRIVE, or SPACE (~0.6 mm thickness) acts as a 3D cisternography sequence, and the high-resolution images obtained are very useful in the evaluation of the fluid-filled inner ear structures and cisternal and intracanalicular segments of the VII and VIII cranial nerves (Fig. 2.5). Sagittal oblique reformatted images perpendicular to the internal acoustic meatus (IAC) clearly delineate the relations of the VII and VIII nerve complexes within the IAC (Fig. 2.6).

FIESTA (GE)/TrueFISP (Siemens) is a balanced steady-state gradient echo sequence that is highly sensitive to magnetic field inhomogeneities and may produce band like artifacts especially at sites like the skull base. FIESTA-C/CISS sequence is a modification of the above and is composed of two consecutive runs of the True FISP sequence with varied excitation levels, which are combined subsequently to form an image where the phase errors cancel out. CUBE/SPACE is a 3D turbo spin echo sequence with variable flip angles. 3D T2-SPACE has been found to be superior to 3D CISS sequence in the evaluation of cranial nerves near the skull base as it is less prone to susceptibility artifacts through RF refocusing [5].

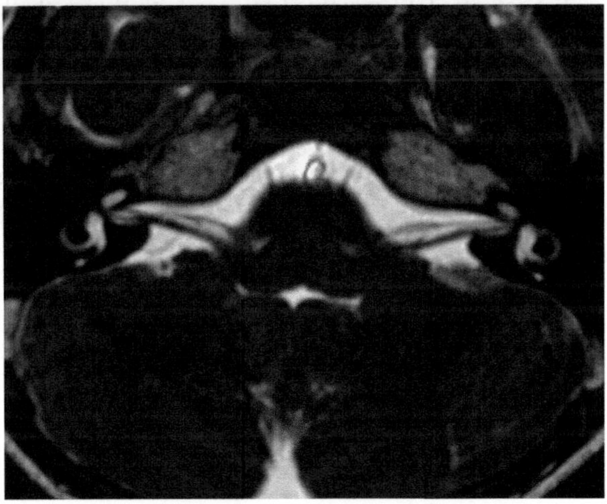

Fig. 2.5 Axial FIESTA-C image through the CP angle and IAC depicting inner ear structures and VII/VIII nerve complexes on both sides

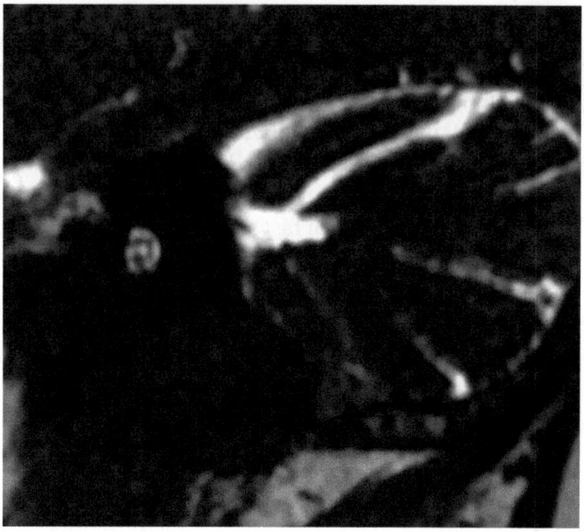

Fig. 2.6 Oblique sagittal FIESTA-C image though the IAC depicting four nerves within—facial nerve, cochlear nerve, and superior and inferior vestibular nerve

A 2 mm thickness axial T1-weighted images help in characterization of lesions such as cholesterol granulomas in the petrous apex or IAC lipomas which appear hyperintense on T1.

In suspected cases of cholesteatoma, 3 mm thickness axial diffusion-weighted imaging (DWI) with b-factor of 0 and 1000 s/mm^2 and ADC maps are essential in identifying the pathology. DWI can be done using echo planar imaging (EPI) or non-EPI-based sequences. Turbo spin-echo (TSE)-based DWI is a spin-echo-based single-shot (SS) or multi-shot (MS) non-EPI technique with longer echo time and a higher signal-to-noise ratio than conventional SS EPI-DWI. It has been reported to be less prone to geometric distortion, susceptibility artifacts, and chemical shift and provide better spatial resolution and thinner slices than that can be obtained with EPI-based sequences [6].

Fat-saturated T1-weighted images with 2 mm thickness done before and after intravenous injection of gadolinium are useful in the evaluation of tumors, infections, and vascular complications. Contrast-enhanced MRI can also discriminate between the non-enhancing cholesteatoma and other contrast-enhancing findings, e.g., inflammation, scar, or granulation tissue.

Post processing techniques such as volume rendering can create a 3-dimensional model of the membranous labyrinth with accurate depiction of the cochlear and semicircular canal anatomy (Figs. 2.7 and 2.8).

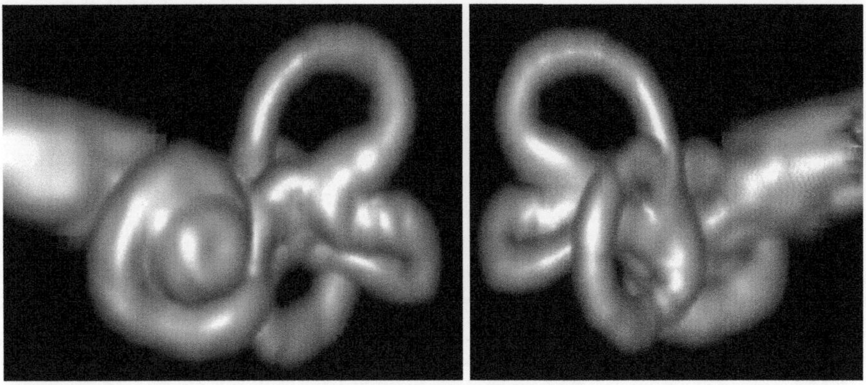

Figs. 2.7 and 2.8 3D-reconstructed volume-rendered reconstruction of the FIESTA-C images depicting the semicircular canals and cochlea

References

1. ACR–ASNR–SPR Practice Parameter For The Performance Of Computed Tomography (CT) Of The Extracranial Head And Neck, revised 2021. Available at: https://www.acr.org/-/media/ACR/Files/Practice-Parameters/CT-Head-Neck.pdf
2. Niu Y, Wang Z, Liu Y, Liu Z, Yao V. Radiation dose to the lens using different temporal bone CT scanning protocols. Am J Neuroradiol. 2010;31(2):226–9.
3. Yang N. On the importance of proper window and level settings in temporal bone CT imaging. Philipp J Otolaryngol Head Neck Surg. 2020;35(2):51.
4. Quintas-Neves M, Saraiva J. Recalling the usefulness of conebeam CT in temporal bone imaging: higher resolution with lower radiation dose. Am J Neuroradiol. 2022;43(11):E43–4.
5. Kinger NP, Chien LC, Sharma PS, Gravolet RB, Aiken AH, Baugnon KL, et al. Comparison of 3D constructive interference in steady state (CISS) and T2 sampling perfection with application optimized contrasts using different flip angle evolution MR imaging of the intracranial trigeminal nerve and central skull base neuroforamina. Neuroradiol J. 2022;35(6):678–83.
6. Henninger B, Kremser C. Diffusion weighted imaging for the detection and evaluation of cholesteatoma. World J Radiol. 2017;9(5):217–22.

Chapter 3
CT and MRI Anatomy of Temporal Bone

Harshavardhan Mahalingam

3.1 Imaging Anatomy as Related to Gross Anatomy

3.1.1 External Ear

The external ear comprises the pinna and the external auditory canal (EAC). The pinna is the part of the external ear which projects out from the head. It is composed primarily of elastic cartilage covered by skin. It has an outermost elevated rim called the helix and a parallel inner elevated rim called the antihelix. The anterior part of the helix above the EAC is called the crus helix while the anterior part of the antihelix splits into two crura. The central hollow area in the pinna is called the concha. Anterior to the lateral end of the EAC is a cartilaginous projection called the tragus, while posteroinferior to it lies the antitragus. The inferiormost part of the pinna lacks cartilage and is called the lobule. Anatomy of the pinna is represented in Fig. 3.1.

The EAC has an outer cartilaginous and inner bony part. It is well represented on axial and coronal HRCT images (Figs. 3.2 and 3.3). The cartilaginous part is better evaluated on the soft tissue window (Figs. 3.4 and 3.5). Cerumen can be visualized as a soft tissue density structure within the lumen of the EAC. Fissures of Santorini which are defects in the cartilaginous part of EAC cannot be visualized on imaging. The foramen of Huschke can be occasionally seen as a defect in the anteroinferior part of the bony EAC.

Supplementary Information The online version contains supplementary material available at https://doi.org/10.1007/978-981-95-6132-2_3.

H. Mahalingam (✉)
Department of Radiology, SRIHER, Chennai, India
e-mail: drharsha@sriramachandra.edu.in

H. Mahalingam (ed.), *Temporal Bone Imaging*,
https://doi.org/10.1007/978-981-95-6132-2_3

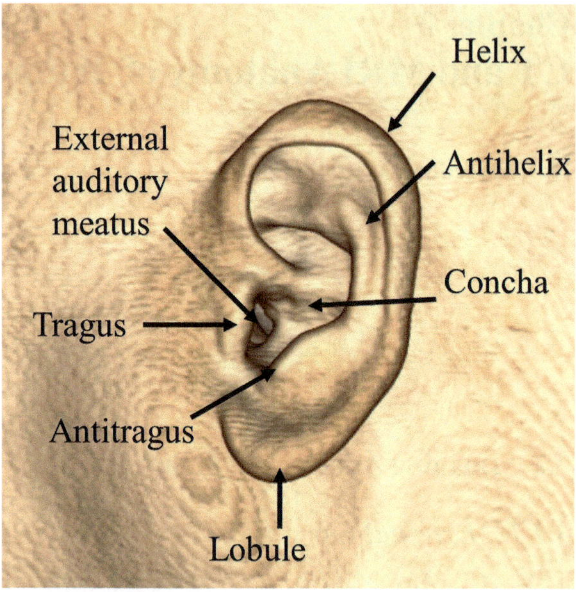

Fig. 3.1 Volume-rendered image of HRCT temporal bone showing the structure of the pinna

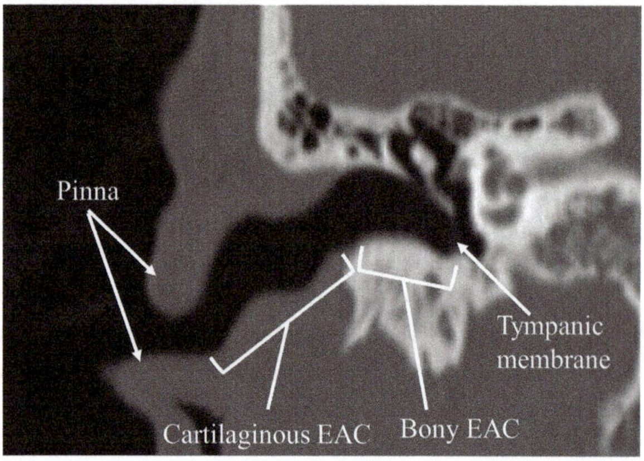

Fig. 3.2 Axial HRCT section of temporal bone showing the outer cartilaginous and inner bony parts of the EAC. Also note the tympanic membrane at medial end of the EAC

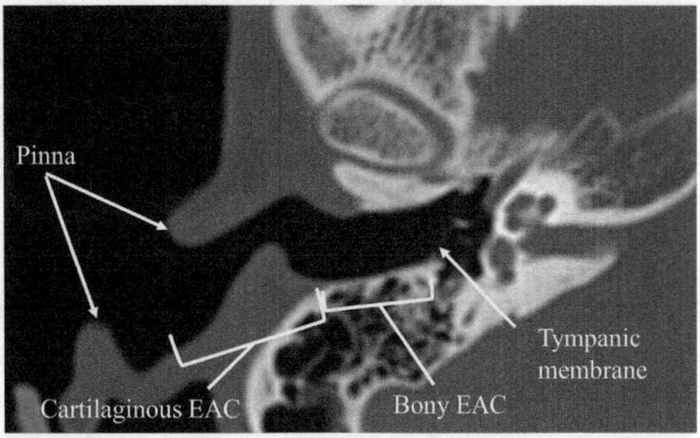

Fig. 3.3 Coronal HRCT section of temporal bone showing the outer cartilaginous and inner bony parts of the EAC. Also note the tympanic membrane at medial end of the EAC with a medial convexity at the tip of the malleus handle called the umbo

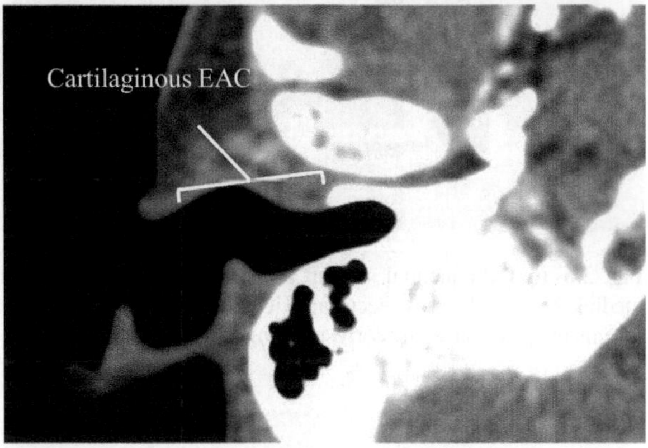

Fig. 3.4 Axial section of temporal bone in soft tissue window better demonstrating the outer cartilaginous part of the EAC

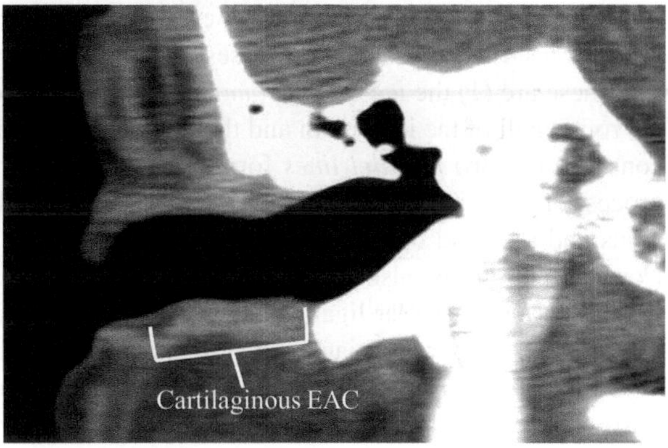

Fig. 3.5 Coronal section of temporal bone in soft tissue window better demonstrating the outer cartilaginous part of the EAC

The tympanic membrane (TM) is normally visualized on the axial and coronal sections as a thin line, approximately 1 mm in thickness. If the middle or external ear is filled with soft tissue, the TM may not be seen separately.

Sagittal sections can be used to visualize the walls of the EAC circumferentially to assess for thickening and bone erosions (Fig. 3.6).

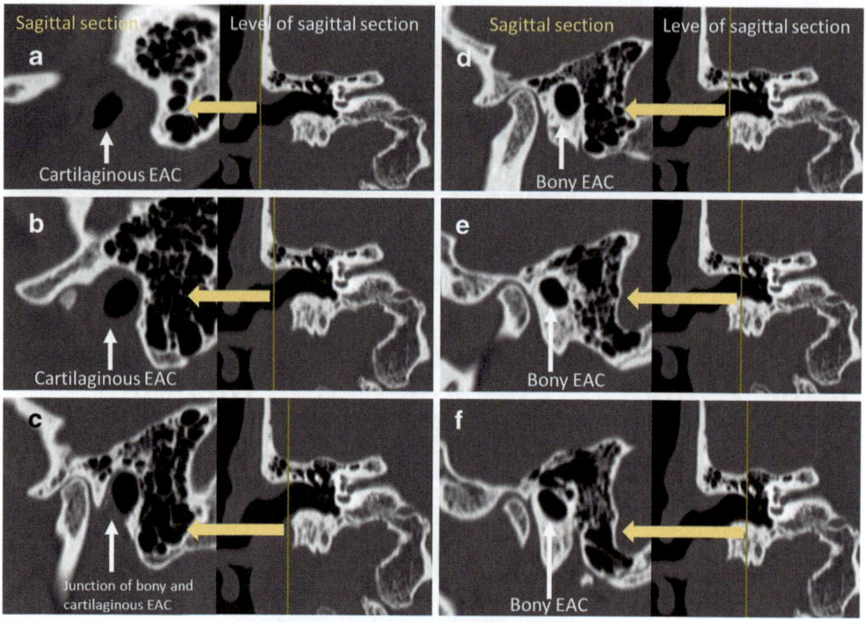

Fig. 3.6 **(a–f)** Sequential sagittal reconstruction of the EAC at different levels from lateral to medial showing the cross-sectional view of the EAC. The yellow line on the coronal sections represents the position of the corresponding reconstructed sagittal section

3.1.2 Middle Ear

The axial plane is routinely used to evaluate the ossicles. Classically, three axial sections need to be evaluated to assess ossicular integrity—from superior to inferior, these are (1) the *ice-cream cone* appearance with the head of malleus forming the round ball of the ice-cream and the body and short process of incus forming the cone, (2) the *two parallel lines* formed by handle of malleus anteriorly and long process of incus posteriorly, and (3) the *two dots* formed by lenticular process of the incus and the head of stapes—represented in Figs. 3.7, 3.8, and 3.9, respectively. Coronal sections are also useful in assessing the ossicles (Figs. 3.10 and 3.11).

The normal ossicular ligaments are inconsistently visualized on HRCT images. They can be better appreciated when thickened or ossified.

On the coronal sections, the middle ear cavity can be divided into *epitympanum* (also called the attic or epitympanic recess), *mesotympanum*, and *hypotympanum* based on lines parallel to superior and inferior margins of the TM. The bony projection seen at the medial end of the EAC where the superior margin of the TM is attached is called the *scutum*. The space between the pars flaccida of TM and scutum laterally and the neck of malleus medially is the *Prussak's space*—a common site for acquired cholesteatomas. Blunting of the scutum is an important imaging feature to recognize in cases of attic cholesteatoma.

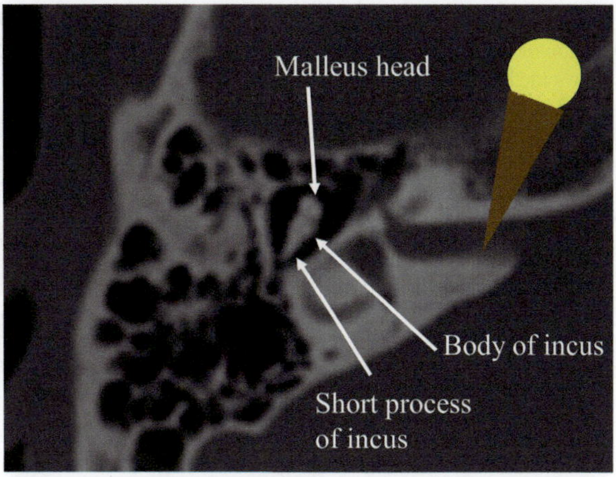

Fig. 3.7 Axial HRCT section having the ice cream cone appearance—formed by head of malleus and the body and short process of incus

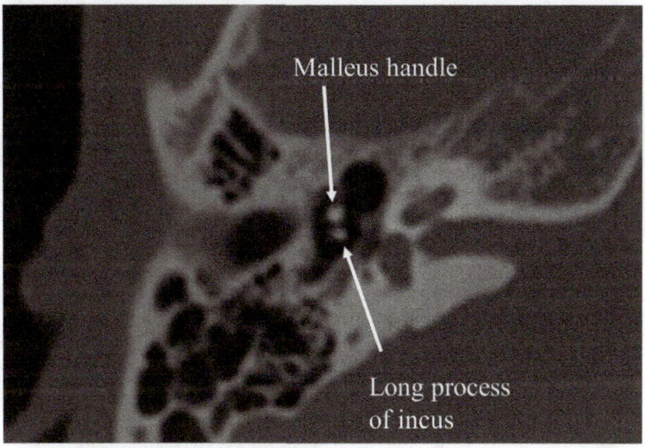

Fig. 3.8 Axial HRCT section showing the two parallel lines—formed by handle of malleus and long process of incus

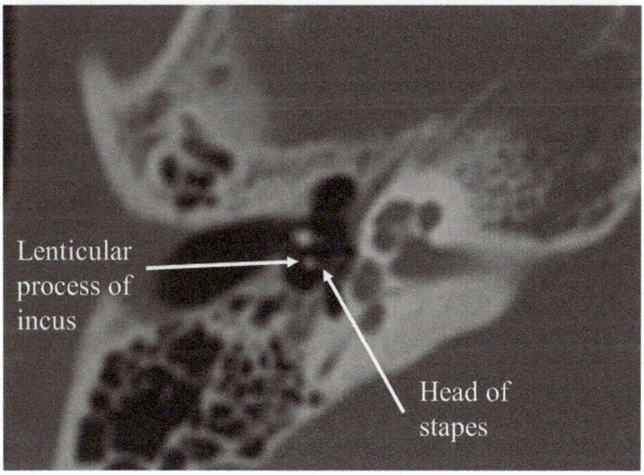

Fig. 3.9 Axial HRCT section showing the two dots—formed by lenticular process of the incus and the head of stapes. Also note the stapes crura and footplate on the oval window

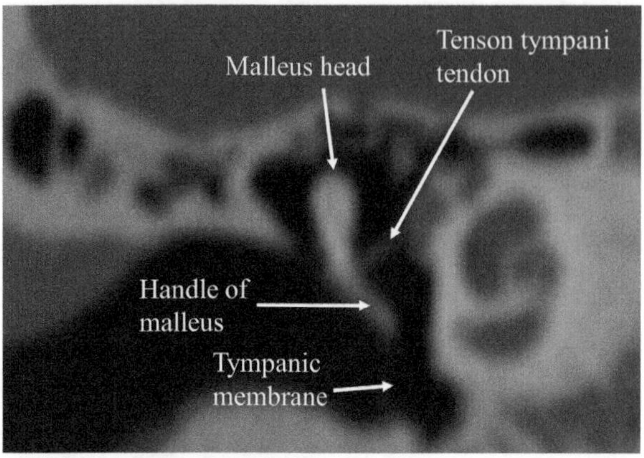

Fig. 3.10 Coronal HRCT section of temporal bone shows the head and handle of the malleus. Note the handle of malleus lying on the tympanic membrane. Also note the tendon of tensor tympani attached to the neck of malleus

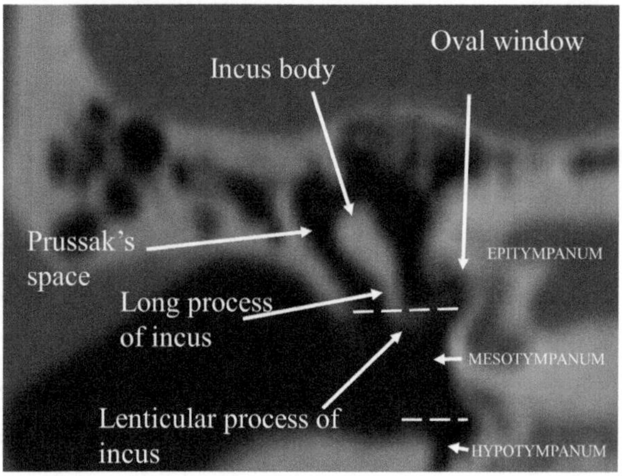

Fig. 3.11 Coronal HRCT section of temporal bone shows the body, long process, and lenticular process of the incus with the stapes lying opposite the oval window

The anterior wall of the middle ear is marked superiorly by *hemicanal for tensor tympani* (Fig. 3.12) and inferiorly by the opening for the *Eustachian tube* (Fig. 3.13). Medial to the Eustachian tube opening lies the impression of the *carotid canal* along the junction of the anterior and medial walls of the middle ear.

The medial wall of middle ear is marked by multiple structures. From superior to inferior, these are the lateral semicircular canal (SCC), the tympanic segment of the facial nerve, the oval window with stapes footplate, the promontory formed by basal turn of cochlea, and the round window niche (Figs. 3.14, 3.15, 3.16 and 3.17).

Coronal plane shows all these structures in cross section in a single image (Fig. 3.18). The walls of the tympanic segment of the facial nerve are less than 1 mm thick. Microscopic studies have shown that more than half of all temporal bones may have dehiscence in the tympanic segment of the facial nerve canal. HRCT demonstration of such dehiscence is complicated by issues of spatial resolution and partial volume effect (the course of the canal is oblique to the coronal plane). Facial nerve course variants are not uncommon. Sometimes, the nerve can

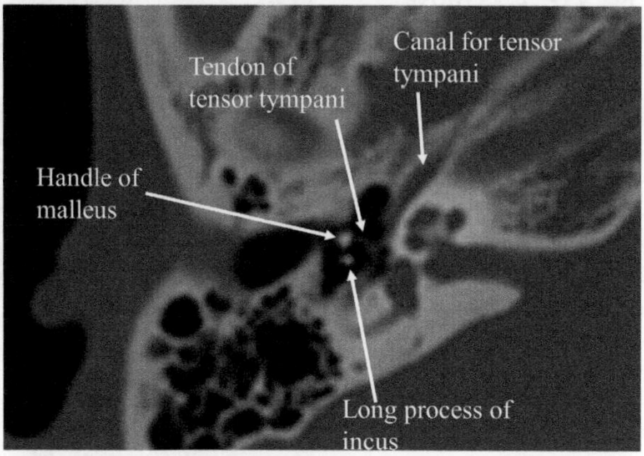

Fig. 3.12 Axial HRCT section showing the canal for tensor tympani. Also note the tendon of tensor tympani taking a right angle turn within the middle ear to insert on the malleus

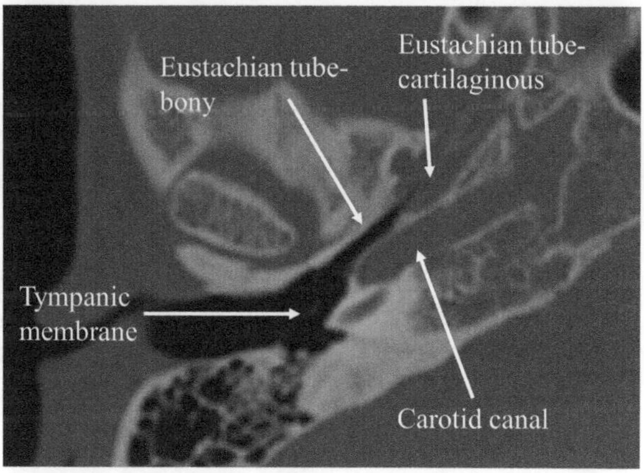

Fig. 3.13 Axial HRCT section showing the Eustachian tube opening into the middle ear cavity. Note the lateral part of the tube is bony while the more medial part is cartilaginous. Also note the carotid canal with thin plate of bone separating it from the middle ear cavity

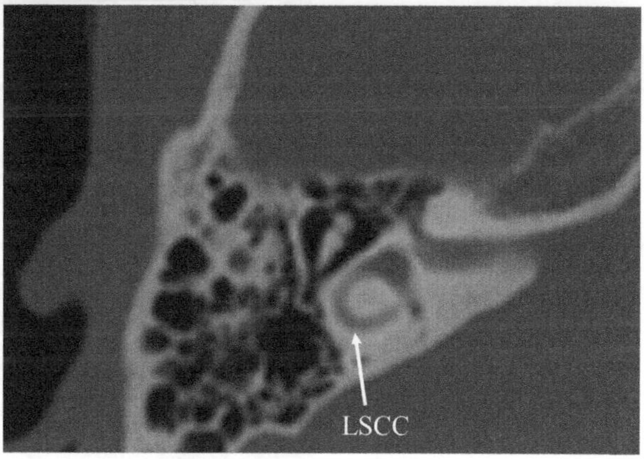

Fig. 3.14 Axial HRCT section showing the anterior limb of the lateral semicircular canal lying just medial to the medial wall of middle ear. The thin plate of bone separating the two can be eroded by disease processes leading to a labyrinthine fistula

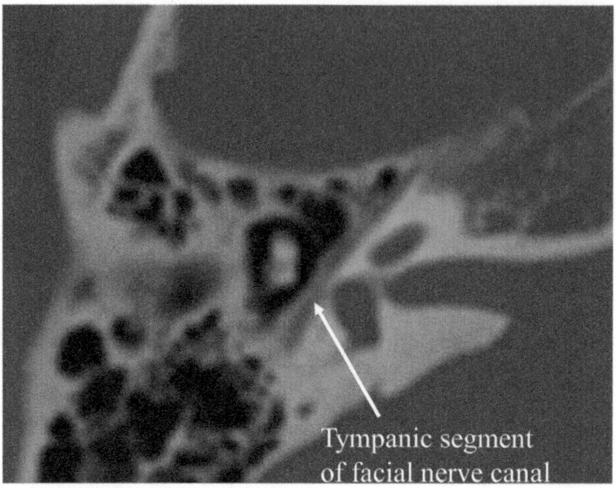

Fig. 3.15 Axial HRCT section showing the tympanic segment of the facial nerve canal running along the medial wall of middle ear

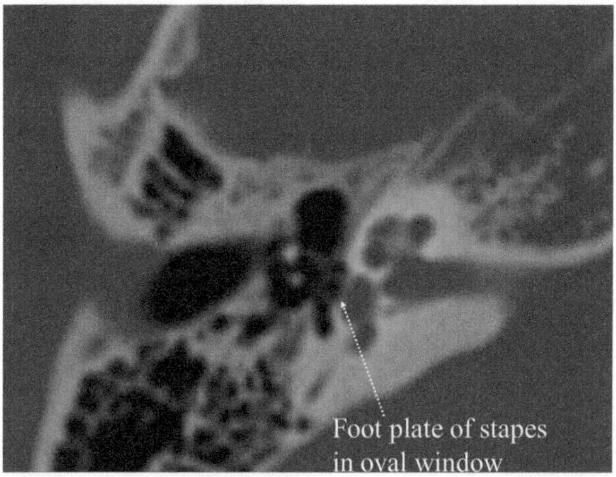

Fig. 3.16 Axial HRCT section just below the level of the facial nerve showing the oval window with the footplate of stapes

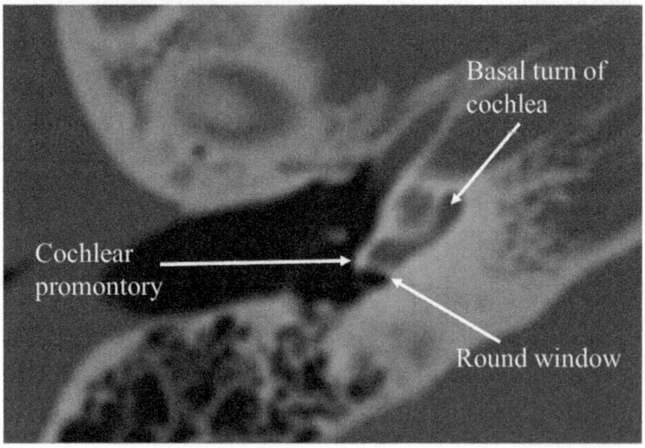

Fig. 3.17 A more inferior axial HRCT section showing the basal turn of cochlea indenting on the medial wall of middle ear forming the cochlea and the round window seen more posteroinferiorly

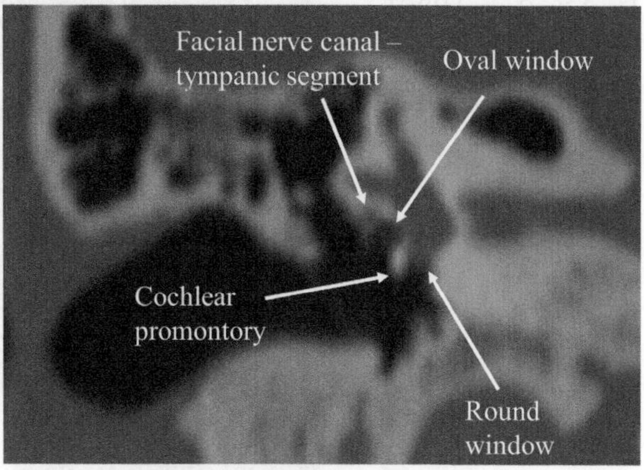

Fig. 3.18 Coronal HRCT section showing lateral semicircular canal (SCC), the tympanic segment of the facial nerve, oval window, promontory, and round window niche along the medial wall of the middle ear

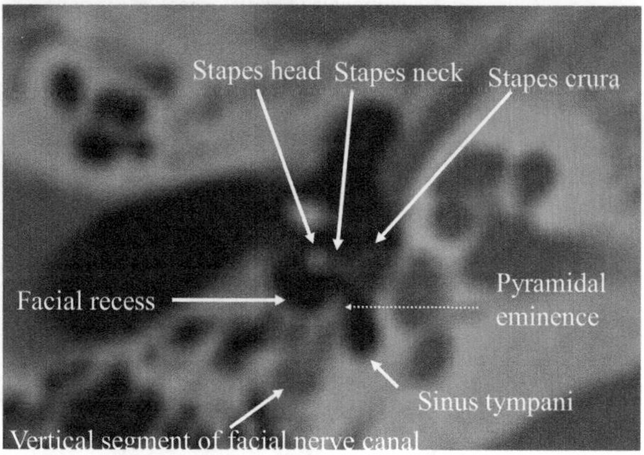

Fig. 3.19 Axial HRCT section showing the pyramidal eminence along the posterior wall of middle ear with the sinus tympani and facial recess. Note the facial nerve canal at region of the second genu lying posterior to the posterior wall

course directly lateral to the oval window and lie on the stapes. Lack of the facial nerve canal notch on coronal plane just below the lateral SCC should raise suspicion of anomalous course of the nerve. Recognition of such anomalous course can help in preventing iatrogenic injury of the facial nerve during middle ear surgery.

The posterior wall is marked by the *pyramidal eminence*. Lateral to the pyramidal eminence is the *facial recess* while medial to it is the *sinus tympani* (Fig. 3.19). The stapedius tendon can be seen arising from tip of the pyramidal eminence to attach to neck of stapes. The 2nd genu of the facial nerve lies medial to the facial recess and can be visualized as a round radiolucency.

The coronal plane is also useful to assess the roof and floor of the middle ear cavity (Figs. 3.20, 3.21, 3.22 and 3.23). The roof of the middle ear cavity is formed by plate of bone called tegmen tympani. More posteriorly, the roof of the mastoid antrum is formed by plate of bone called tegmen mastoideum. The tegmen can show varying degrees of pneumatization. Any defect or erosion in the tegmen can facilitate spread of infection from middle ear into intracranial compartment.

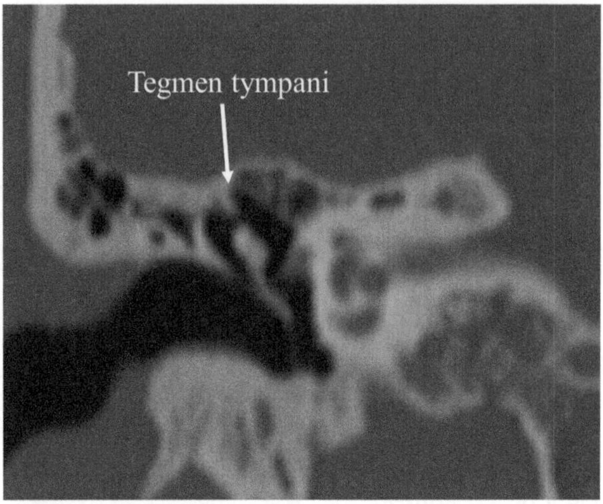

Fig. 3.20 Coronal HRCT section showing the tegmen tympani

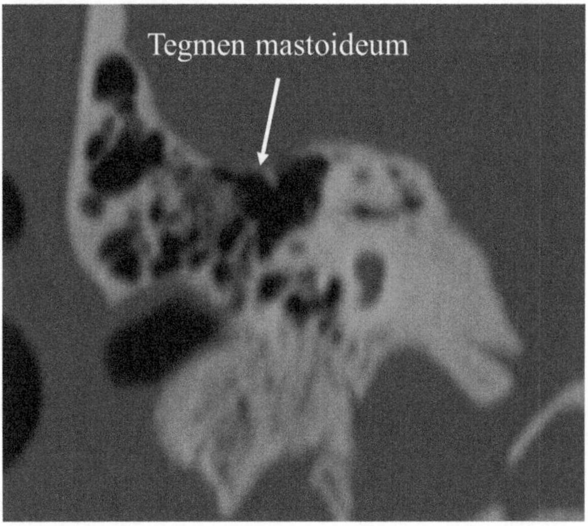

Fig. 3.21 Coronal HRCT section more posterior to Fig. 20 showing the tegmen mastoideum

The floor of the middle ear is a plate of bone which separates it from the jugular fossa posteriorly and carotid canal anteriorly. The thickness of this bone is variable depending on the size of the jugular fossa. In case of large or high-riding jugular bulb, this bone can be very thin or dehiscent. Sometimes, the internal jugular vein can course through the middle ear with no intervening bone. Such a variant can be evident even on otoscopic examination. Anteriorly, the jugular foramen is separated from the carotid canal by the caroticojugular spine (Fig. 3.24).

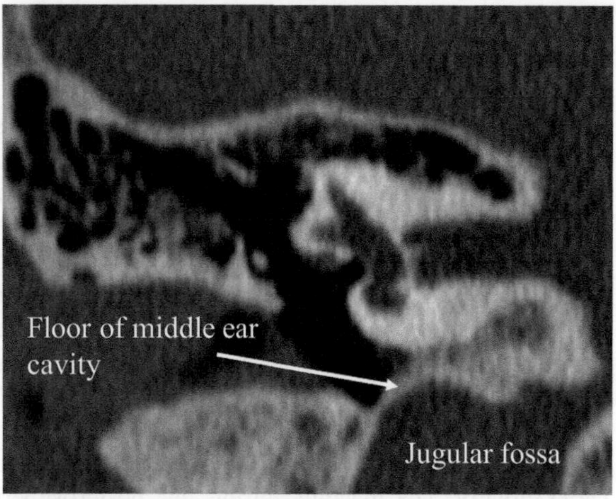

Fig. 3.22 Coronal HRCT section showing a thin plate of bone forming the floor of the middle ear and separating it from the jugular fossa

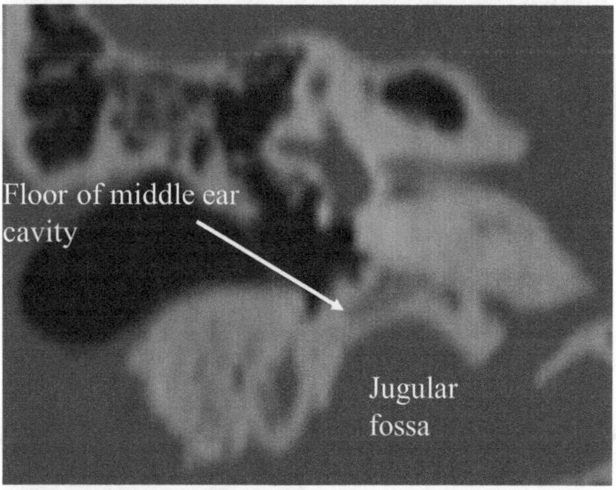

Fig. 3.23 Coronal HRCT section in a different patient showing a thick plate of bone forming the floor of the middle ear

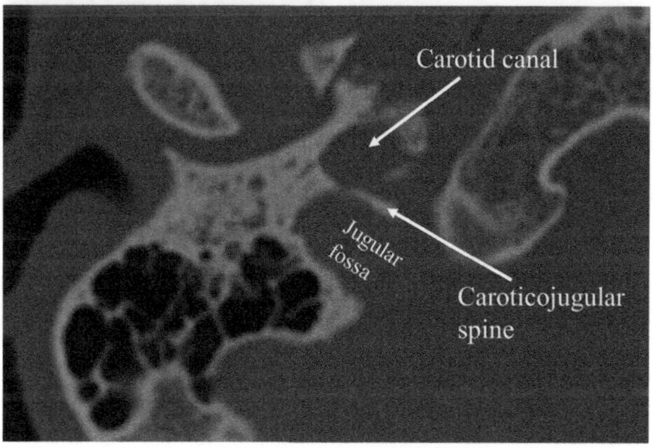

Fig. 3.24 Axial HRCT section showing the jugular fossa. Note the thin plate of bone separating it from the carotid canal (caroticojugular spine)

The *facial nerve* has a meandering course within the temporal bone. The facial canal (also called the fallopian canal) is visualized on HRCT (Fig. 3.25). The *labyrinthine segment* and 1st genu are best visualized on axial sections as it travels anteriorly from the IAC and then forms an acute turn at the first genu. At the first genu, it is covered by a thin plate of bone with a hiatus for the greater superficial petrosal nerve. On coronal section at the level just posterior to the 1st genu, the nerve is seen as two round lucent areas above the cochlea—this appearance has been called "snake eyes." The 2nd part or tympanic segment courses in the medial wall of middle ear as described above. The 2nd genu lies at the junction of the nearly horizontal tympanic segment and the vertical mastoid segment. The mastoid segment lies posterior to the posterior wall of the middle ear and finally exits via the stylomastoid foramen. The nerve itself is not visualized on HRCT.

The mastoid in adults consists of a central mastoid antrum and multiple peripheral intercommunicating air cells (Fig. 3.26). The degree of mastoid pneumatization varies greatly. The mastoid antrum lies posterosuperior to the epitympanum to which it communicates via the aditus ad antrum (Fig. 3.27).

Potential routes of infection spread from the mastoid are the subarcuate canal (Fig. 3.28) and the mastoid emissary vein (Fig. 3.29). These structures are not constant and can sometimes be absent on imaging.

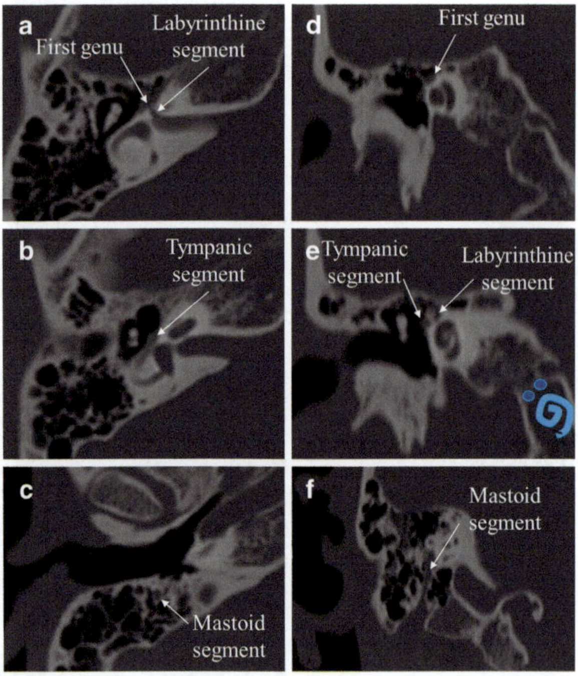

Fig. 3.25 Axial (**a–c**, from superior to inferior) and coronal (**d–f**, from anterior to posterior) sections of HRCT temporal bone showing the different segments of the facial nerve canal

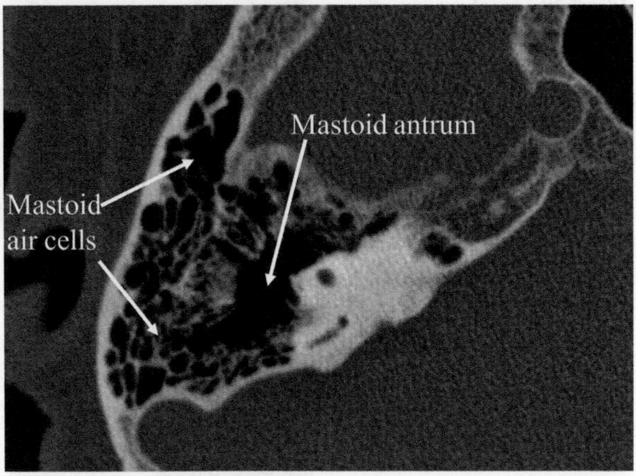

Fig. 3.26 Axial section of HRCT temporal bone showing the mastoid antrum and surrounding mastoid air cells

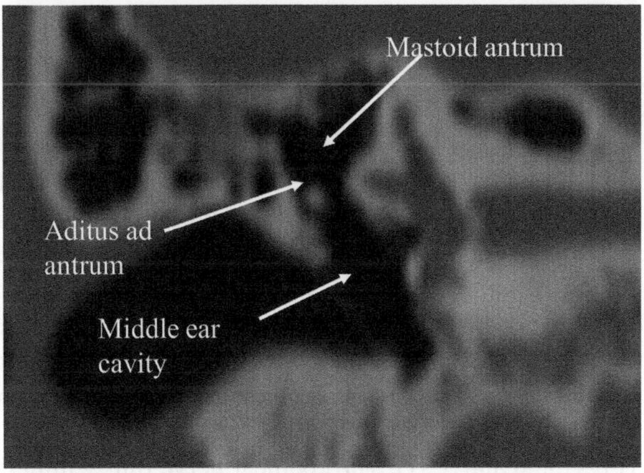

Fig. 3.27 Coronal section of HRCT temporal bone showing the aditus ad antrum between the epitympanum and the mastoid antrum

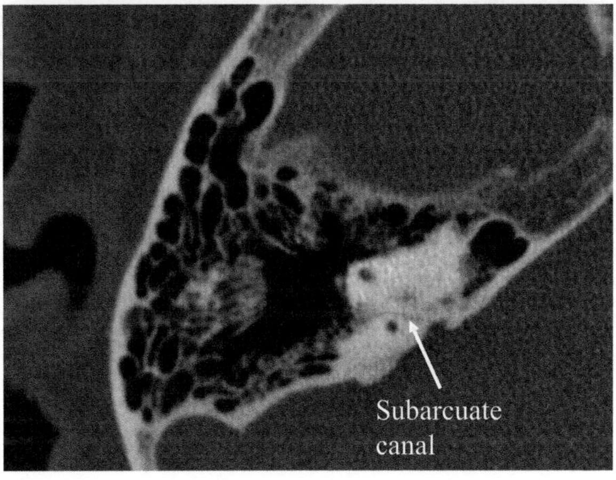

Fig. 3.28 Axial section of HRCT temporal bone showing a curvilinear lucency extending from the mastoid to posterior aspect of the petrous temporal bone at level inferior to the superior SCC. This canal transmits the subarcuate artery and vein

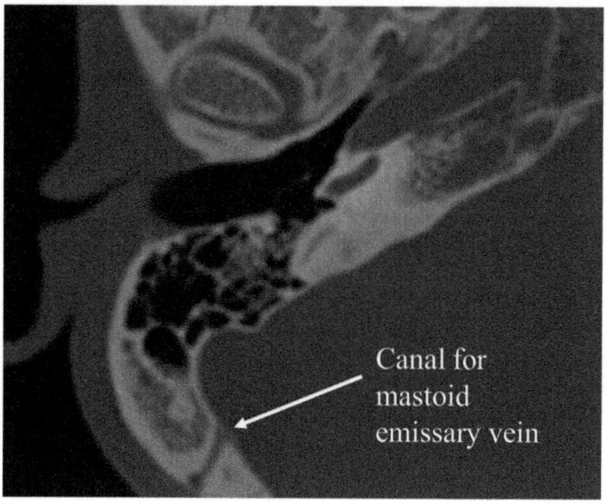

Fig. 3.29 Axial section of HRCT temporal bone showing a linear lucency traversing entire thickness of the calvarium just posterior to the mastoid. This represents canal for mastoid emissary vein which connects sigmoid sinus to the occipital vein

3.1.3 Inner Ear

The inner ear consists of an outer bony labyrinth and an inner membranous labyrinth. The space between the bony and membranous labyrinth is filled by a fluid called the perilymph, and the space within the membranous labyrinth is filled with a fluid called the endolymph. The bony labyrinth is well visualized on HRCT sections. The anterior component of the bony labyrinth is the cochlea, while the posterior component is the vestibule with semicircular canals (SCC).

The cochlea is seen on axial HRCT sections as a snail shell-like structure with around two and a half to two and three-fourth turns. It has a basal turn, middle turn, and apical turn with a central branching bony structure called the modiolus (Figs. 3.30 and 3.31). The cochlear nerve runs within the modiolus. A central aperture or lucency within the modiolus can be seen on HRCT corresponding to location of the cochlear nerve. The osseous spiral lamina branches out from the modiolus into the cochlear turns. The interscalar septum separates one turn of cochlea from the next. The rest of the internal cochlear structure (the cochlear duct/scala media, scala tympani, scala vestibuli, and basilar membrane) cannot be visualized on HRCT.

An oblique sagittal reconstruction parallel to the basal turn of the cochlea can be used to measure the cochlear width (distance from the round window to farthest point of the cochlea). This can be used to calculate the cochlear duct length using a formula which helps in planning cochlear implant surgery (Fig. 3.32).

The three semicircular canals are oriented in different planes and are usually evaluated on routine axial and coronal HRCT sections. Visualization of each complete canal in a single image requires special double oblique reconstructions (Fig. 3.33) which are not routinely used. Superior SCC dehiscence may be demonstrated on such a reconstruction.

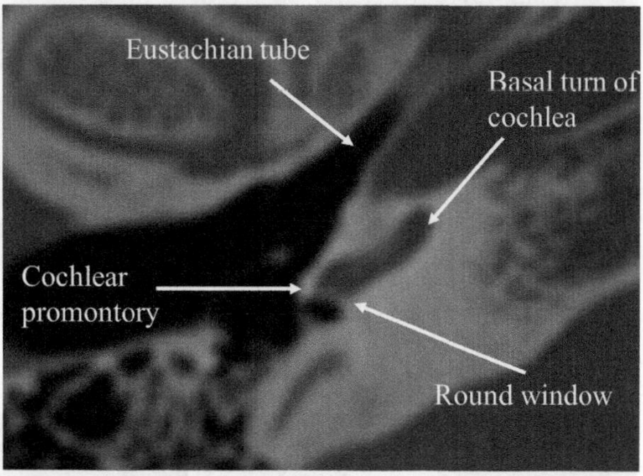

Fig. 3.30 Axial HRCT section showing the basal turn of the cochlea. Also noted are the round window niche and Eustachian tube opening into middle ear

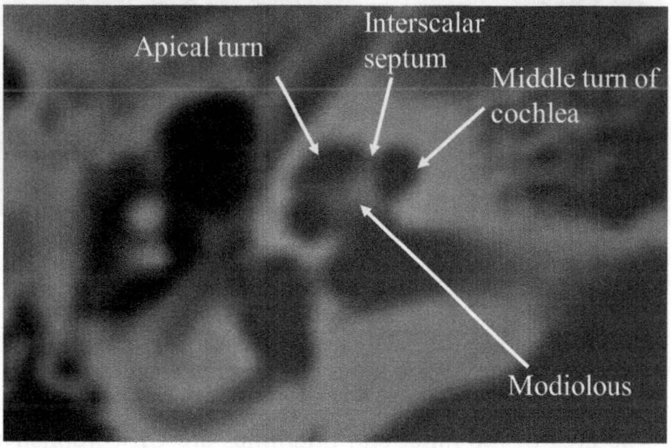

Fig. 3.31 Axial HRCT section showing the middle and apical turns of the cochlea with the central modiolus. Note the interscalar septum radiating from the modiolus and separating the cochlear turns

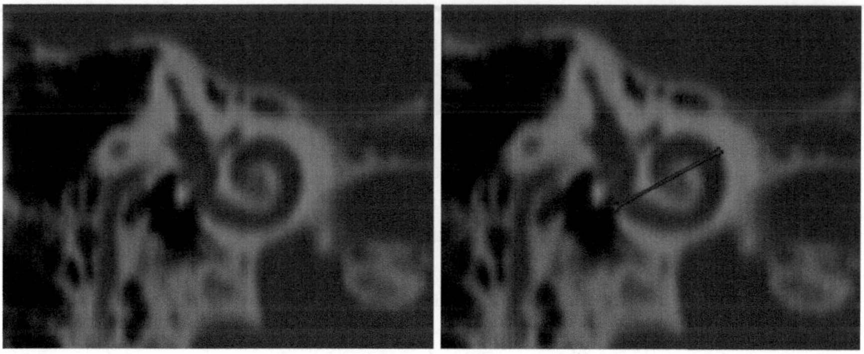

Fig. 3.32 Oblique sagittal HRCT section of the cochlea with the round window. The distance from the round window to farthest point of cochlea can be used to calculate the cochlear duct length (in mm) using a formula 4.16 x A - 2.7 where is A is the measured distance in mm

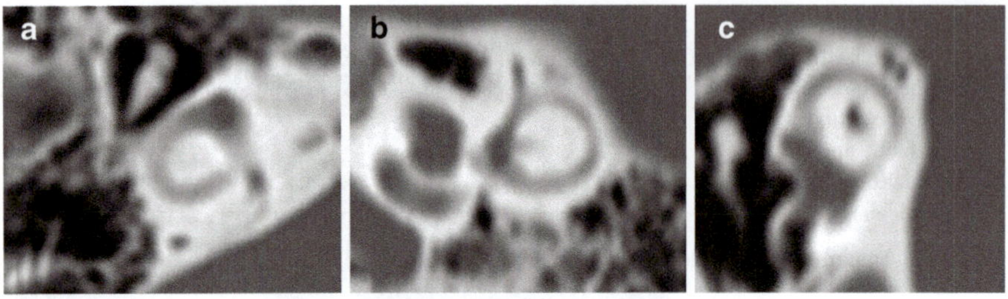

Fig. 3.33 Double oblique HRCT sections demonstrating the lateral (**a**), posterior (**b**), and superior (**c**) semicircular canals

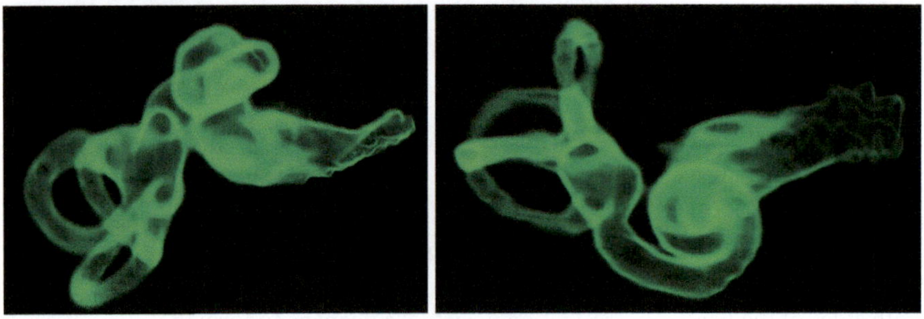

Fig. 3.34 Volume-rendered reconstructions of the inner ear structures and the internal auditory canal

Heavily T2-weighted 3D MRI sequences can be used to visualize the fluid-filled structures of the inner ear. Examples are CISS (constructive interference in steady state), FIESTA (fast imaging employing steady-state acquisition), and T2 SPACE (sampling perfection with application-optimized contrasts using flip angle evolution). The endolymph and perilymph, though physiologically different, appear similar in intensity to CSF on MRI sequences. The scala tympani and scala vestibuli can be seen as separate compartments on MRI separated by the spiral lamina. The scala media or cochlear duct and its internal structures are however not clearly visualized on images obtained in clinical 3T MRI scanners. The visualization of the membranous labyrinth (cochlear duct, saccule, utricle, and semicircular ducts) is currently not possible on routine clinical imaging and is a subject of research.

Heavily T2-weighted MRI sequences are also useful in performing volume rendered (VR) and maximum intensity projections (MIP) of inner ear structures (Figs. 3.34 and 3.35).

A clear advantage of MRI over CT is in evaluating the structures of the internal auditory canal. The VII/VIII cranial nerve complex is visualized in good detail on heavily T2-weighted 3D MRI sequences (Fig. 3.36). In superior sections of the axial MRI, the facial and superior vestibular nerve can be seen as two parallel lines while in inferior sections, the cochlear and inferior vestibular nerve can be seen forming a

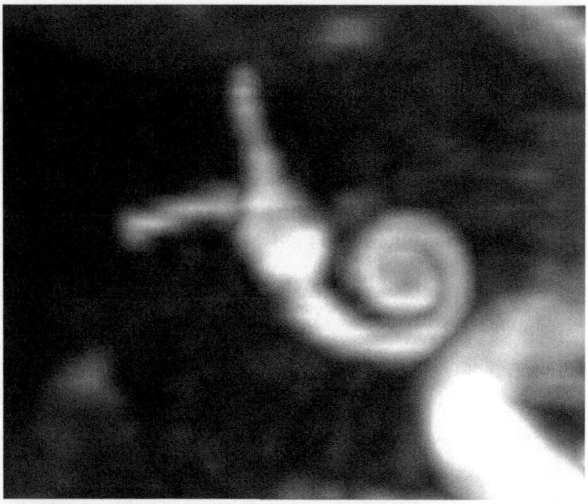

Fig. 3.35 MIP MR image of inner ear showing the cochlear turns, vestibule, and semicircular canals

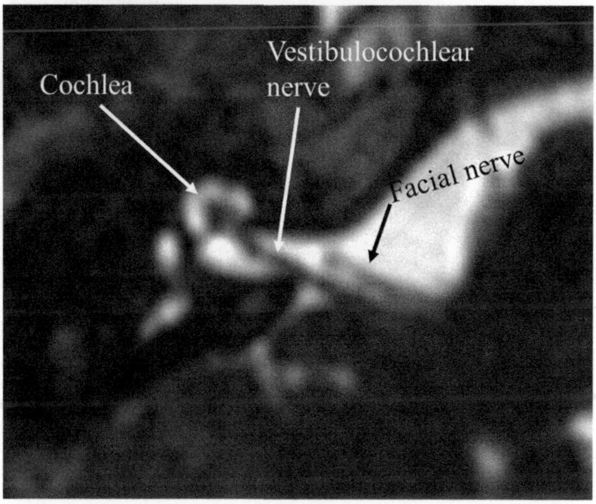

Fig. 3.36 Axial heavily T2-weighted image through the IAC shows the anteriorly placed facial nerve and posteriorly placed vestibulocochlear nerve. Also note the cochlea with modiolus and spiral lamina within

"Y." Oblique sagittal reconstructions perpendicular to the orientation of the IAC offer the best images of the VII/VIII nerve complex from origin from the brainstem up to inner ear level (Fig. 3.37). On the oblique sagittal images, the VIII nerve is twice as thick as the VII nerve. Thin section pre- and post-contrast fat-saturated T1-weighted images are used to look for enhancement along the nerves.

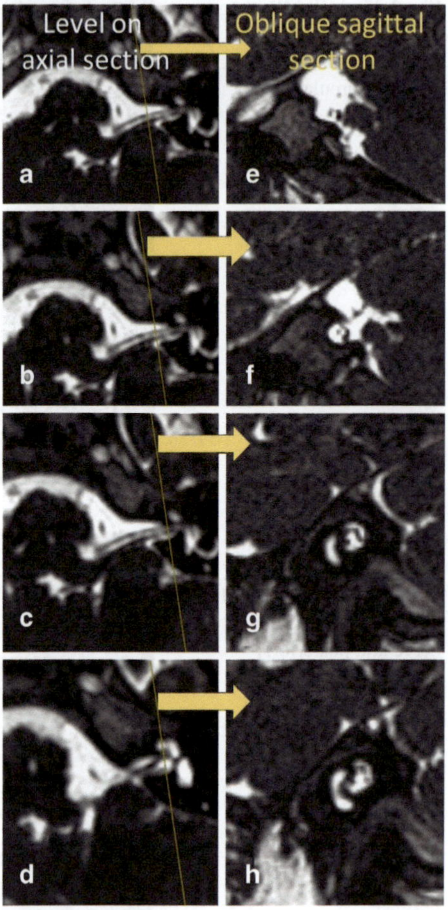

Fig. 3.37 Oblique sagittal T2-weighted image from medial to lateral (**e**–**h**) through the IAC shows the facial nerve, cochlear nerve, and superior and inferior vestibular nerves. The yellow line on the axial images (**a**–**d**) shows the level of the corresponding oblique sagittal sections

3.2 Imaging Anatomy on Scan Images

Standard HRCT of the temporal bone is acquired in the axial plane with scan done parallel to a line connecting the inferior orbital rim to the midpoint of the external auditory meatus (orbitomeatal line). Reconstruction of the axial and coronal planes are done parallel and perpendicular to the lateral semicircular canal.

Anatomy on axial HRCT sections from cranial to caudal is presented below in Figs. 3.38–3.57.

Anatomy on coronal HRCT sections from anterior to posterior is presented below in Figs. 3.58–3.71.

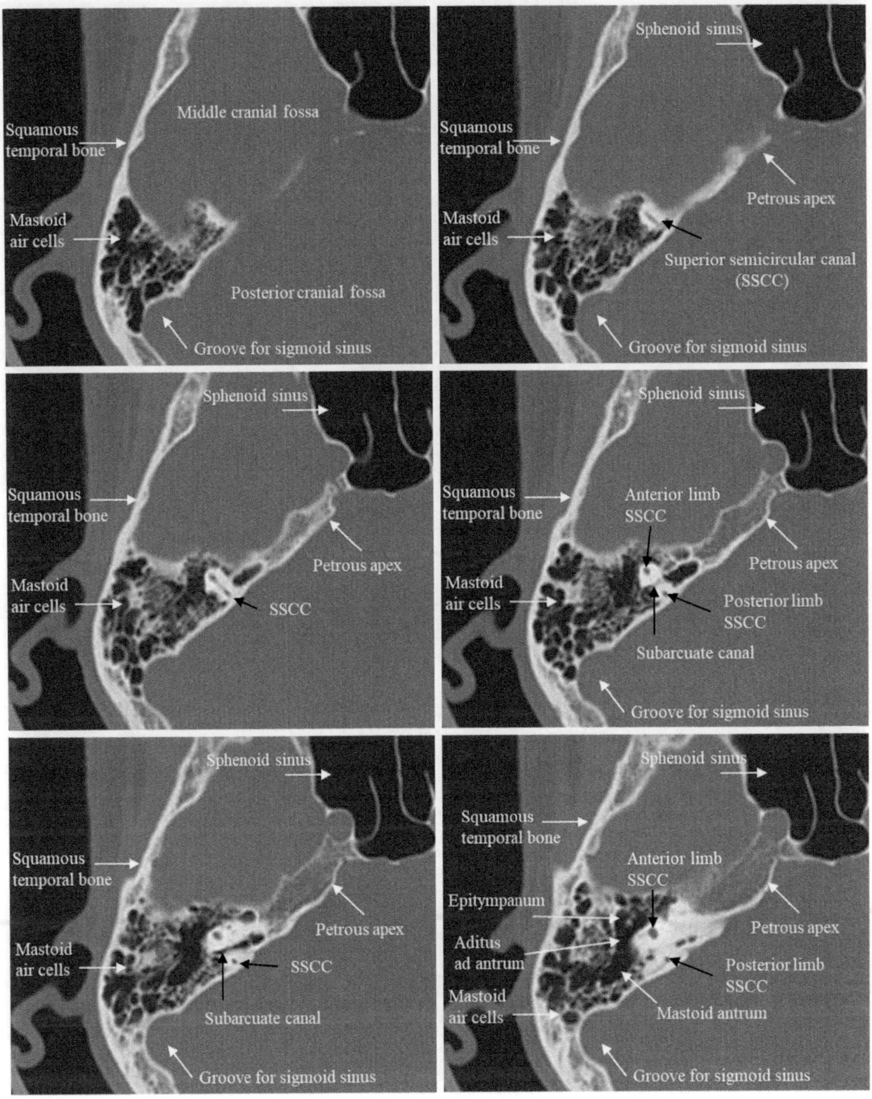

Figs. 3.38–3.57 Labelled sequential axial sections of HRCT temporal bone from cranial to caudal

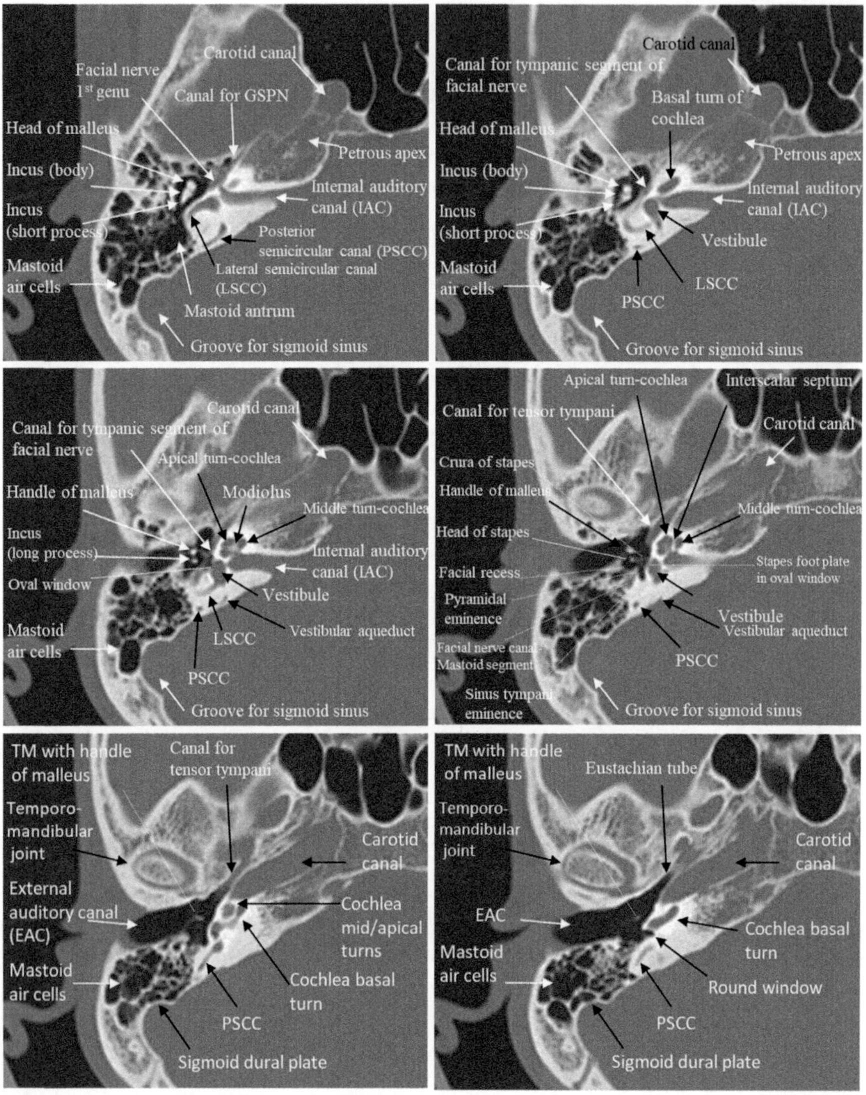

Figs. 3.38–3.57 (continued)

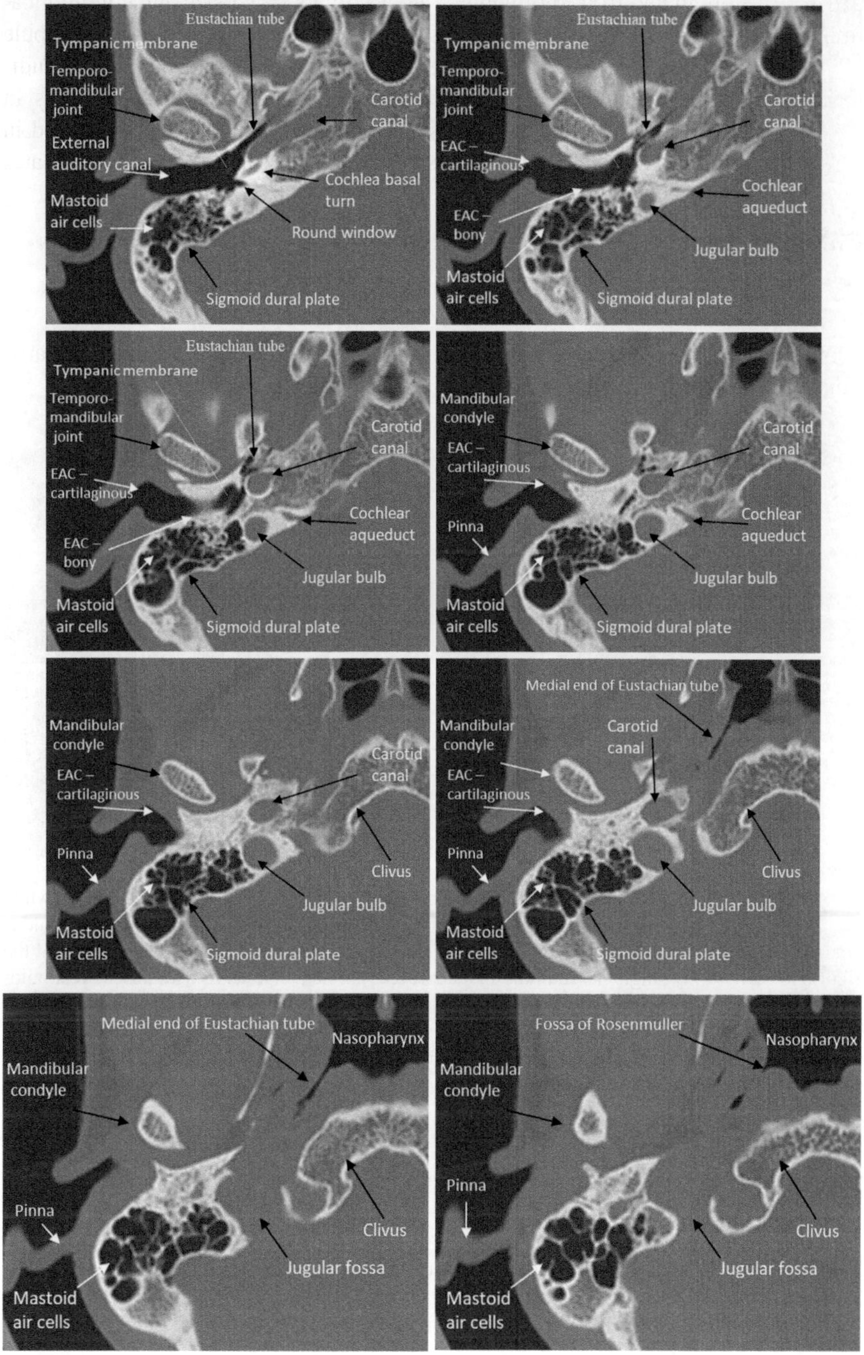

Figs. 3.38–3.57 (continued)

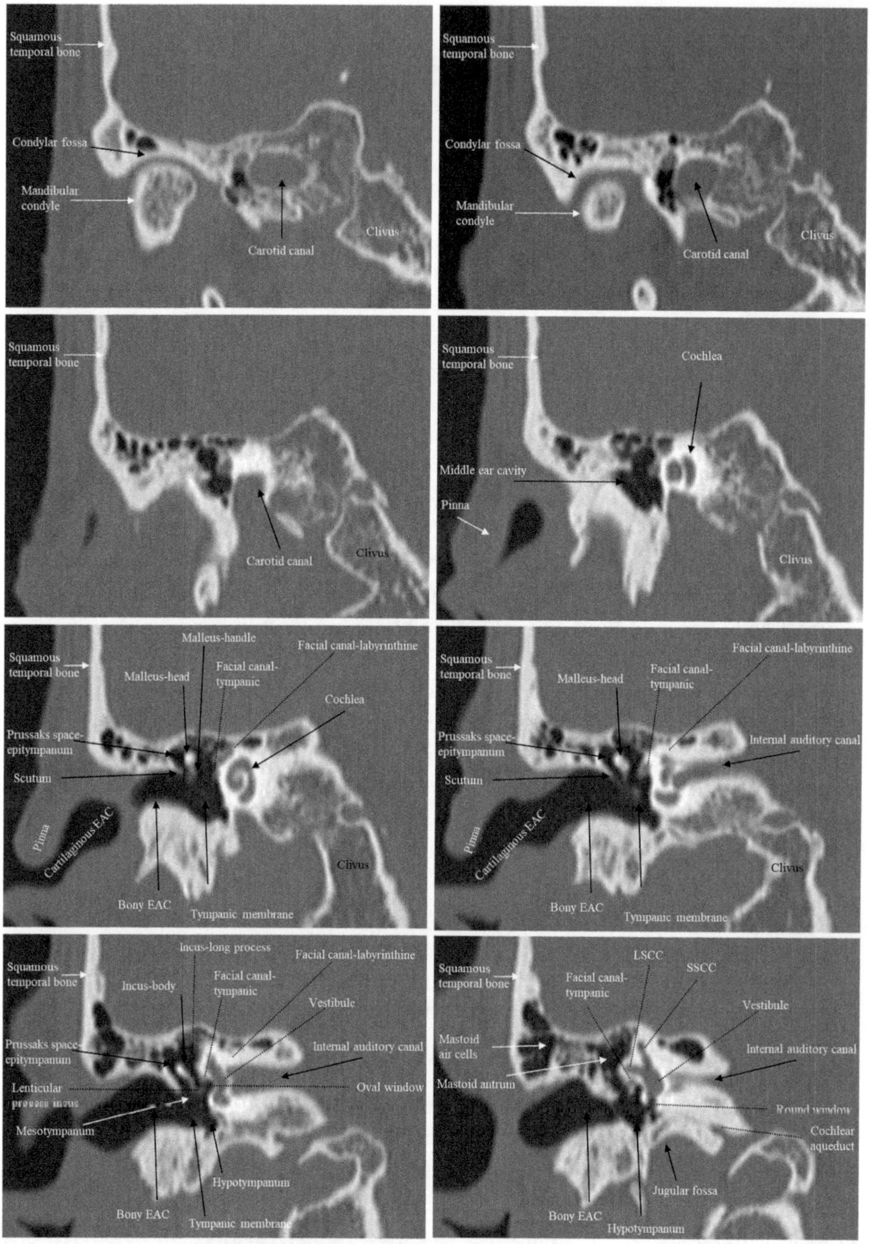

Figs. 3.58–3.71 Labelled sequential coronal sections of HRCT temporal bone from anterior to posterior

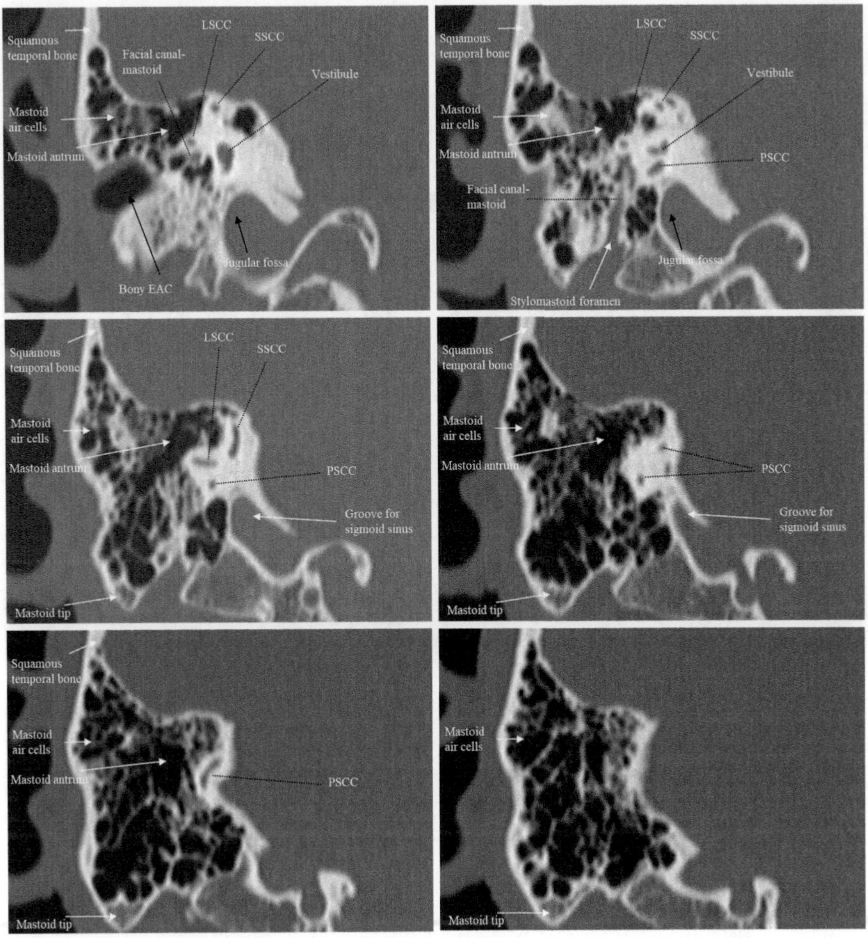

Figs. 3.58–3.71 (continued)

Poschl plane—Reconstruction is done in an oblique sagittal plane around 45 degrees oblique to midsagittal plane. The Poschl plane lies perpendicular to long axis of the petrous temporal bone (Fig. 3.72).

Stenver plane—Reconstruction is done in an oblique coronal plane parallel to long axis of the petrous temporal bone (Fig. 3.73).

Anatomy on axial heavily T2-weighted MR images from cranial to caudal is presented below in Figs. 3.74–3.88.

Anatomy on oblique heavily T2-weighted MR images from cranial to caudal is presented below in Figs. 3.89–3.103. The oblique sagittal images are acquired in direction perpendicular to the internal auditory canal.

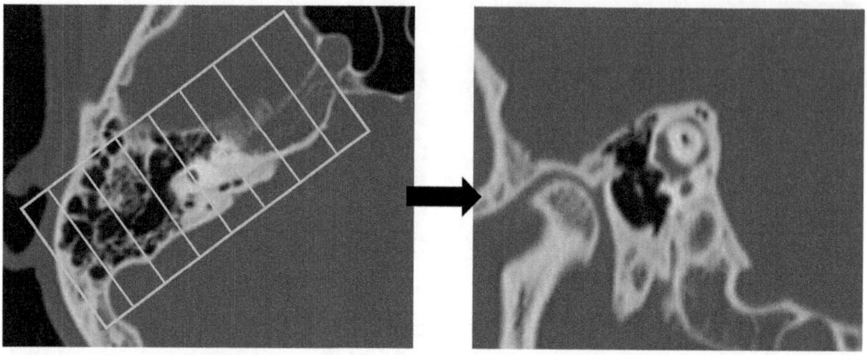

Fig. 3.72 Reconstructed image of HRCT temporal bone in the Poschl plane.

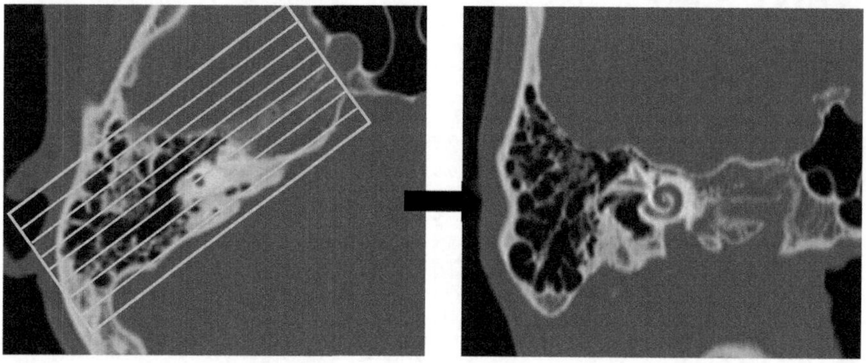

Fig. 3.73 Reconstructed image of HRCT temporal bone in the Stenver plane.

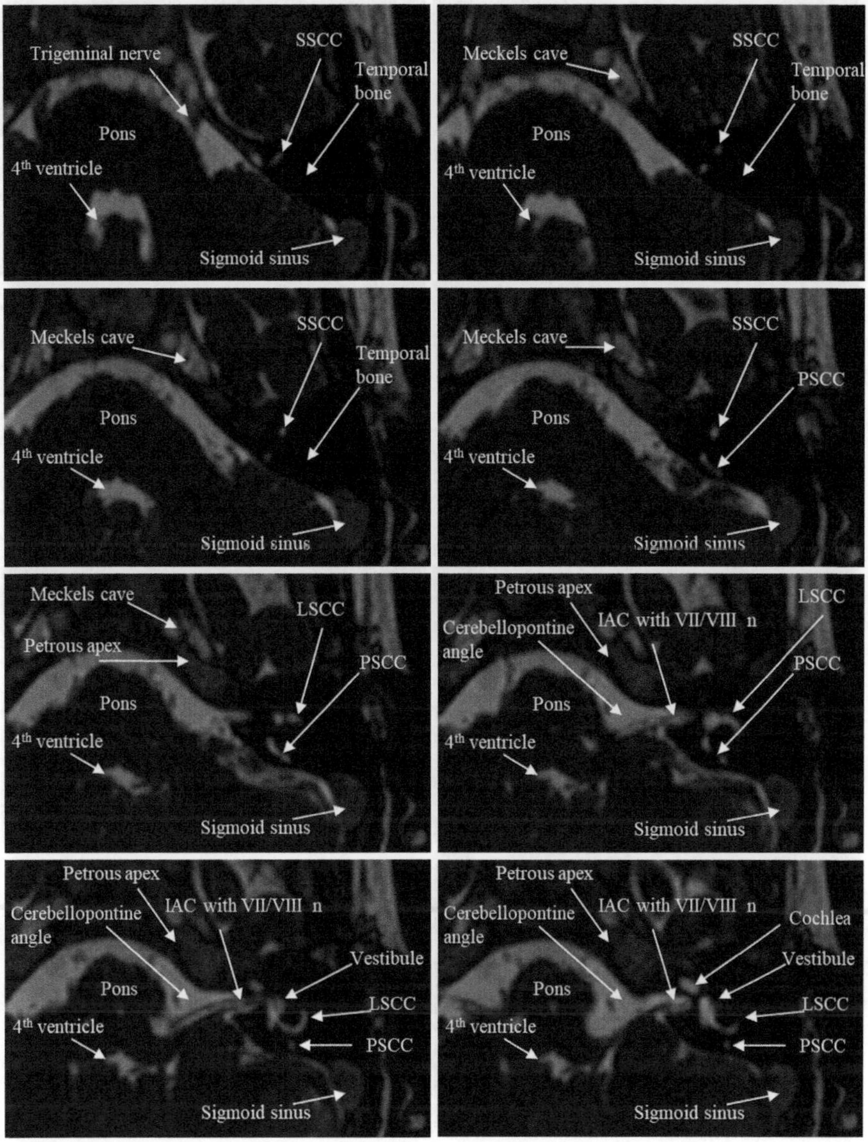

Figs. 3.74–3.88 Labelled sequential axial heavily T2-weighted MR images of the temporal bone from cranial to caudal

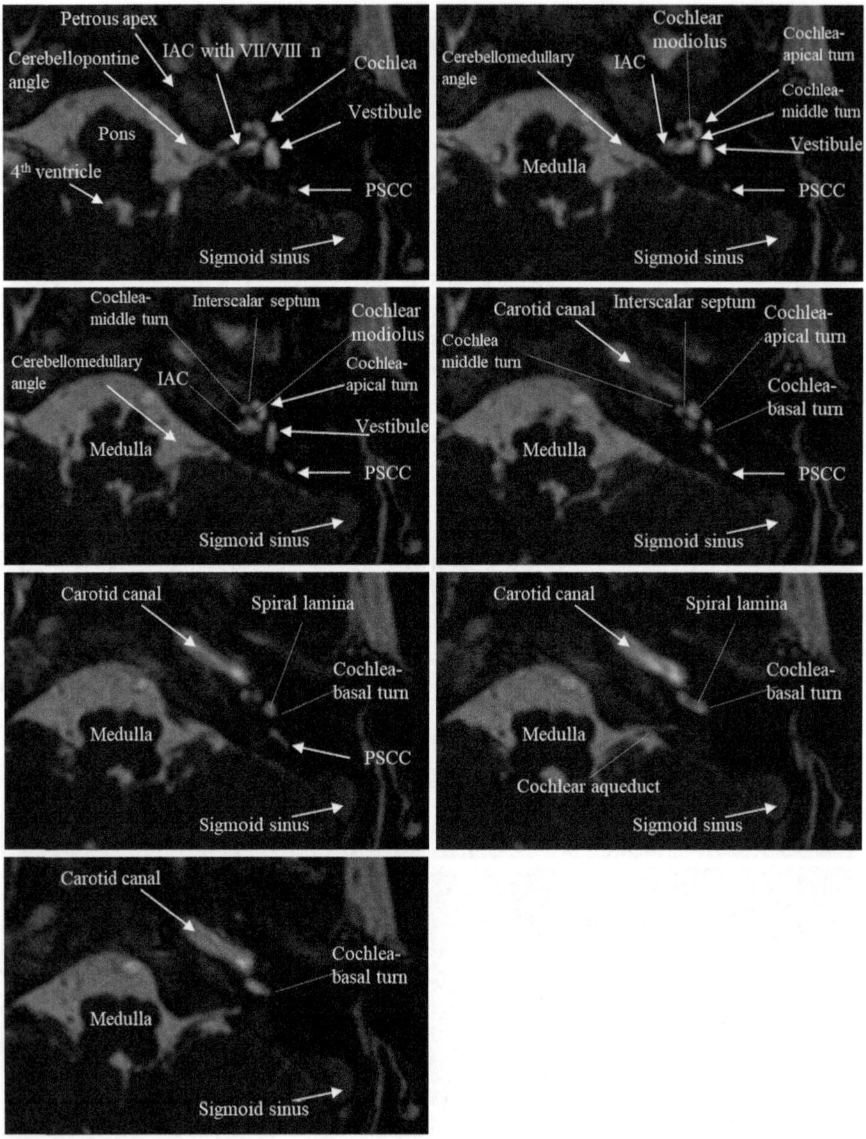

Figs. 3.74–3.88 (continued)

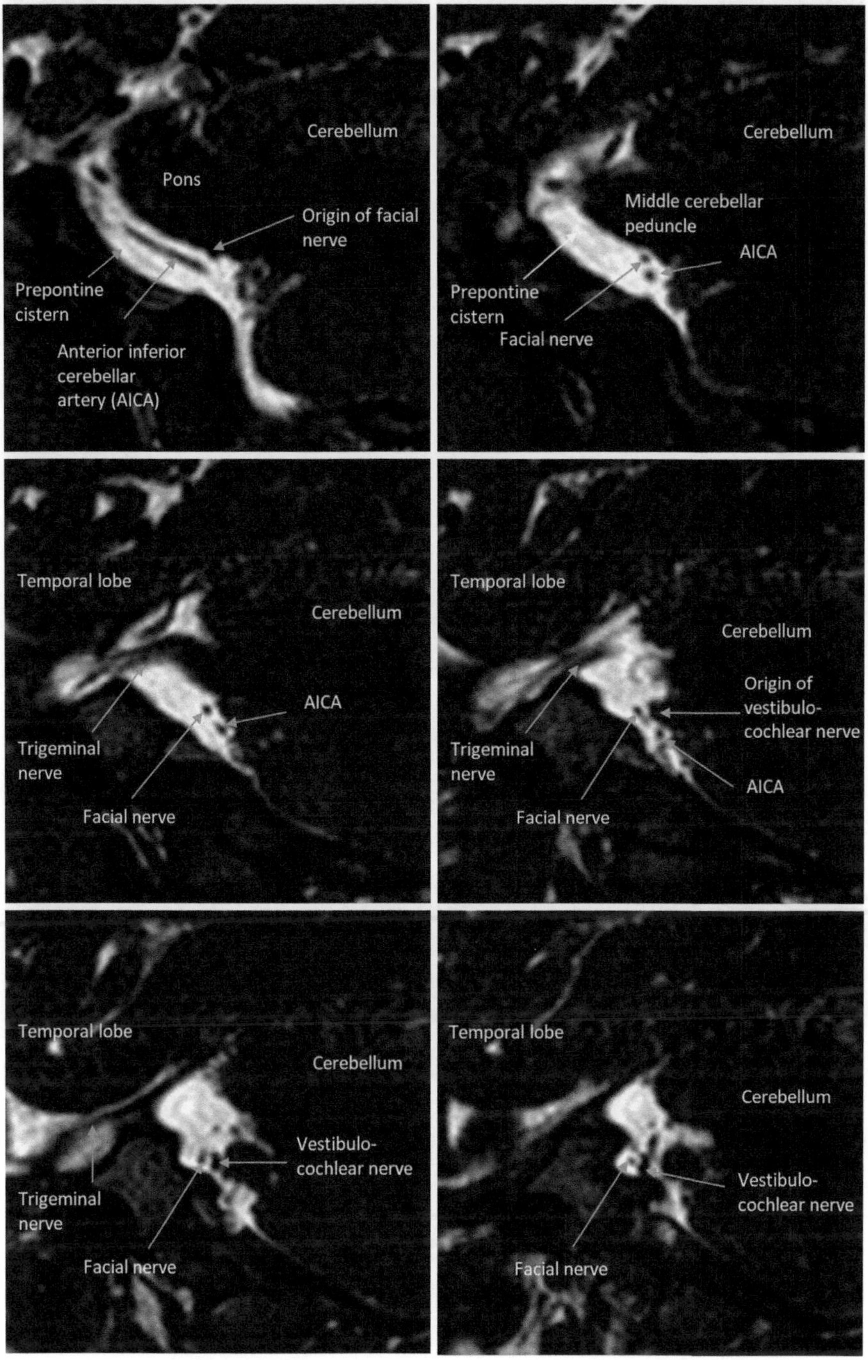

Figs. 3.89–3.103 Labelled sequential oblique sagittal heavily T2-weighted MR images of the temporal bone from medial to lateral

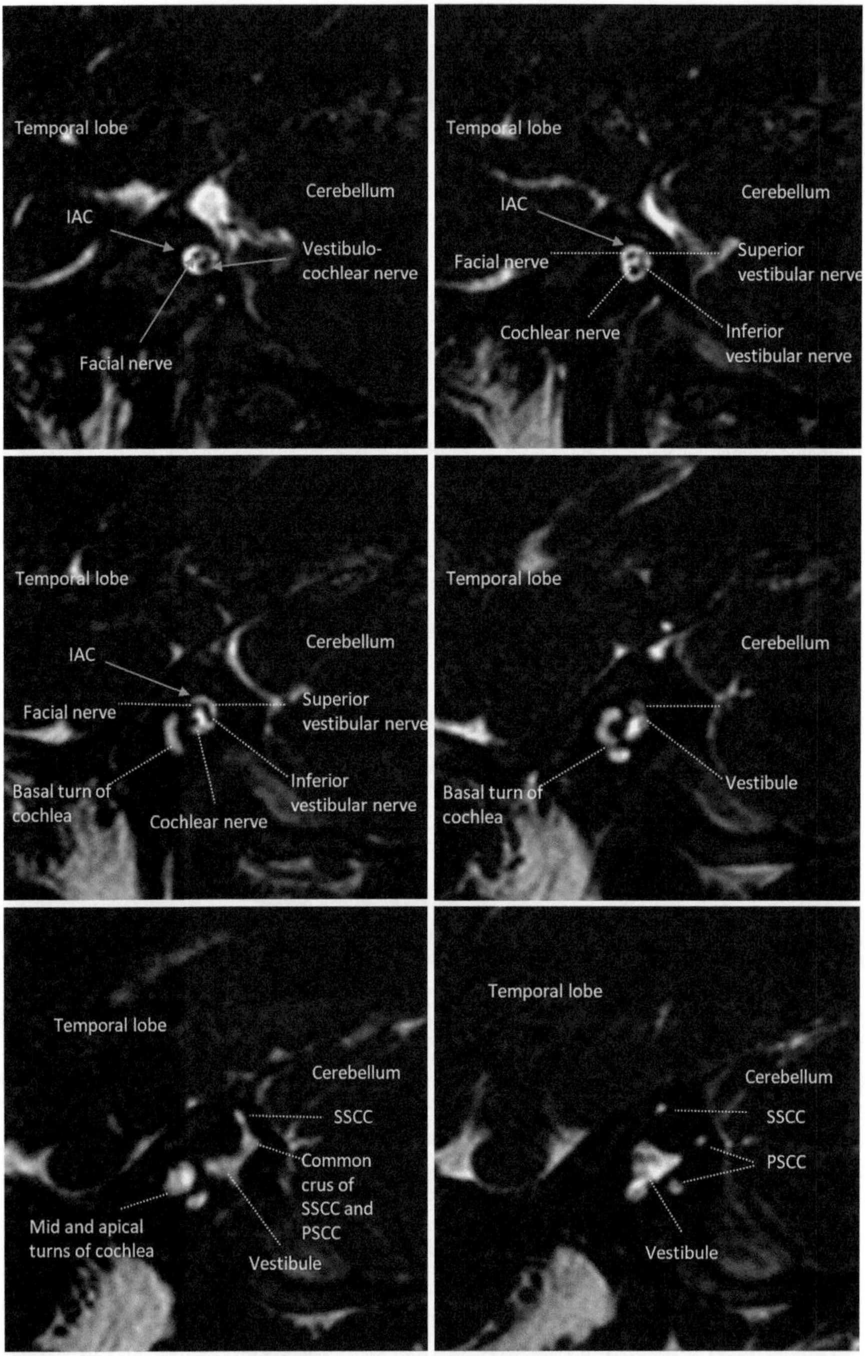

Figs. 3.89–3.103 (continued)

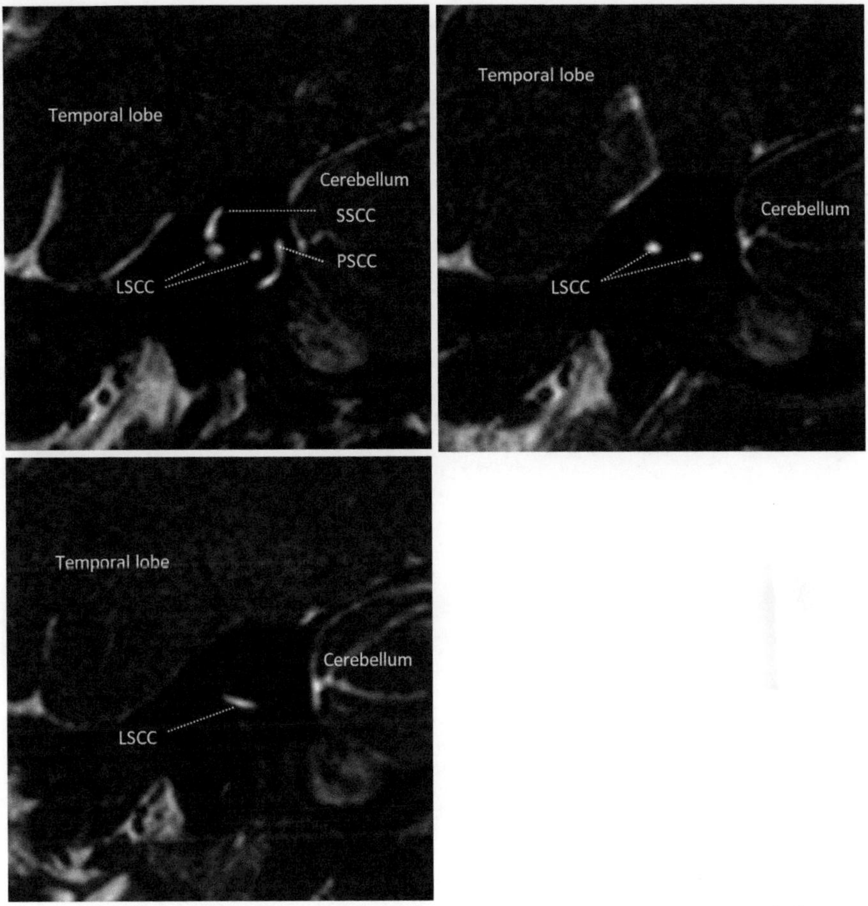

Figs. 3.89–3.103 (continued)

Part II
Case Based Approach to Temporal Bone Pathologies

Chapter 4
Congenital Anomalies of Temporal Bone: External Auditory Canal Atresia

Nikshita Jain and Aparna Irodi

Clinical History A 7-year-old boy with bilateral microtia.

Supplementary Information The online version contains supplementary material available at https://doi.org/10.1007/978-981-95-6132-2_4.

N. Jain (✉) · A. Irodi
Department of Radiology, CMC, Vellore, India

H. Mahalingam (ed.), *Temporal Bone Imaging*,
https://doi.org/10.1007/978-981-95-6132-2_4

Radiological Findings (Fig. 4.1)

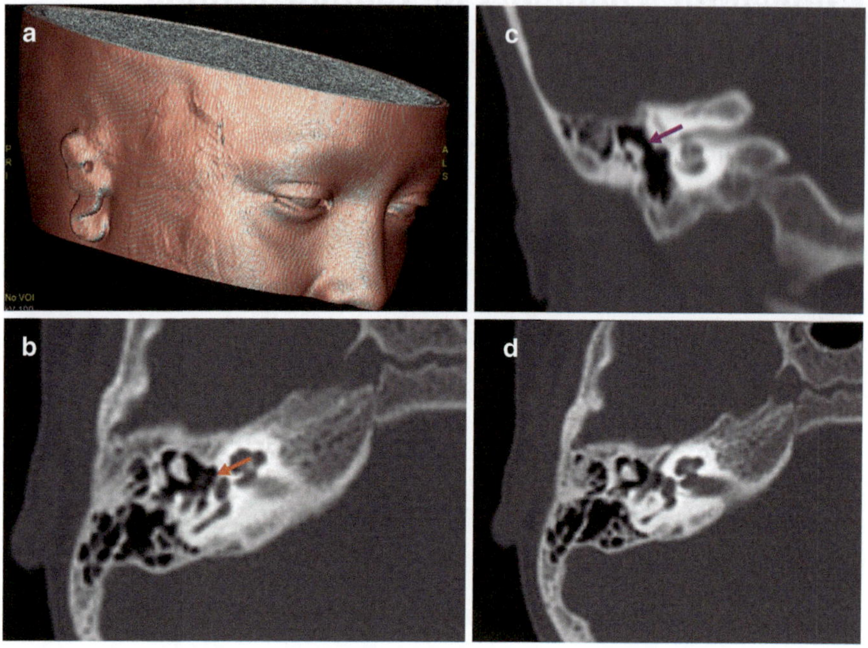

Fig. 4.1 Right ear: A rudimentary handle of malleus is noted. The head of malleus and short process of incus appear dysplastic; however, incudomalleolar articulation (purple) is maintained. The long process of incus, crus, and footplate of stapes (orange arrow) are normal. Width of middle ear cavity is 4–7 mm. Volume-rendered image (**a**) shows the microtia

Radiological Findings (Fig. 4.2)

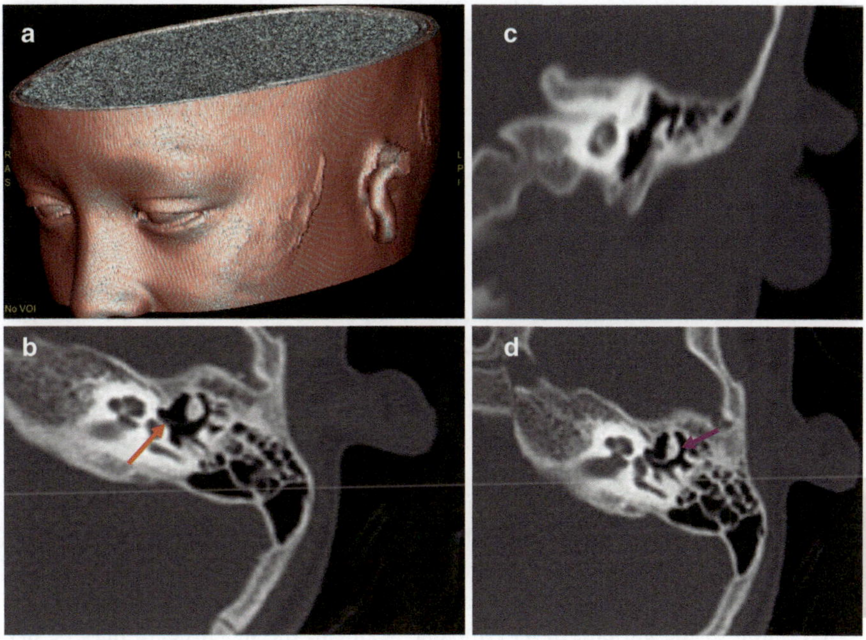

Fig. 4.2 Left ear: The handle of malleus is not seen. The head of malleus and short process of incus appear dysplastic; however, incudomalleolar articulation is maintained (purple arrow). The long process of incus, crus, and footplate of stapes are dysplastic (orange arrow). The width of middle ear cavity is 3.5–3.9 mm

Diagnosis Bilateral external auditory canal atresia, microtia, and dysplastic ossicles

Differential Diagnosis (If Applicable) Nil

Discussion

External auditory canal atresia (EACA) can be an isolated phenomenon or can be associated with various syndromes such as Goldenhar syndrome (craniofacial anomaly spectrum with malformation of the first and second branchial arch derivatives, characterized by facial and temporal bone hypoplasia, also involving ectodermal structures such as the otic placode), Treacher Collins syndrome (craniofacial dysplasia complex caused by a malformation of the first and second branchial arch derivatives and characterized by bilateral midface hypoplasia, micrognathia, and external and middle ear deformity), and Pierre Robin sequence (bilateral cleft palate, retrognathia, and glossoptosis) [1].

Usual presentation is with conductive hearing loss, and given the preserved sensorineural hearing, surgical restoration of the hearing can be achieved. A systematic approach in evaluating temporal bone HRCT in the EACA patient is essential. The grading scale introduced by Jahrsdoerfer et al. [2] is commonly used. According to this scale, the presence or absence of nine anatomical structures yields a score from 0 to 10. The higher the Jahrsdoerfer score, the higher is the probability of a good postoperative hearing outcome. In general, patients with a Jahrsdoerfer score <6 are not considered surgical candidates. An important perquisite for using the grading scale is that cochlear function and inner ear structures must be normal.

The Jahrsdoerfer grading scale:

1. Stapes: Two points are assigned if the stapes is present, 0 if it is absent.
2. Oval window: The oval window diameter should be ≥2 mm where the oval window enters the vestibule (1 point). A diameter <2 mm gives 0 points.
3. Middle ear cavity: In the coronal plane, the width of the middle ear cavity is measured from the promontory to the atretic bone. A measure ≥3 mm receives 1 point, whereas measures <3 mm receive 0 points.
4. Facial nerve: If the course of the facial nerve is unfavorable for surgical approach, it receives 0 points. Otherwise, 1 point is assigned. The descending segment is frequently displaced in the ventral and lateral directions resulting in the facial nerve passing along or through the atretic plate. Anterolateral displacement of the stylomastoid foramen may lead to extracranial facial nerve injury during elevation of the auricle. In its tympanic segment, the facial nerve may be displaced caudally, overlying the oval window. Typically, the pyramidal eminence with the second genu is displaced anteriorly in the tympanic cavity.
5. Incudomalleolar articulation: Usually normal (1 point is assigned), with a rudimentary hammer handle attached to the atretic plate. Severe incudomalleolar dysplasia and integrity of the incudostapedial joint is best evaluated in the coronal planes.
6. Mastoid pneumatization: A sclerotic, poorly or non-aerated mastoid receives 0 points. Otherwise, 1 point is assigned.
7. Incudostapedial articulation: If the joint is well defined, 1 point is assigned. In case of joint discontinuity, rotation or fusion to adjacent bony structures, 0 points are assigned.
8. Round window: If the round window diameter is <1 mm in diameter, it is considered stenotic and assigned 0 points. Otherwise, 1 point is assigned.
9. External ear: A normal and fairly developed auricle is assigned 1 point, but when configuration is poorer (microtia), 0 points are assigned.

References

1. Gassner EM, Mallouhi A, Jaschke WR. Preoperative evaluation of external auditory canal atresia on high-resolution CT. Am J Roentgenol. 2004;182(5):1305–12.
2. Yeakley JW, Jahrsdoerfer RA. CT evaluation of congenital aural atresia: what the radiologist and surgeon need to know. J Comput Assist Tomogr. 1996;20(5):724–31.

Chapter 5
Congenital Anomalies of Temporal Bone: Goldenhar Syndrome

Harshavardhan Mahalingam and Asthik Biswas

Clinical Data A 2-year-old male child with previous diagnosis of Goldenhar syndrome referred for evaluation of reduced hearing.

Radiological Findings (Fig. 5.1)

Diagnosis Microtia, stenotic EAC, dysplastic ossicles, otitis media, and right C1 hemivertebra – Goldenhar syndrome (ocular-auriculo-vertebral spectrum, OAVS)

Differential Diagnosis (If Applicable) Nil

Discussion

Goldenhar syndrome is a rare congenital disorder characterized by anomalies of development of the 1st and 2nd branchial arches. It is thought to be sporadic in most cases, with a few isolated reports of autosomal dominant or autosomal recessive pattern of inheritance. Prevalence is reported to be around 1 in 3500 births with a 3:2 male predominance.

Ear anomalies are the most common manifestation and include preauricular tags/appendages and microtia often accompanied by hemifacial microsomia/mandibular hypoplasia. Ocular abnormalities are next most common manifestation and include microphthalmia, anophthalmia, coloboma, and an epibulbar dermoid. The triad is

Supplementary Information The online version contains supplementary material available at https://doi.org/10.1007/978-981-95-6132-2_5.

H. Mahalingam (✉)
Department of Radiology, SRIHER, Chennai, India

A. Biswas
Department of Pediatric Neuroradiology, Great Ormond Street Hospital, London, UK

H. Mahalingam (ed.), *Temporal Bone Imaging*,
https://doi.org/10.1007/978-981-95-6132-2_5

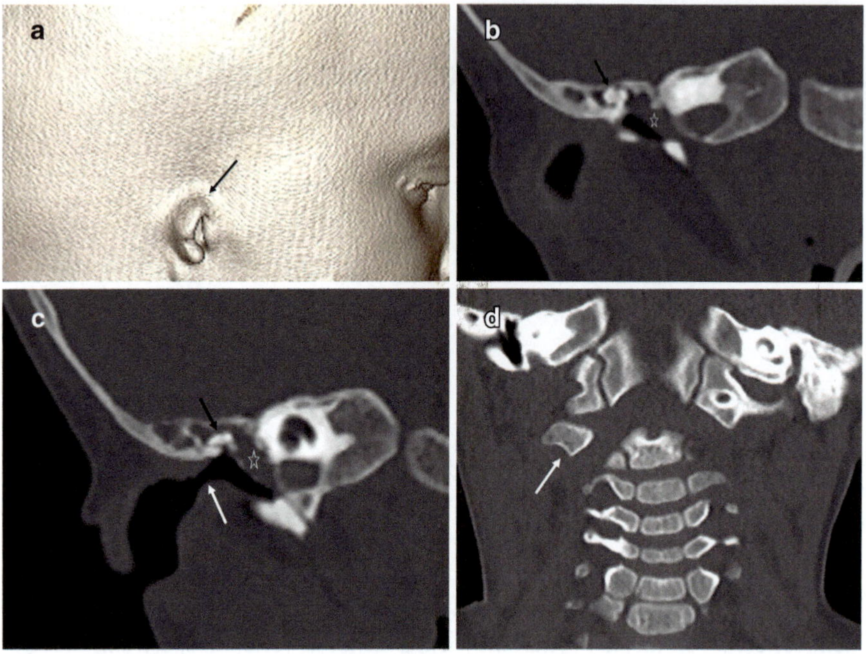

Fig. 5.1 (**a**) Volume-rendered image of the soft tissue reconstruction of temporal bone CT shows small deformed pinna suggestive of microtia. (**b**) Coronal reconstruction of temporal bone HRCT shows dysplastic malleus and incus (black arrow). (**c**) Coronal reconstruction of temporal bone HRCT shows narrowing at the external auditory meatus (white arrow) and soft tissue density filling the middle ear and mastoid antrum (star) with dysplastic malleus and incus (black arrow). (**d**) Coronal reconstruction of cervical spine CT shows C1 hemivertebra on the right side (arrow) with the left half of the C1 vertebra not being visualized

completed by abnormalities of the cervical spine such as hemivertebra, block vertebra, scoliosis, and spinal dysraphism. These manifestations are usually unilateral and are more common on the right side. Bilateral involvement has also been reported.

Other associated anomalies described include cleft lip/cleft palate, congenital heart disease, radial ray anomalies, and anomalies of the urogenital system, central nervous system, and upper aerodigestive tract [1].

In the temporal bone, external and middle ear anomalies are more common, and include microtia, anotia, EAC stenosis/atresia, and ossicular dysplasia. Inner ear anomalies have been reported in up to one-third of these patients and include narrowing or enlargement of the IAC, semicircular canal dysplasia (with lateral SCC being most commonly affected), vestibular dysplasia, and rarely cochlear anomalies. Anomalies in course of facial nerve can also be seen [2].

References

1. Strömland K, Miller M, Sjögreen L, Johansson M, Joelsson BE, Billstedt E, et al. Oculo-auriculo-vertebral spectrum: associated anomalies, functional deficits and possible developmental risk factors. Am J Med Genet A. 2007;143A(12):1317–25.
2. Hennersdorf F, Friese N, Löwenheim H, Tropitzsch A, Ernemann U, Bisdas S. Temporal bone changes in patients with Goldenhar syndrome with special emphasis on inner ear abnormalities. Otol Neurotol. 2014;35(5):826–30.

Chapter 6
Congenital Anomalies of Temporal Bone: Inner Ear Anomalies

Hiren Panwala, Asthik Biswas, Harshavardhan Mahalingam, and Sonal Garg

Clinical History A 3-month-old child detected to have congenital hearing loss.

Supplementary Information The online version contains supplementary material available at https://doi.org/10.1007/978-981-95-6132-2_6.

H. Panwala (✉) · S. Garg
Department of Radiology, SRCC, Mumbai, India

A. Biswas
Department of Pediatric Neuroradiology, Great Ormond Street Hospital, NHS Foundation Trust, London, UK

H. Mahalingam
Department of Radiology, SRIHER, Chennai, India

H. Mahalingam (ed.), *Temporal Bone Imaging*,
https://doi.org/10.1007/978-981-95-6132-2_6

Radiological Findings (Fig. 6.1)

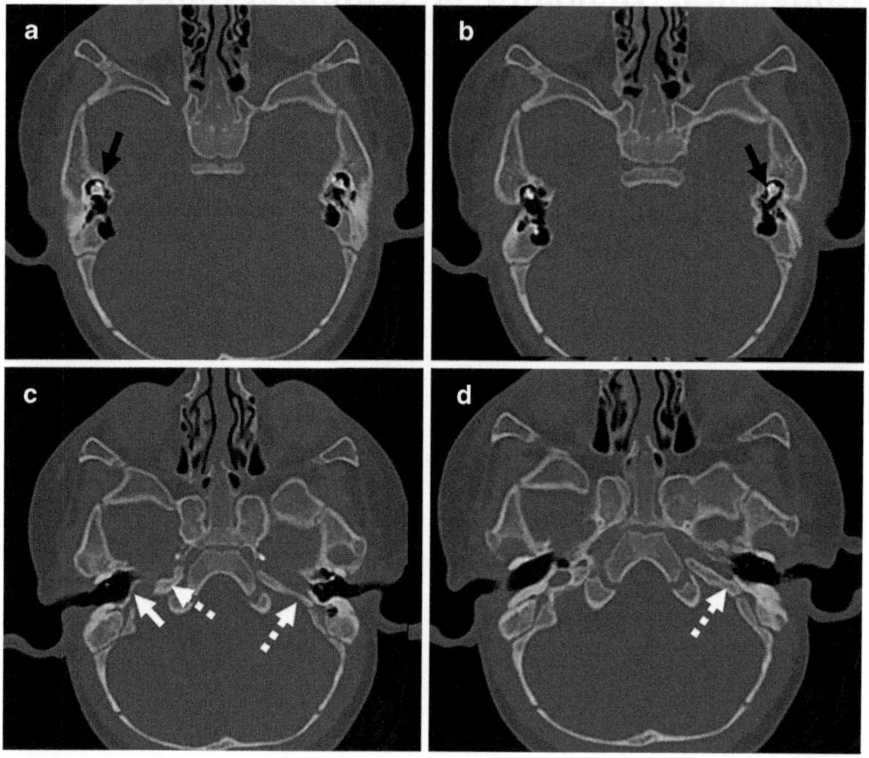

Fig. 6.1 (**a** and **b**) Axial sections of HRCT temporal bone at more cranial level show small bilateral middle ear cavities with dysplastic ossicles (black arrows). (**c** and **d**) Axial sections of HRCT temporal bone at more caudal levels show complete absence of the otic capsule and severely hypoplastic petrous apices (dashed arrows). Note the flattened medial wall of middle ear (white arrow). Bilateral IAC were absent and the facial canal could not be clearly delineated

Diagnosis Complete labyrinthine aplasia (CLA) on both sides

Discussion

CLA is a rare inner ear malformation (accounting for around 1% of inner ear anomalies) characterized by absent inner ear structures. It is also known as Michel's deformity. It is caused by arrest in development of the otic placode early in embryonic life during or before the 3rd week of gestation.

It is usually accompanied by petrous apex hypoplasia. The otic capsule (represented by an island of dense sclerotic bone in the petrous pyramid) may be hypoplastic or absent. Based on these features, CLA can be classified into three types: (1) CLA with hypoplastic or aplastic petrous temporal bone, (2) CLA with aplastic otic capsule, and (3) CLA with otic capsule [1].

The internal auditory canal when present contains only the facial nerve. The IAC may also be completely absent. Hypoplasia of the middle ear cavity and hypoplasia/dysplasia of the stapes can be observed. Other associated anomalies described include absent round and oval windows, anomalous course of the facial nerve, and skull base and craniovertebral junction anomalies.

CLA with otic capsule can sometimes by misdiagnosed as labyrinthitis ossificans which in late stages can show complete obliteration of inner ear structures. It can be distinguished from CLA by the clinical history of prior inner ear infection/meningitis and a well-formed promontory seen as a convex bulge along the medial wall of middle ear [2].

CLA is obviously a contraindication for cochlear implantation. Auditory brainstem implantation (ABI) is the only option for hearing rehabilitation in these patients.

Clinical History A 7-month-old boy detected to have congenital hearing loss

Radiological Findings (Fig. 6.2)

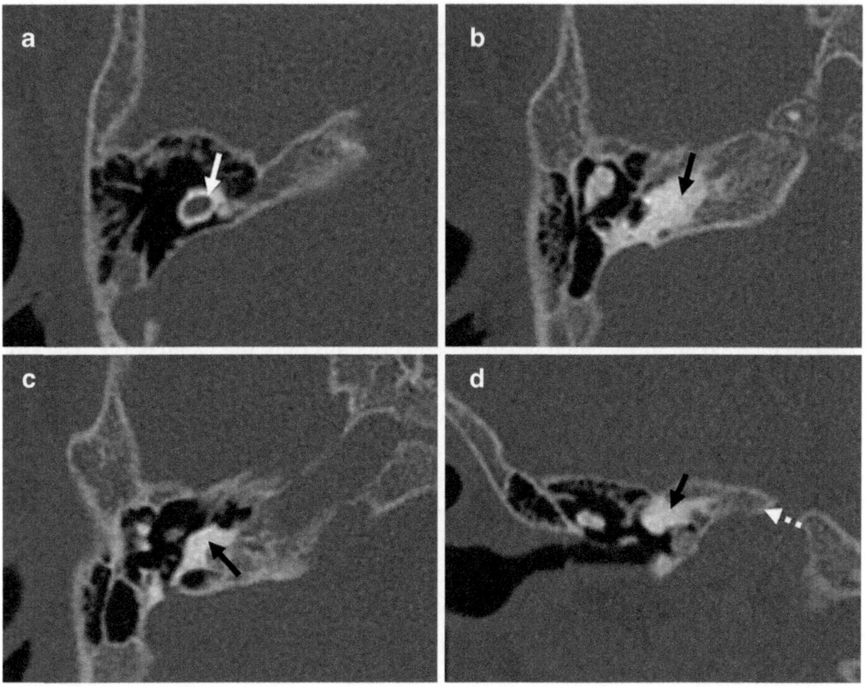

Fig. 6.2 (**a–c**) Axial HRCT sections of the right temporal bone (from cranial to caudal) show a small cystic structure (white arrow) within the otic capsule of the petrous temporal bone with no discernible bony labyrinthine structure. The right internal auditory canal is absent. (**d**) Coronal HRCT section of the right temporal bone shows normal external and middle ear with hypoplastic petrous apex (dashed arrow). The black arrows point to the dense sclerotic bone of the otic capsule. (Case courtesy Dr. Sonal Garg Consultant radiologist, SRCC hospital, Mumbai)

Diagnosis Rudimentary otocyst (right ear)

Discussion

Rudimentary otocyst refers to a small cystic structure within the otic capsule (usually measuring only a few mm in size) with no intracranial communication. It occurs due to developmental arrest at stage of otic vesicle in 3rd to 4th week of embryonic life. The internal auditory canal (IAC) is absent. Hypoplasia of the petrous bone may be present. Similar to CLA, these patients are also not candidates for cochlear implantation.

Clinical History A 9-month-old girl detected to have congenital hearing loss

Radiological Findings (Fig. 6.3)

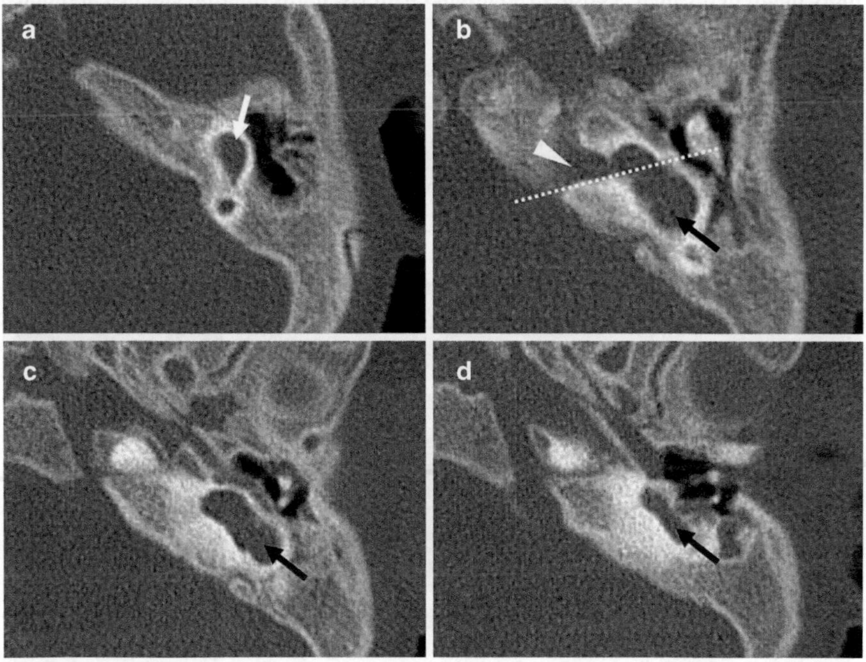

Fig. 6.3 (**a**) Axial HRCT section of temporal bone shows a dilated dysplastic superior semicircular canal. (**b–d**) Axial sections at more caudal levels show an ovoid cystic structure (black arrow) within the otic capsule with no definite differentiation into the cochlea and vestibule. Note the internal auditory canal (arrowhead) opening into the cystic structure. A line drawn along the posterior border of the internal auditory canal passes through the cystic structure

Diagnosis Common cavity malformation

Discussion

Common cavity (CC) malformation refers to an ovoid or round cystic structure in the otic capsule which represents undifferentiated cochlea and vestibule. It occurs due to developmental arrest of inner ear at 4th week of embryonic life. The common cavity shows communication with the IAC. Superior semicircular canal may be present and is often dysplastic.

CC is differentiated from rudimentary otocyst by its larger size and communication with the IAC. Differentiation of CC from cochlear aplasia dilated vestibule (CADV) is important. A line drawn along the posterior border of the internal auditory canal passes through the cystic structure in CC malformation, whereas in CADV, the cystic structure is wholly posterior to this line. CADV is discussed in more detail in the next section [3]. Patients with CC malformation can be candidates for cochlear implantation.

Clinical History A 17-month-old boy detected to have congenital hearing loss

Radiological Findings (Fig. 6.4)

Diagnosis Cochlear aplasia with dilated vestibule (right ear) and incomplete partition type 1 (left ear)

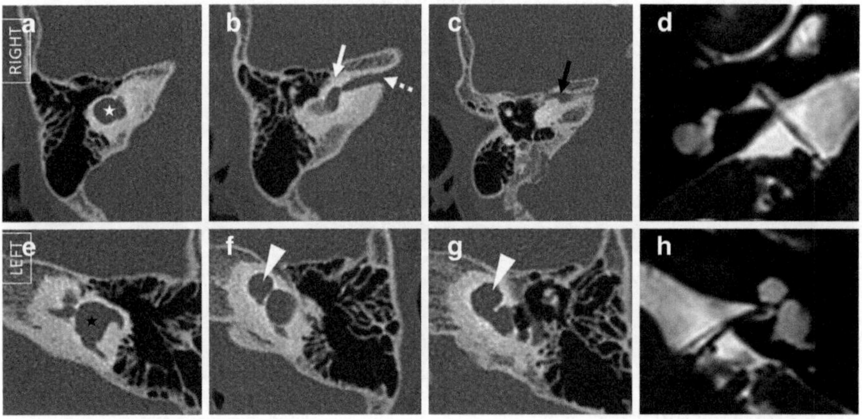

Fig. 6.4 (**a–c**) Axial HRCT sections of right temporal bone show dilated cystic vestibule (white star) with absent cochlea (white arrow) and narrow IAC (dashed arrow). Note the anomalous course of facial nerve with obtuse angle at first genu (black arrow). (**d**) CISS image at level of the right IAC shows only single nerve in the IAC representing the facial nerve with absent vestibulocochlear nerve. (**e–g**) Axial HRCT sections of left temporal bone show dilated vestibule (black star) with a cystic dilated cochlea with no modiolus (white arrowheads). (**h**) CISS image at level of the left IAC shows normal IAC dimensions with normal 7th and 8th cranial nerves. (Case courtesy Dr. Sonal Garg Consultant radiologist, SRCC hospital, Mumbai)

Discussion

Cochlear aplasia (CA) is characterized by complete absence of cochlea with the usual location of the cochlea being occupied by dense sclerotic bone. The cochlear nerve is also absent in this anomaly. IAC is usually narrow with obtuse angle at 1st genu of facial nerve.

CA occurs when there is interruption of inner ear development between the 3rd and 5th week of embryonic life. It is a rare inner ear malformation accounting for around 3%. Two types are described: CA with a normal vestibule and CA with dilated vestibule, the latter being more common.

CA with dilated vestibule (CADV) needs to be differentiated from common cavity malformation as both conditions show a dilated cystic structure in the petrous bone connected to the IAC. This differentiation on imaging is important as patients with common cavity malformation may benefit from a cochlear implantation while patients with CADV are typically not candidates for cochlear implantation. These two conditions can be differentiated by the relation of the lateral end of the IAC to the cystic structure in inner ear. In CADV, the cystic structure is wholly posterior to the posterior border of IAC while in CC malformation, the IAC opens into the center of the cystic structure.

Incomplete partition (IP) refers to a group of anomalies in which the cochlea and vestibule are seen as two separate structures with normal external dimensions but have various defects in their internal structure. Three different types of IP are described based on status of the modiolus and the interscalar septa.

In incomplete partition type 1 (IP-1), the cochlea is located normally and appears entirely cystic with complete absence of the modiolus and interscalar septa. This is usually accompanied by an enlarged vestibule giving a "figure of 8" appearance. Vestibular aqueduct is usually normal in dimension. Defects may also be seen between the IAC and cochlea and at the stapes footplate. Due to these defects, there is high risk of CSF gusher during cochlear implantation surgery. These patients are also at high risk of recurrent meningitis with infection spreading from middle ear to the inner ear and the CSF compartment [1].

Clinical History A 6-year-old boy with SNHL

Radiological Findings (Fig. 6.5)

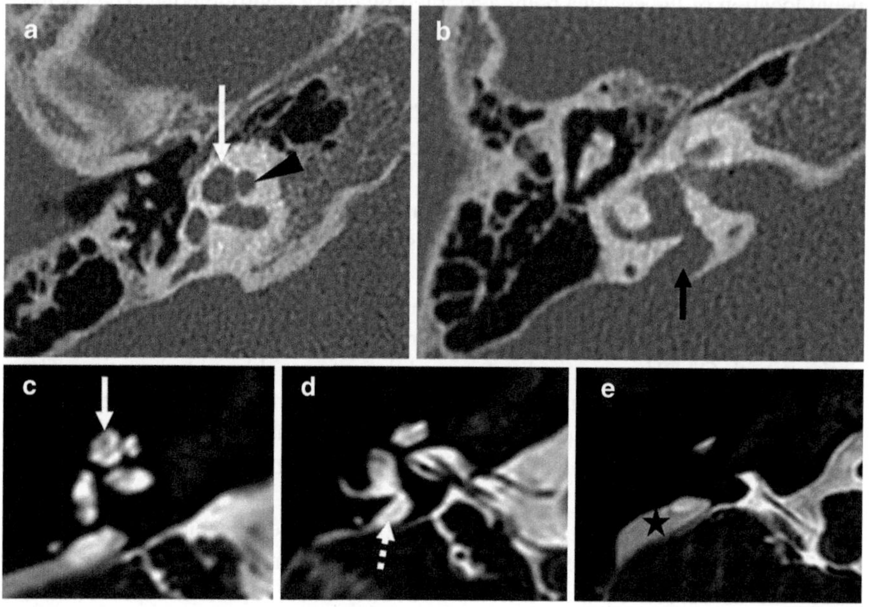

Fig. 6.5 (**a** and **b**) Axial HRCT sections of right temporal bone show dilated cystic cochlear apex (white arrow) with normal basal turn of cochlea (arrowhead). Note the dilated vestibular aqueduct (black arrow). (**c**–**e**) Axial sections of heavily T2-weighted images of right inner ear show the cystic cochlear apex (white arrow), dilated vestibular aqueduct (dashed arrow), and endolymphatic sac (star). (Case courtesy Dr. Shruti Bansal, pediatric otorhinolaryngologist, Mumbai)

Diagnosis Incomplete partition type 2 (IP-2)

Discussion
In incomplete partition type 2 (IP-2) anomaly, the apical part of the modiolus and corresponding interscalar septae are defective resulting in the cochlear apex appearing cystic. The basal turn of cochlea appears normal and external diameter of the cochlea is maintained.

The triad of cystic cochlear apex, minimally dilated vestibule, and enlarged vestibular aqueduct is called the Mondini deformity. It is to be noted that all patients with IP-2 need not have Mondini deformity.

It is hypothesized that this condition develops due to the dilated endolymphatic duct which allows high pressure to be transmitted to other inner ear structures [4]. This results in variable findings in severity with dilatation of the vestibule, scala vestibule, superior/partial/complete defect of the modiolus. CSF oozing and gusher sometimes may be observed in cochlear implant surgery due to the modiolar defect; however, the chances of CSF gusher in IP-2 are lesser than that in IP-1 and IP-3 malformations.

Clinical History A 1-year-old boy with poor response to sound

Radiological Findings (Fig. 6.6)

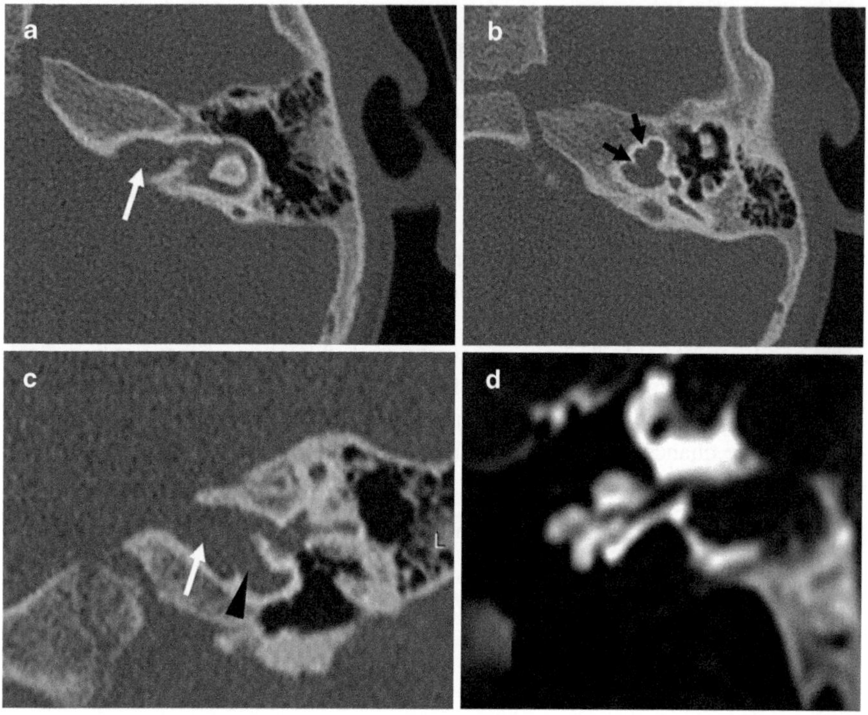

Fig. 6.6 (**a** and **b**) Axial HRCT sections of left temporal bone show dilated internal auditory canal (white arrow) and a normal-sized cochlea with interscalar septa (black arrows) but no modiolus (corkscrew appearance). (**c**) Coronal reconstruction of HRCT temporal bone showing dilated internal auditory canal (white arrow) with a patulous communication with the cochlea (black arrowhead). (**d**) Sagittal reconstruction of heavily T2-weighted image of left cochlea shows cochlea with no modiolus and cochlear nerve entering the cochlea. (Case courtesy Dr. Shruti Bansal, pediatric otorhinolaryngologist, Mumbai)

Diagnosis Incomplete partition type 3 (IP-3)

Discussion

IP-3 anomaly is seen in X-linked deafness. It is the rarest form of IP group of anomalies (~2% of all inner ear malformations). In IP-3, there is complete absence of modiolus with normal interscalar septa. The IAC is bulbous with incomplete separation of cochlear turns from the IAC. The external dimension of the cochlea is normal. A hypointense spiral structure is seen within the apparently empty cochlea on MRI which is hypothesized to represent the membranous labyrinth. Other recognized imaging features include irregular outline of the vestibule and thin otic capsule [5]. The wide communication between the IAC and cochlea with deficient lamina cribrosa in IP-3 results in high incidence of the meningitis, CSF gusher, and electrode misplacement into IAC during cochlear implantation.

References

1. Sennaroğlu L, Bajin MD. Classification and current management of inner ear malformations. Balk Med J. 2017;34(5):397.
2. Ozgen B, Oguz KK, Atas A, Sennaroglu L. Complete labyrinthine aplasia: clinical and radiologic findings with review of the literature. Am J Neuroradiol. 2009;30(4):774–80.
3. Weiss NM, Langner S, Mlynski R, Roland P, Dhanasingh A. Evaluating common cavity cochlear deformities using CT images and 3D reconstruction. Laryngoscope. 2021;131(2):386–91.
4. Sennaroglu L. Histopathology of inner ear malformations: do we have enough evidence to explain pathophysiology? Cochlear Implants Int. 2016;17(1):3–20.
5. Hong R, Du Q, Pan Y. New imaging findings of incomplete partition type III inner ear malformation and literature review. Am J Neuroradiol. 2020;41(6):1076–80.

Chapter 7
Congenital Anomalies of Temporal Bone: Congenital Cholesteatoma

Harshavardhan Mahalingam and Asthik Biswas

Clinical Data An 8-year-old male with reduced hearing in right ear. There was no history of ear discharge or fever. Otoscopy revealed an intact TM with pearly mass seen behind the tympanic membrane.

Supplementary Information The online version contains supplementary material available at https://doi.org/10.1007/978-981-95-6132-2_7.

H. Mahalingam (✉)
Department of Radiology, SRIHER, Chennai, India

A. Biswas
Department of Pediatric Neuroradiology, Great Ormond Street Hospital, NHS Foundation Trust, London, UK

H. Mahalingam (ed.), *Temporal Bone Imaging*,
https://doi.org/10.1007/978-981-95-6132-2_7

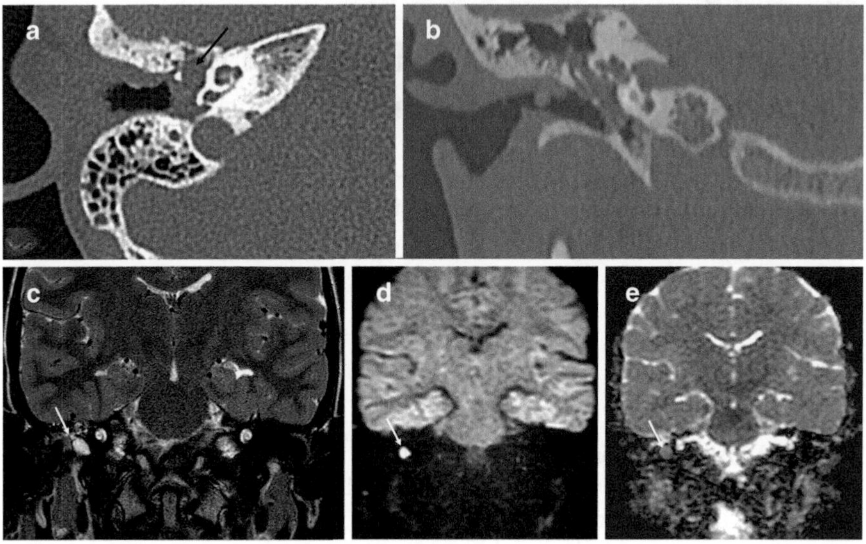

Fig. 7.1 (**a**) Axial HRCT section of the temporal bone shows soft tissue density completely filling the middle ear cavity (arrow). (**b**) Coronal HRCT section of the temporal bone shows soft tissue density filling the middle ear cavity. No erosion of ossicles or mastoid noted. (**c**) Coronal T2-weighted MR image shows T2 hyperintense content within the middle ear cavity. (**d**) Diffusion-weighted magnetic resonance image shows bright signal within the middle ear cavity. (**e**) ADC map showing relatively dark signal corresponding to region of high signal seen on DWI image

Radiological Findings (Fig. 7.1)

Diagnosis Middle ear cholesteatoma. In view of intact TM and the absence of clinical features of otitis media, this is likely to represent a congenital cholesteatoma (Potsic stage 2)

Differential Diagnosis (If Applicable) Acquired cholesteatoma, otitis media without cholesteatoma

Discussion

Cholesteatoma is a sac-like structure lined by squamous epithelium with keratin debris within. Cholesteatomas can be congenital or acquired. A general discussion about cholesteatoma is presented in Chap. 13. The following discussion is about congenital cholesteatomas.

Congenital cholesteatomas are rare compared to acquired ones. Congenital cholesteatomas account for only 2% of all cholesteatomas. They may occur in any site in the temporal bone, with the external auditory canal, middle ear, mastoid and petrous apex being the more common sites. They are believed to arise from persistent embryonic epithelial cell rests in these regions. They are usually encountered in children. Clinical presentation can be in form of incidentally detected mass on otoscopy or may manifest with hearing loss, otalgia, tinnitus, and facial palsy [1].

Table 7.1 Staging of congenital cholesteatoma

Stage	Feature seen
1	Single quadrant involvement; no mastoid or ossicular erosion
2	Multiple quadrant involvement; no mastoid or ossicular erosion
3	Ossicular involvement present with no mastoid erosion
4	Mastoid extension

The imaging appearance of congenital cholesteatoma of the middle ear is similar to that of acquired cholesteatoma. On HRCT, it is seen as an expansile soft tissue density lesion, with or without bone erosions. Bone erosion is less common in congenital cholesteatomas compared to acquired cholesteatomas. On MRI, these appear T2 hyperintense, T1 hypointense and do not show any enhancement within. They show intense diffusion restriction on diffusion-weighted MRI sequences. This imaging appearance combined with clinical features such as an intact tympanic membrane, whitish mass in middle ear cavity, absence of a previous history of otorrhea, and absence of prior otologic surgery, clinches the diagnosis of congenital cholesteatoma [2].

The surgical staging of congenital cholesteatoma according to Potsic et al. [3] is presented in Table 7.1. Note that the quadrants in this staging system correspond to the four quadrants of the tympanic membrane, namely the anterosuperior, anteroinferior, posterosuperior, and posteroinferior. These quadrants are separated by two imaginary lines - a vertical line along the handle of the malleus and a horizontal line perpendicular to the first line at the level of the umbo.

Advanced stages of cholesteatoma require more extensive surgery and have a higher risk of residual disease at end of surgery.

References

1. Park KH, Park SN, Chang KH, Jung MK, Yeo SW. Congenital middle ear cholesteatoma in children; retrospective review of 35 cases. J Korean Med Sci. 2009;24(1):126–31.
2. Baráth K, Huber AM, Stämpfli P, Varga Z, Kollias S. Neuroradiology of cholesteatomas. AJNR Am J Neuroradiol. 2011;32(2):221–9.
3. Potsic WP, Samadi DS, Marsh RR, Wetmore RF. A staging system for congenital cholesteatoma. Arch Otolaryngol Head Neck Surg. 2002;128(9):1009–12.

Chapter 8
Congenital Anomalies of Temporal Bone: Vascular Variants

Harshavardhan Mahalingam

Clinical Data A 30-year-old male with features of sinusitis and ear pain. Otoscopy revealed a pulsatile middle ear mass.

Supplementary Information The online version contains supplementary material available at https://doi.org/10.1007/978-981-95-6132-2_8.

H. Mahalingam (✉)
Department of Radiology, SRIHER, Chennai, India

H. Mahalingam (ed.), *Temporal Bone Imaging*,
https://doi.org/10.1007/978-981-95-6132-2_8

Radiological Findings (Fig. 8.1)

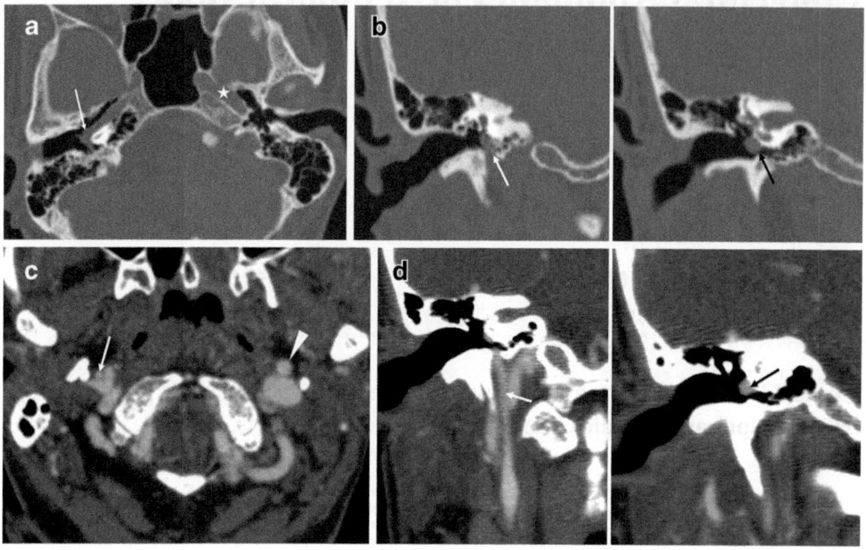

Fig. 8.1 (**a**) Axial section of HRCT temporal bone shows anomalous right internal carotid artery (ICA) within the middle ear cavity with no bony wall between the carotid artery and the middle ear cavity (arrow). Note the normal position of the left carotid canal (star). (**b**) Coronal reconstruction sections of HRCT temporal bone show right ICA entering the middle ear cavity via an enlarged inferior tympanic canaliculus (white arrow) and a more anterior section showing intratympanic part of the ICA (black arrow) nearly abutting the tympanic membrane. (**c**) Axial contrast-enhanced CT shows smaller caliber of the right cervical ICA (arrow) compared to left side (arrowhead indicating left ICA). (**d**) Coronal reconstructions of contrast-enhanced CT shows cervical ICA (white arrow) entering the middle ear cavity via the inferior tympanic canaliculus and its middle ear course (black arrow)

Diagnosis Aberrant right internal carotid artery with intratympanic course

Differential diagnosis (if applicable) Lateralized internal carotid artery

Discussion

Aberrant ICA is a congenital anomaly characterized by replacement of its normal distal cervical and proximal petrous course by a collateral pathway via the inferior tympanic and caroticotympanic arteries.

It is essential to review the course of the normal ICA to understand this anomaly. The normal ICA enters the cranium through a carotid canal in the petrous temporal bone. Going from proximal to distal, this canal has a vertical segment, an anteromedially directed horizontal segment, and a second vertical segment. The first vertical segment is separated from the middle and inner ear by a thin carotid plate. Here, it gives off a tiny branch (caroticotympanic artery) which traverses the carotid plate to enter the middle ear and anastomose with inferior tympanic branch of ascending pharyngeal artery (a branch of external carotid artery) which enters the middle ear via the inferior tympanic canaliculus.

Regression of the distal cervical segment of the ICA during embryogenesis is hypothesized to lead to development of this aberrant ICA. The aberrant ICA is a collateral pathway between the proximal cervical and distal petrous segments of the ICA via the inferior tympanic and caroticotympanic anastomosis. The aberrant ICA enters the middle ear cavity via an enlarged inferior tympanic canaliculus which lies within the caroticojugular spine. It lies lateral to the cochlear promontory within the middle ear cavity and courses anteriorly to enter the horizontal part of petrous carotid canal [1].

Aberrant ICA can be encountered as an incidental finding during evaluation for other pathologies or may present with tinnitus (usually pulsatile) and/or conductive hearing loss. It is seen as a vascular (red or bluish) retrotympanic mass. The otoscopic appearance is similar to highly vascular tumors such as a glomus tumor. Misdiagnosis of an aberrant ICA as a tumor can have catastrophic consequences. HRCT with CT/MR angiography readily demonstrates the diagnosis.

A lateralized ICA can sometimes be confused with an aberrant ICA. Lateralized ICA is characterized by a more lateral entry the of carotid canal in the skull base which can protrude into the anterior middle ear cavity. The carotid canal in this case enters lateral to a mid-cochlear anteroposterior line. The lateralized ICA does not course close to the cochlear promontory and has no relation to inferior tympanic canaliculus [2].

A Short Discussion on Vascular Tinnitus

Tinnitus is an abnormal perception of sound in absence of external stimuli. A wide variety of local and systemic conditions can result in tinnitus, and evaluation of tinnitus requires a multidisciplinary approach. A subset of patients with tinnitus can have pulsatile tinnitus which is characterized by tinnitus in synchrony with the subject's pulse. The causes of vascular tinnitus can be classified as arterial, arteriovenous, or venous (Table 8.1). HRCT temporal bone and contrast-enhanced MRI along with CT/MR angiogram have a crucial role in evaluation of pulsatile tinnitus [3].

Table 8.1 Differential diagnosis of vascular tinnitus

Category	Diagnosis	Diagnosis/imaging features
Arteriovenous	Glomus tympanicum/ jugulotympanicum	Intensely enhancing mass lesion in middle ear. Larger lesion can show permeative bone destruction. "Salt and pepper" appearance on MRI. Imaging of glomus tympanicum is discussed in chapter 23 and imaging of glomus jugulare is discussed in Chap. 25
	Dural AVF/brain AVM	Multiple tortuous and abnormal flow voids in relation to the temporal bone
	Otosclerosis	Rarefaction of bone at fissula ante fenestram. Discussed in chap. 27
	Paget's disease	Areas of mixed lysis and sclerosis with cortical thickening and bone expansion. Resorption of optic capsule can occur. Discussed in Chap. 31
Venous	Non-regional causes	Conditions associated with hyperdynamic circulation like anemia and thyrotoxicosis. Idiopathic intracranial hypertension is a common cause of pulsatile tinnitus and can be accompanied by venous sinus stenosis.
	Jugular bulb variations	High riding/dehiscent jugular bulb can be encountered in patients in pulsatile tinnitus but its association with symptoms is controversial. Extension of the jugular bulb above floor of internal acoustic meatus or basal turn of cochlea have been used to define high-riding jugular bulb in literature.
	Sigmoid sinus diverticulum	An outpouching of the sigmoid sinus projecting into mastoid or middle ear cavity through defect inner table of temporal bone (Fig. 8.2)
	Venous sinus stenosis/thrombosis	Isolated transverse sinus stenosis can rarely cause tinnitus. Incidental arachnoid granulations are common at this location and can mimic venous sinus stenosis.
Arterial	Aberrant ICA	Refer to discussion above.
	Persistent stapedial artery	HRCT temporal bone shows absent foramen spinosum with a canal connecting the petrous carotid canal to the tympanic segment of the facial canal. The artery then traverses anteriorly from the facial canal and gives rise to middle meningeal artery.
	Other carotid artery pathologies	Atherosclerosis/vasculitis/fibromuscular dysplasia/ petrous carotid aneurysm

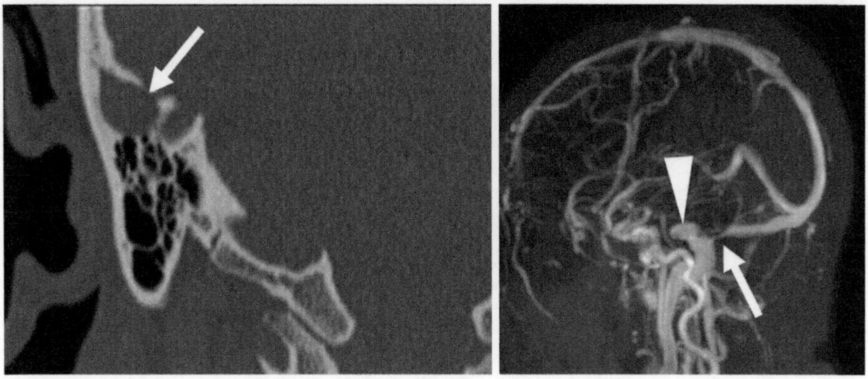

Fig. 8.2 A 36-year-old female presented with right-sided tinnitus. (**a**) Coronal section of the HRCT temporal bone showing a defect in the inner table of the skull in the region of sigmoid plate with soft tissue density projecting into the mastoid air cells. (**b**) MR venogram shows focal severe stenosis of the transverse sinus (arrow) with a diverticulum of the sigmoid sinus (arrowhead)

References

1. Nicolay S, De Foer B, Bernaerts A, Van Dinther J, Parizel PM. Aberrant internal carotid artery presenting as a retrotympanic vascular mass. Acta Radiol Short Rep. 2014;3(10):2047981614553695.
2. Glastonbury CM, Harnsberger HR, Hudgins PA, Salzman KL. Lateralized petrous internal carotid artery: imaging features and distinction from the aberrant internal carotid artery. Neuroradiology. 2012;54(9):1007–13.
3. Pegge SAH, Steens SCA, Kunst HPM, Meijer FJA. Pulsatile tinnitus: differential diagnosis and radiological work-up. Curr Radiol Rep. 2017;5(1):5.

Chapter 9
Congenital Anomalies of Temporal Bone: Dehiscences

Harshavardhan Mahalingam

Clinical Data A 36-year-old female with left ear pain for 1 week. Otoscopy revealed retracted inflamed tympanic membrane with a possible bluish mass in the posterior retrotympanic region.

H. Mahalingam (✉)
Department of Radiology, SRIHER, Chennai, India

H. Mahalingam (ed.), *Temporal Bone Imaging*,
https://doi.org/10.1007/978-981-95-6132-2_9

Radiological Findings (Fig. 9.1)

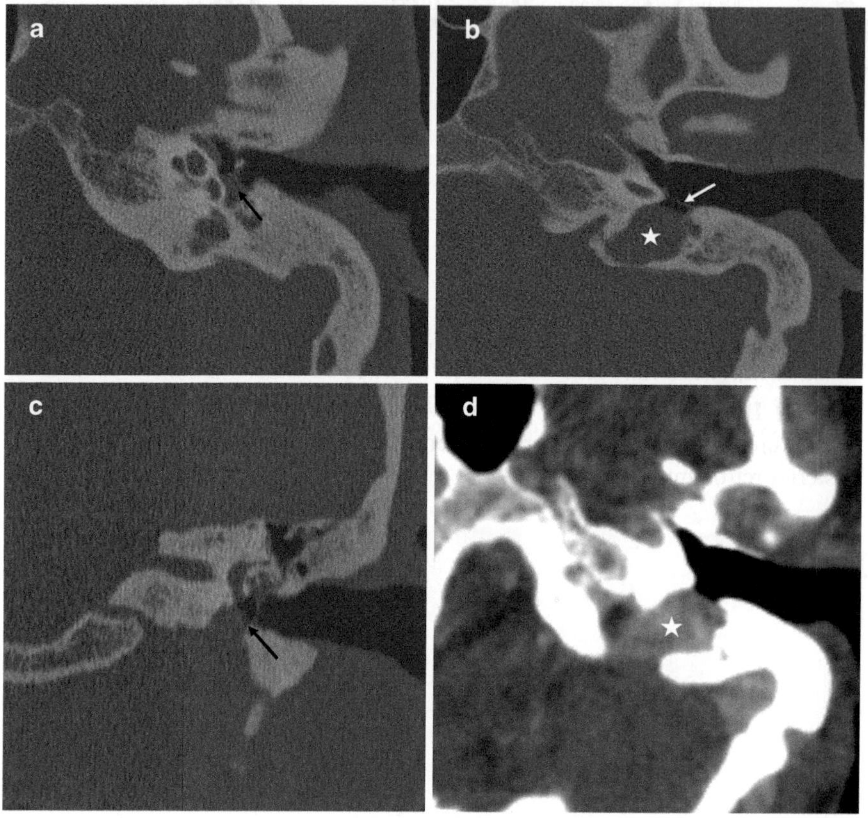

Fig. 9.1 (**a**) Axial section of HRCT temporal bone shows soft tissue density within the middle ear cavity in the mesotympanum. (**b**) More caudal axial section of HRCT temporal bone at level of hypotympanum shows defect in bony plate with jugular bulb (star) seen close to the tympanic membrane (white arrow). (**c**) Coronal reconstruction section of HRCT temporal bone shows the defect in bony plate of the jugular bulb (arrow). (**d**) Axial section of contrast-enhanced CT shows enhancement in the jugular bulb (star). The soft tissue density within the middle ear cavity did not show any enhancement

Diagnosis Acute otitis media with dehiscent jugular bulb

Differential diagnosis (if applicable) High-riding jugular bulb with no dehiscence

Discussion

Jugular bulb refers to the prominent cranial portion of the internal jugular vein situated in the jugular fossa of the skull base. It is located in close proximity to the inner and middle ear structures. "High-riding" jugular bulb and dehiscent jugular bulb are common anatomic variants which can be encountered in temporal bone imaging studies with a prevalence of around 8% and 2.5%, respectively [1].

Multiple anatomic landmarks have been suggested to define a "high-riding" jugular bulb. Extension of the jugular bulb above the level of the floor of the internal acoustic meatus or basal turn of the cochlea or inferior rim of the round window have been used to define high-riding jugular bulb. This is best assessed on coronal reconstructed HRCT images.

A "high-riding" jugular bulb is usually covered by a thin plate of bone separating it from the middle ear cavity. When this bony plate covering the jugular bulb is absent, it is termed as a dehiscent jugular bulb which can protrude into the middle ear cavity and can be seen as a vascular retrotympanic "mass" on otoscopic examination. The presence of a distinct outpouching from the jugular bulb into the middle ear can also be encountered and is termed a jugular bulb diverticulum [2].

Bony dehiscence can also be encountered in other temporal bone structures. These are discussed briefly in the following paragraphs.

Third window phenomenon refers to the characteristic symptoms of sound- or pressure-induced vertigo with air-bone gap on audiogram in the low frequencies. This occurs due to bony defects in inner ear structures. Some examples of pathologies associated with third window phenomenon are perilabyrinthine fistula, superior semicircular canal dehiscence (SSCCD), and X-linked deafness with CSF gusher. Perilabyrinthine fistula, perhaps the most common of these, develops as a complication of middle ear infection eroding the walls of inner ear structures, most commonly the lateral semicircular canal. SSCCD is an idiopathic defect in the roof of the SSCC which is best demonstrated on thin section HRCT images reconstructed in Stenver and Poschl planes. Figure 9.2 demonstrates SSCCD in the Poschl plane. X-linked deafness is characterized by absent modiolus and lamina cribrosa which act as a third window [3].

Another clinical scenario where dehiscence in temporal bone structures assumes importance is recurrent meningitis with no other apparent cause and spontaneous CSF rhinorrhea/otorrhea. Dehiscence in the middle or inner ear structures can act as a route for infection spread from the ear into the CSF compartment and can also be

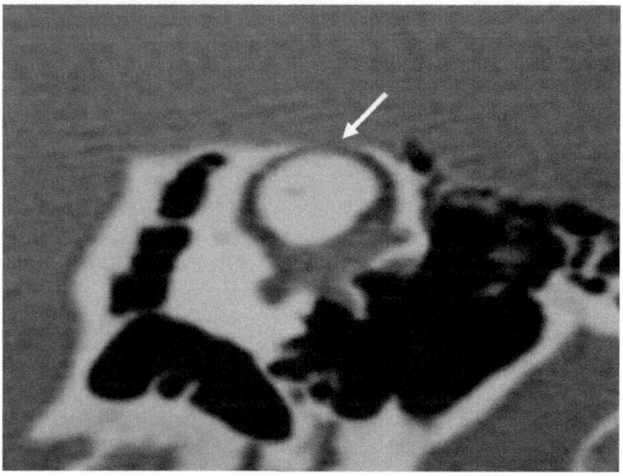

Fig. 9.2 HRCT temporal bone reconstruction in Poschl plane demonstrates dehiscence of the superior semicircular canal (arrow)

a site of CSF leak [4]. The congenital defects associated with CSF leaks can be translabyrinthine (examples include inner ear anomalies with absent modiolus or enlarged vestibular aqueduct) or extra-labyrinthine (examples include a defect in the tegmen, a persistent petromastoid canal and Hyrtl's fissure) [5].

Facial canal dehiscence is a variant where the facial canal is covered by fibrous tissue with an absent bony covering. It is of clinical significance as a dehiscent facial canal makes the nerve more susceptible to injury due to inflammatory processes or during surgery. The prevalence of a dehiscent facial canal is estimated to be as high as 50% with the tympanic segment of the facial canal being the most commonly affected. The dehiscence of the facial canal is best assessed on CT in a plane perpendicular to the course of the facial canal. Ultrahigh-resolution CT with 0.1 mm spatial resolution may be better at identifying facial canal dehiscence than routine HRCT [6].

References

1. Friedmann DR, Eubig J, Winata LS, Pramanik BK, Merchant SN, Lalwani AK. Prevalence of jugular bulb abnormalities and resultant inner ear dehiscence: a histopathologic and radiologic study. Otolaryngol Head Neck Surg. 2012;147(4):750–6.
2. Sayit AT, Gunbey HP, Fethallah B, Gunbey E, Karabulut E. Radiological and audiometric evaluation of high jugular bulb and dehiscent high jugular bulb. J Laryngol Otol. 2016;130(11):1059–63.
3. Ho ML, Moonis G, Halpin CF, Curtin HD. Spectrum of third window abnormalities: semicircular canal dehiscence and beyond. AJNR Am J Neuroradiol. 2017;38(1):2–9.
4. Rupa V. Diagnosis and management of Congenital Perilymph Fistula causing recurrent meningitis: a review. Ann Otol Neurotol. 2018;01(01):040–2.
5. Thomeer HG, Schreurs C, van Doormaal TP, Straatman LV. Management and outcomes of spontaneous cerebrospinal fluid otorrhoea. Front Surg. 2020;7:21.
6. Tang R, Zhang Z, Zhao P, Zhao L, Xu N, Yin H, et al. A novel imaging scoring method for identifying facial canal dehiscence: an ultra-high-resolution CT study. Eur Radiol. 2023;33(4):2830–9.

Chapter 10
Infections and Inflammatory Disease of Temporal Bone: Otitis Externa

Harshavardhan Mahalingam

Clinical Data A 69-year-old male with left ear pain and discharge for 1 month. Patient also had difficulty in mouth opening and chewing.

Radiological Findings (Fig. 10.1)

Supplementary Information The online version contains supplementary material available at https://doi.org/10.1007/978-981-95-6132-2_10.

H. Mahalingam (✉)
Department of Radiology, SRIHER, Chennai, India

H. Mahalingam (ed.), *Temporal Bone Imaging*,
https://doi.org/10.1007/978-981-95-6132-2_10

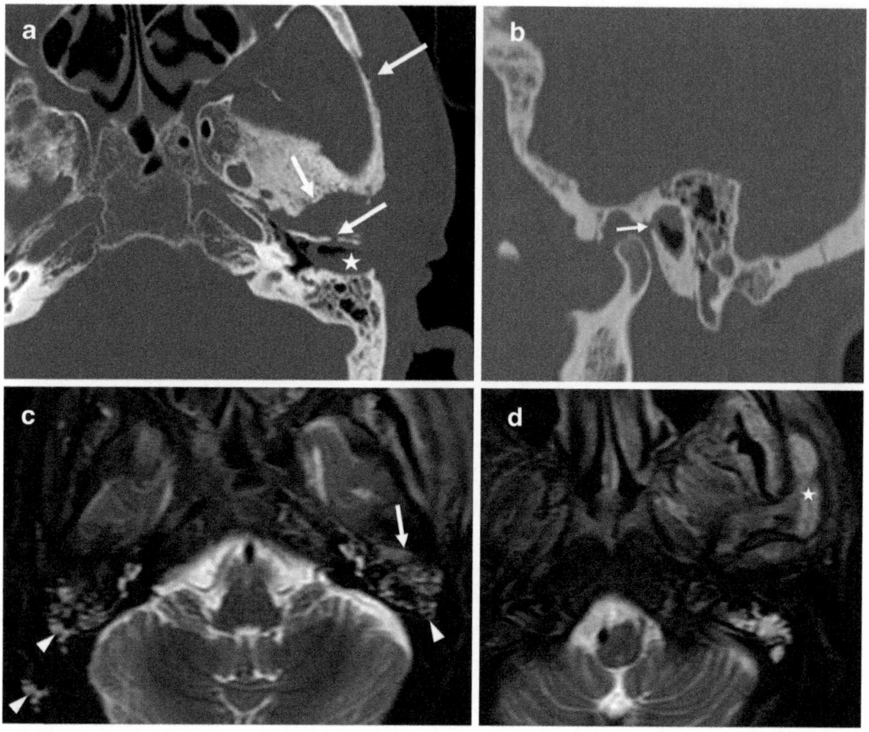

Fig. 10.1 (**a**) Axial HRCT image of the temporal bone shows soft tissue thickening in the left external auditory canal (EAC) (star) with multiple erosions seen in the bony EAC, condylar fossa, and zygomatic process of the left temporal bone (arrows). (**b**) Sagittal reconstructed image of the left temporal bone shows erosion in the anterior wall of EAC (arrow) with circumferential soft tissue thickening within. (**c**) Axial fat-saturated T2-weighted MR image shows fluid signal in the left EAC (arrow) and bilateral mastoids (arrowheads). (**d**) Axial fat-saturated T2-weighted MR image shows fluid collection (star) in close relation to the left temporomandibular joint and the zygomatic process of the temporal bone with adjacent soft tissue edema

Diagnosis Necrotizing otitis externa

Differential diagnosis (if applicable) Squamous cell carcinoma of EAC

Discussion

Necrotizing otitis externa (NOE), formerly called malignant otitis externa, is an invasive infection of the external ear. Pseudomonas aeruginosa is the most commonly implicated causative agent in this infection. It is more common in diabetics. Patients typically present with severe otalgia. The disease begins in the external ear and spreads to the infratemporal soft tissues via the fissures of Santorini. It can also involve the mastoid, TM joint, and skull base.

The diagnosis of NOE is based on clinical findings, elevated serum inflammatory markers, and imaging evidence of soft tissue thickening with/without bone erosion in the EAC and the infratemporal fossa [1].

CT shows soft tissue thickening along the walls of the cartilaginous and bony EAC with adjacent fat stranding and displacement of fat planes. Complete occlusion of the EAC lumen due to soft tissue swelling or granulation tissue can be seen. Bone erosions in the EAC and adjacent skull base are typically present [2].

MRI is helpful in identifying extent of soft tissue and marrow involvement. Post gadolinium images are helpful in identifying abscesses. The presence of retrocondylar fat pad edema/enhancement is an important clue to diagnosis [3].

Skull base osteomyelitis is a dreaded complication of NOE and can result in multiple cranial nerve palsies and ICA/IJV thrombosis.

References

1. Rubin Grandis J, Branstetter BF, Yu VL. The changing face of malignant (necrotising) external otitis: clinical, radiological, and anatomic correlations. Lancet Infect Dis. 2004;4(1):34–9.
2. Grandis JR, Curtin HD, Yu VL. Necrotizing (malignant) external otitis: prospective comparison of CT and MR imaging in diagnosis and follow-up. Radiology. 1995;196(2):499–504.
3. Tsuno NSG, Tsuno MY, Coelho Neto CAF, Noujaim SE, Decnop M, Pacheco FT, et al. Imaging the external ear: practical approach to normal and pathologic conditions. Radiographics. 2022;42(2):522–40.

Chapter 11
Infections and Inflammatory Disease of Temporal Bone: Otomastoiditis Without Complications

Harshavardhan Mahalingam

Clinical Data A 3-year-old child with fever, cough, and nasal discharge for 5 days and persistent crying for 1 day. Otoscopic examination revealed congestion of bilateral tympanic membranes and mastoid tenderness.

Radiological Findings (Fig. 11.1)

Diagnosis Bilateral acute otomastoiditis

Differential diagnosis (if applicable) Otitis media with effusion

Discussion

Acute otitis media is the second most common infection of childhood after upper respiratory tract infections. It can also occur in adults, although less commonly. It most often occurs following a viral respiratory tract infection that compromises mucosal integrity and predisposes to bacterial infection (Streptococcus pneumoniae, Moraxella catarrhalis, and Haemophilus influenzae are the most common causative organisms). Infection from the upper respiratory tract spreads to middle ear and mastoid via the Eustachian tube. In fact, Eustachian tube dysfunction is one of the important causative factors in development of otitis media.

Supplementary Information The online version contains supplementary material available at https://doi.org/10.1007/978-981-95-6132-2_11.

H. Mahalingam (✉)
Department of Radiology, SRIHER, Chennai, India

H. Mahalingam (ed.), *Temporal Bone Imaging*,
https://doi.org/10.1007/978-981-95-6132-2_11

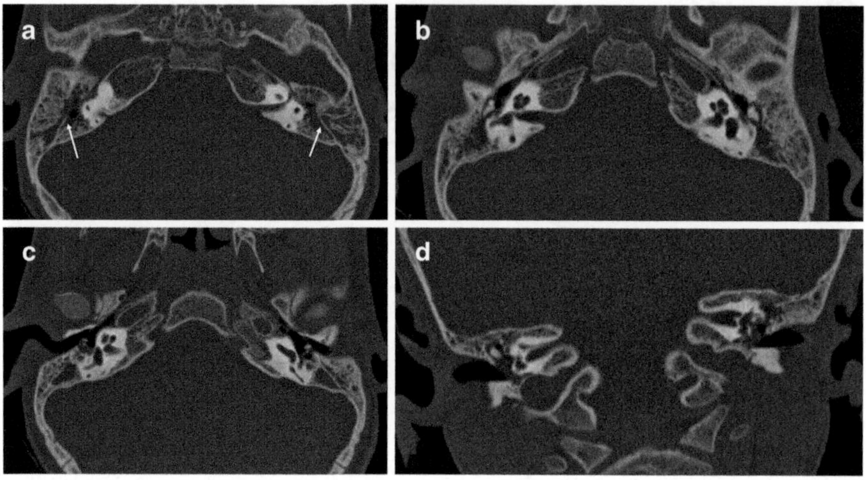

Fig. 11.1 (**a–c**) Axial HRCT sections of the temporal bones show soft tissue density in bilateral middle ear and mastoids with no bone erosion. (**d**) Coronal HRCT section showing soft tissue density in the middle ear and mastoids. No bone erosions were noted

Acute otitis media/acute otomastoiditis (AOM) is characterized by acute-onset symptoms, middle ear effusion, and signs of middle ear inflammation on examination. AOM usually responds to antibiotic therapy within 48–72 h [1].

Imaging is required in suspected complicated AOM. Possible complications include coalescent mastoiditis, subperiosteal abscess, facial nerve palsy, acute labyrinthitis, sigmoid sinus thrombosis, venous infarction of brain, meningitis, brain abscess, and otitic hydrocephalus. The prevalence of complications in AOM is reported to be approximately 1–5%.

CT in uncomplicated AOM shows soft tissue density filling the middle ear and mastoid. Bone erosions are not present in the early stages. Persistent infection for more than a few days can result in demineralization, which manifests as erosions of the ossicles, mastoid, or middle ear walls. Resorption of septae between the mastoid air cells results in formation of a cavity within the mastoid, a condition known as coalescent mastoiditis [2]. An example of coalescent mastoiditis is presented in Fig. 11.2.

This can progress to a subperiosteal abscess in the mastoid with cortical erosion. Bezold abscess refers to a pus collection in the neck tracking from mastoid into digastric sulcus and further into digastric/sternocleidomastoid muscles.

Contrast-enhanced MRI is better at demonstration of intracranial complications of AOM like meningitis, abscess, and venous thrombosis. *Examples of other complications of otomastoiditis are presented in the subsequent chapters.*

Diagnostic Pitfalls

- The diagnosis of acute or chronic otitis media is based on clinical signs and symptoms. Presence of sclerosis suggests chronicity of the condition, but lack of sclerosis does not rule out a chronic disease process.

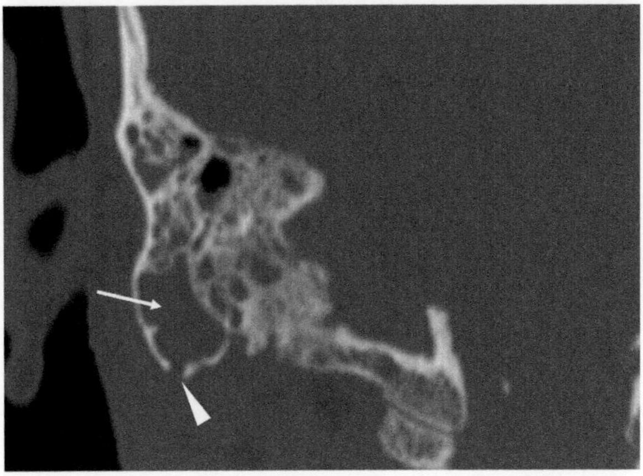

Fig. 11.2 Coalescent mastoiditis. Coronal HRCT section showing resorption of walls of mastoid air cells with a fluid-filled cavity within the mastoid (arrow) with erosion in mastoid tip (arrowhead)

- Otitis media with effusion (serous otitis media) is characterized by finding of middle ear effusion on examination combined with lack of inflammatory signs. Imaging findings will be similar to those of AOM without bone erosions. Presence of otitis media with effusion in adults should prompt a search for nasopharyngeal mass lesion.
- Imaging, especially MRI, often reveals incidental fluid/soft tissue within the mastoid and middle ear in patients undergoing scans for other indications. This cannot be diagnosed as otomastoiditis based on just imaging findings and needs to be correlated with clinical features.

References

1. Gotcsik M. Otitis media. In: Textbook of clinical pediatrics. Springer Science & Business Media; 2012. p. 863–71.
2. Trojanowska A, Drop A, Trojanowski P, Rosińska-Bogusiewicz K, Klatka J, Bobek-Billewicz B. External and middle ear diseases: radiological diagnosis based on clinical signs and symptoms. Insights Imaging. 2011;3(1):33–48.

Chapter 12
Infections and Inflammatory Disease of Temporal Bone: Otomastoiditis with Ossicular Erosion

Harshavardhan Mahalingam

Clinical Data A 28-year-old male with history of right ear discharge and reduced hearing for 6 months.

Radiological Findings (Fig. 12.1)

Supplementary Information The online version contains supplementary material available at https://doi.org/10.1007/978-981-95-6132-2_12.

H. Mahalingam (✉)
Department of Radiology, SRIHER, Chennai, India

H. Mahalingam (ed.), *Temporal Bone Imaging*,
https://doi.org/10.1007/978-981-95-6132-2_12

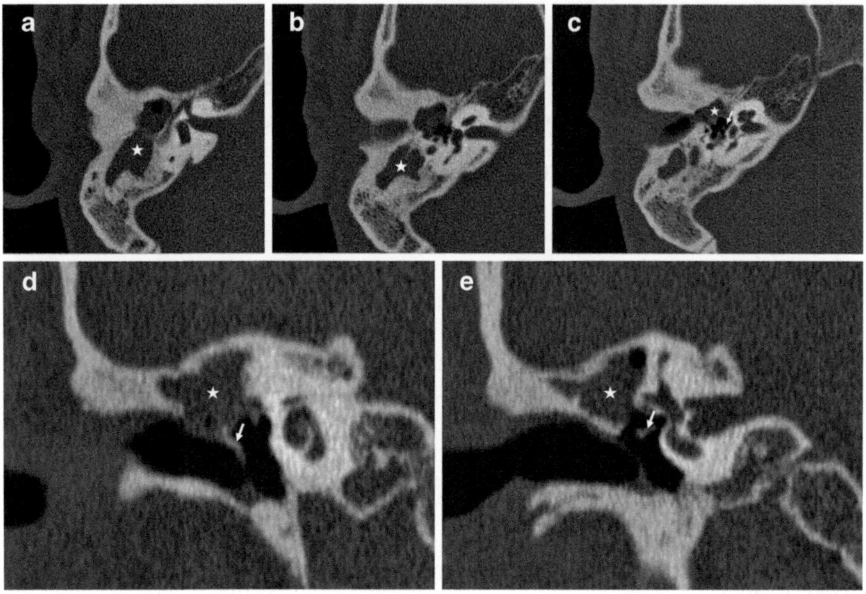

Fig. 12.1 (**a–c**) Axial HRCT sections of the right temporal bone show soft tissue density (star) filling the mastoid antrum and the middle ear with a non-visualized head of malleus and body of incus. The stapes crura are intact (arrow). (**d**, **e**) Coronal HRCT sections of the right temporal bone show the remnant handle of the malleus and distal long process of incus (arrows) with rest of the malleus and incus being eroded. The soft tissue is seen localized to the epitympanum (star)

Diagnosis Chronic otomastoiditis with ossicular erosions.

Differential diagnosis (if applicable) Cholesteatoma, congenital anomaly of ossicles

Discussion

Conductive hearing loss in chronic suppurative otitis media (CSOM) can be due to ossicular fixation or erosions. Ossicular fixation is a clinical diagnosis. It can be supported by imaging evidence of soft tissue density encasing ossicles, punctate calcifications in middle ear, and ligamentous calcifications. The key role of HRCT in the context of conductive hearing loss in CSOM is to rule out ossicular chain erosions and to rule out other causes of conductive hearing loss like otosclerosis [1].

On axial images, the key structures to recognize ossicular integrity are (from superior to inferior sections):

- Ice cream cone appearance—head of malleus and body of incus
- Two parallel lines—handle of malleus and long process of incus
- Two dots—lenticular process of incus and head of stapes

Normal imaging appearance of ossicles has been highlighted in Chap. 3 in Figs. 3.7, 3.8, and 3.9. Erosions of ossicles in CSOM can be non-cholesteatomatous (also called post-inflammatory ossicular erosions) or cholesteatomatous. The most commonly involved ossicle in CSOM is the incus with its lenticular process being the most commonly affected. The malleus and stapes footplate are less frequently eroded [2].

References

1. Trojanowska A, Drop A, Trojanowski P, Rosińska-Bogusiewicz K, Klatka J, Bobek-Billewicz B. External and middle ear diseases: radiological diagnosis based on clinical signs and symptoms. Insights Imaging. 2011;3(1):33–48.
2. Varshney S, Nangia A, Bist SS, Singh RK, Gupta N, Bhagat S. Ossicular chain status in chronic suppurative otitis media in adults. Indian J Otolaryngol Head Neck Surg. 2010;62(4):421–6.

Chapter 13
Infections and Inflammatory Disease of Temporal Bone: Otomastoiditis with Tegmen/Middle Ear Erosions

Harshavardhan Mahalingam

Clinical Data A 41-year-old female with history of right ear pain and otorrhea for 4 months. On examination, there was tympanic membrane perforation with an attic retraction pocket.

Radiological Findings (Fig. 13.1)

Diagnosis Chronic otomastoiditis with bone erosions, possible cholesteatoma

Differential diagnosis (if applicable) Chronic otomastoiditis without cholesteatoma

Discussion
Chronic suppurative otitis media (CSOM) is a chronic infection of the middle ear and mastoid characterized by tympanic membrane perforation and otorrhea lasting more than 12 weeks. It is characterized by irreversible inflammatory changes in the mucosa of middle ear and mastoid and is often accompanied by ossicular damage. The causative agents of CSOM could be aerobic or anaerobic bacteria—the common ones being Pseudomonas, Staphylococcus, Klebsiella, Bacteroides, etc. [1].

HRCT of the temporal bone is the first-line imaging investigation. The purpose of imaging in this clinical context is to assess the extent of ossicular and other bone erosion and to rule out other complications.

Supplementary Information The online version contains supplementary material available at https://doi.org/10.1007/978-981-95-6132-2_13.

H. Mahalingam (✉)
Department of Radiology, SRIHER, Chennai, India

H. Mahalingam (ed.), *Temporal Bone Imaging*,
https://doi.org/10.1007/978-981-95-6132-2_13

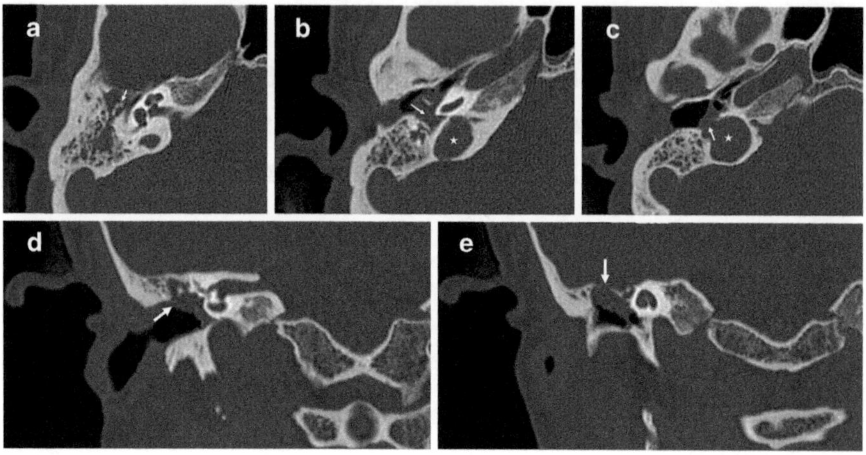

Fig. 13.1 (**a**) Axial HRCT section of the right temporal bone shows soft tissue density filling the middle ear and mastoid with erosion of the malleus and incus (arrow). (**b**) Axial HRCT section of the right temporal bone shows soft tissue density filling the middle ear (arrow). Also note the high-riding jugular bulb (star) seen at the level of the basal turn of the cochlea. (**c**) Axial HRCT section of the right temporal bone shows dehiscence of the sigmoid dural plate (arrow). (**d**) Coronal HRCT section of the right temporal bone shows erosion of the scutum (arrow). (**e**) Coronal HRCT section of the right temporal bone shows erosion of the tegmen tympani (arrow)

HRCT shows opacification of middle ear and mastoid with varying degrees of *mastoid sclerosis/underpneumatization. Ossicular chain fixation* may be suggested by findings of soft tissue density encasing the ossicles or calcific densities (tympanosclerosis) in the middle ear cavity and tympanic membrane (TM). Calcifications of the ossicular ligaments and tendons can occur. Diagnosis of ossicular chain fixation is difficult on imaging in the absence of calcifications. *Ossicular chain erosion* can be easily detected on HRCT [2].

Presence of erosions in walls of middle ear cavity on HRCT can raise suspicion of *cholesteatomatous CSOM*. Cholesteatoma is a sac-like structure formed by squamous epithelium with keratin debris within. Acquired cholesteatomas develop in the middle ear cavity in the context of chronic middle ear infection and a perforated TM.

On HRCT, cholesteatoma is seen as an expansile soft-tissue density lesion. Bone erosion is a key diagnostic clue to presence of cholesteatoma. However, the absence of bone erosions does not rule out cholesteatoma. Diffusion-weighted MRI sequence is the preferred imaging modality for visualizing cholesteatomas, as they typically show intense diffusion restriction (Fig. 13.2). Cholesteatomas appear T2 hyperintense, T1 hypointense and do not show any internal enhancement. These features help differentiate cholesteatoma from granulation tissue or neoplasms [3].

Cholesteatomas can be divided into pars flaccida type (much more common and also called the attic cholesteatoma) and pars tensa type (Table 13.1).

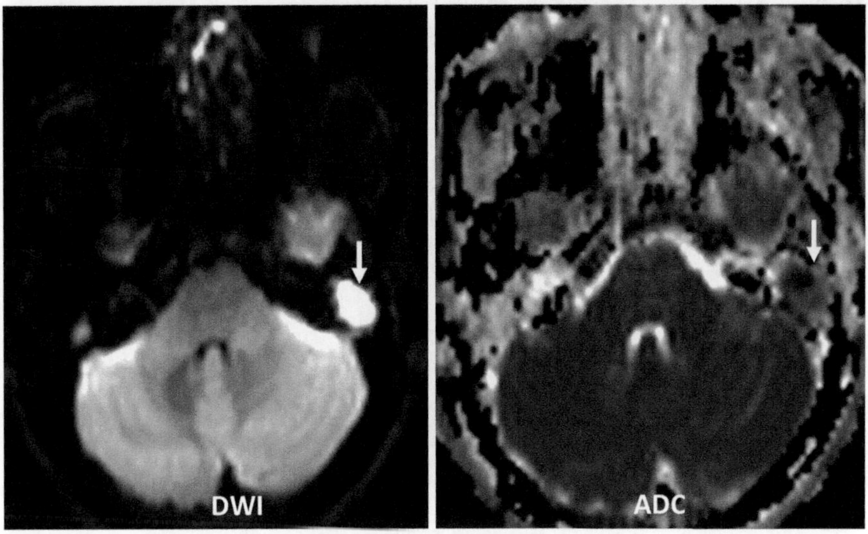

Fig. 13.2 Axial diffusion-weighted images of the temporal bone show intense diffusion restriction (bright on DWI and dark on ADC map) within the left middle ear cavity, suggestive of a cholesteatoma

Table 13.1 Comparison of pars flaccida and pars tensa cholesteatomas

Feature	Pars flaccida cholesteatoma	Pars tensa cholesteatoma
Relation to the TM	Related to upper third of TM	Related to lower two-thirds of TM
Relation to ossicles	Located in Prussak space lateral to ossicles	Located initially in posterior recesses, medial to ossicles
Bone erosion	Erosion of scutum and widening of aditus ad antrum	Erosion of posterior and medial walls of middle ear

Imaging Pitfalls

- Absence of bone erosions does not rule out presence of cholesteatomas.
- Small cholesteatomas (<5 mm) may not be seen on diffusion-weighted imaging.
- Differential diagnosis of soft tissue density in middle ear and mastoid is wide—fluid due to Eustachian tube dysfunction, acute otitis, granulation tissue, cholesteatoma, glomus tumor, cholesterol granuloma, hemotympanum, etc.—hence, correlation with the clinical context is necessary. It may not always be possible to differentiate these entities based on imaging alone.

References

1. Khairkar M, Deshmukh P, Maity H, Deotale V. Chronic suppurative otitis media: a comprehensive review of epidemiology, pathogenesis, microbiology, and complications. Cureus. 2023;15(8):e43729.
2. Mafee MF, Aimi K, Kahen HL, Valvassori GE, Capek V. Chronic otomastoiditis: a conceptual understanding of CT findings. Radiology. 1986;160(1):193–200.
3. Baráth K, Huber AM, Stämpfli P, Varga Z, Kollias S. Neuroradiology of cholesteatomas. AJNR Am J Neuroradiol. 2011;32(2):221–9.

Chapter 14
Infections and Inflammatory Disease of Temporal Bone: Labyrinthitis Ossificans

Nikshita Jain and Aparna Irodi

Clinical Data A 65-year-old gentleman with chronic right otitis media and profound right-sided hearing loss.

Radiological Findings (Fig. 14.1)

Radiological Findings (Fig. 14.2)

Diagnosis Right-sided labyrinthitis ossificans and perforated right tympanic membrane

Differential diagnosis (if applicable) Nil

Discussion

Labyrinthitis ossificans (LO) is an ossification of the inner ear structures, and patients usually present with profound irreversible hearing loss. Labyrinthitis is commonly secondary to infections of the inner ear (viral or bacterial), inflammatory process of the inner ear, temporal bone trauma, hemorrhage, and tumors. Ossification occurs as a sequela to this inflammation and is typically unilateral but can be bilateral and can be found 3–4 months after bacterial meningitis and/or trauma.

Supplementary Information The online version contains supplementary material available at https://doi.org/10.1007/978-981-95-6132-2_14.

N. Jain (✉) · A. Irodi
Department of Radiology, CMC, Vellore, India

H. Mahalingam (ed.), *Temporal Bone Imaging*,
https://doi.org/10.1007/978-981-95-6132-2_14

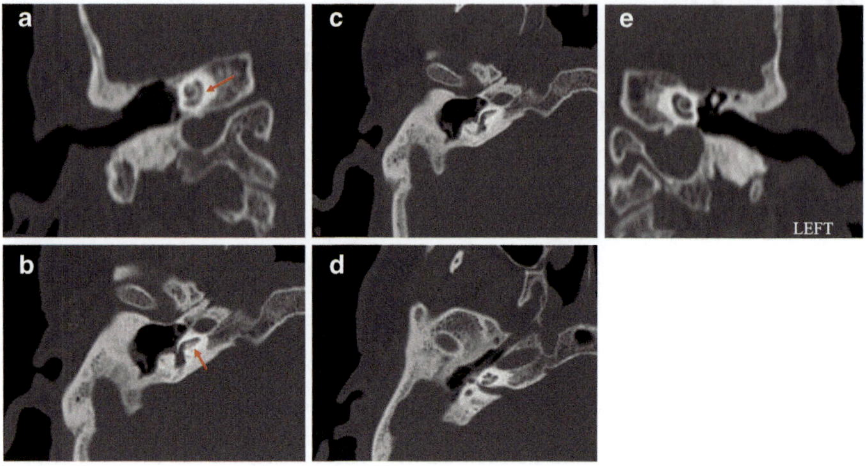

Fig. 14.1 (**a**, **b**) Coronal and axial HRCT sections of the right temporal bone shows calcification in basal turn of cochlea and partly calcified apical turn. (**c**, **d**) Axial HRCT sections of the right temporal bone shows non-visualized ossicles (likely resorbed). The right tympanic membrane is perforated with minimal soft tissue opacity within the middle ear cavity. (**e**) Coronal HRCT section of the left temporal bone shows no significant abnormality

LO can be diagnosed definitively on imaging with CT, which shows sclerosis, irregularities, or obliteration of the cochlea, semicircular canals, or vestibule with different degrees of involvement. CT is specific but has a lower sensitivity with respect to MRI.

It has a spectrum with:

- Mild LO: Hazy increase in density within fluid spaces of the membranous labyrinth.
- Moderate LO: Intermittent ossifications within fluid spaces of the membranous labyrinth.
- Severe LO: Membranous labyrinth is completely obliterated by bone replacing fluid spaces.

MRI shows loss of normal fluid signal in the inner ear, and ossifications may appear as low-intensity foci within the high-signal fluid of inner ear. In the acute/subacute stage of labyrinthitis without ossification, MRI shows enhancement of the membranous labyrinth. Imaging findings are important for treatment guidance (selection of appropriate patients for cochlear implantation) and for prognostication [1].

Differential diagnosis includes cochlear aplasia or labyrinthine aplasia. In labyrinthitis ossificans, the shape/contour of the labyrinth is preserved. However, labyrinthine aplasia is characterized by bilateral absence of differentiated inner ear structures.

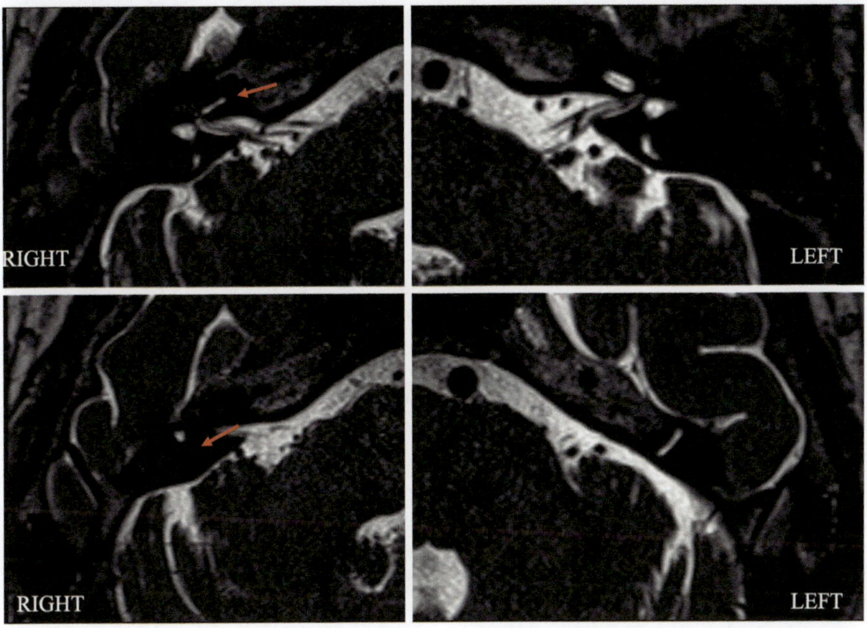

Fig. 14.2 Heavily T2-weighted thin section axial images of right inner ear show partial loss of fluid signal in DRIVE sequence in all the limbs of the semicircular canals. Normal fluid signal in left inner ear is represented on the left side of image for comparison

Reference

1. Taxak P, Ram C. Labyrinthitis and Labyrinthitis Ossificans - a case report and review of the literature. J Radiol Case Rep. 2020;14(5):1–6. https://doi.org/10.3941/jrcr.v14i5.3706.

Chapter 15
Infections and Inflammatory Disease of Temporal Bone: Otomastoiditis with Meningitis/Abscess

Harshavardhan Mahalingam and Karthik Kulanthaivelu

Clinical Data A 61-year-old male with history of fever, headache, and altered sensorium for 3 days. Patient was previously diagnosed with left CSOM 2 years ago.

Radiological Findings (Fig. 15.1)

Supplementary Information The online version contains supplementary material available at https://doi.org/10.1007/978-981-95-6132-2_15.

H. Mahalingam (✉)
Department of Radiology, SRIHER, Chennai, India

K. Kulanthaivelu
Department of Neuroradiology, SRIHER, Chennai, India

H. Mahalingam (ed.), *Temporal Bone Imaging*,
https://doi.org/10.1007/978-981-95-6132-2_15

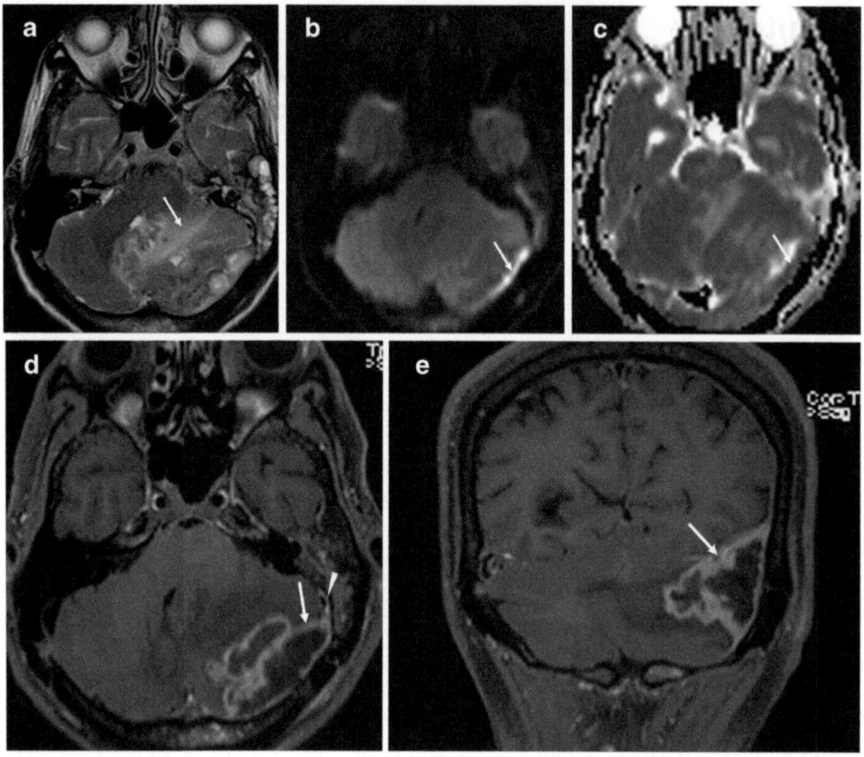

Fig. 15.1 (**a**) Axial T2-weighted MR image showing extensive edema in the left cerebellar hemisphere with mass effect. Also noted is the fluid signal completely filling left mastoid. (**b**, **c**) Diffusion-weighted image and apparent diffusion coefficient map show diffusion restriction along the inner aspect of the calvarium (arrow) along the surface of the left cerebellar hemisphere suggesting abscess formation. (**d**, **e**) Axial and coronal post-contrast T1 fat-saturated images showing subdural and intraparenchymal intercommunicating abscesses in the left cerebellar hemisphere (arrow). Also note the severely narrowed flow void of left sigmoid sinus (arrowhead)

Diagnosis Otomastoiditis with subdural and cerebellar abscess

Differential diagnosis (if applicable) Chronic otomastoiditis without cholesteatoma

Discussion

Intracranial complications of otomastoiditis are the most dreaded with mortality rates ranging from 5% to 25%. Intracranial complications occur in two patient groups: (1) in children and elderly where they often occur in the setting of AOM and (2) in young adults where they occur in the setting of CSOM [1].

MRI is the modality of choice for evaluation of suspected intracranial complications of otitis media [2].The intracranial complications of otitis media and otomastoiditis are presented in the following table with imaging features.

Complication	Imaging features
Meningitis	Leptomeningeal or pachymeningeal enhancement, sulcal FLAIR hyperintensity on non-contrast MRI (Fig. 15.2)
Subdural empyema	Crescentic peripherally enhancing fluid collection typically along the lateral convexities or along tentorium (Fig. 15.3)
Hydrocephalus	Ventricular dilatation usually of communicating type
Encephalitis	Brain parenchymal T2 and FLAIR hyperintensity with intraparenchymal enhancement (Fig. 15.4)
Brain abscess	Peripheral enhancing lesion with central diffusion restriction—most commonly in cerebellum and temporal lobe
Sigmoid sinus thrombosis	Filling defect on post gadolinium gradient echo sequence (empty delta sign). Loss of flow void on spin echo sequences
Venous infarct	T2-FLAIR hyperintensity usually with hemorrhage within in subcortical location—does not correspond to arterial vascular territories

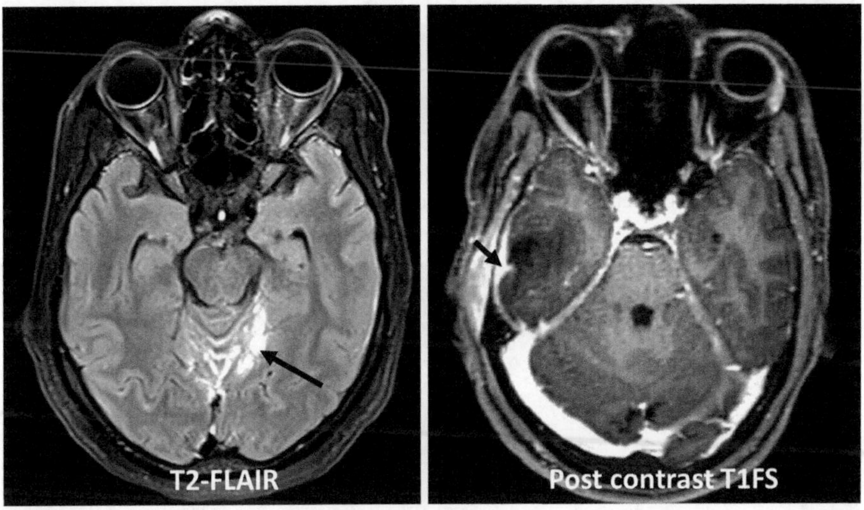

Fig. 15.2 Axial T2-FLAIR image showing hyperintense exudates in the cerebellar sulcal spaces (black arrow). Axial post contrast image showing meningeal enhancement along the lateral convexity of the right temporal lobe

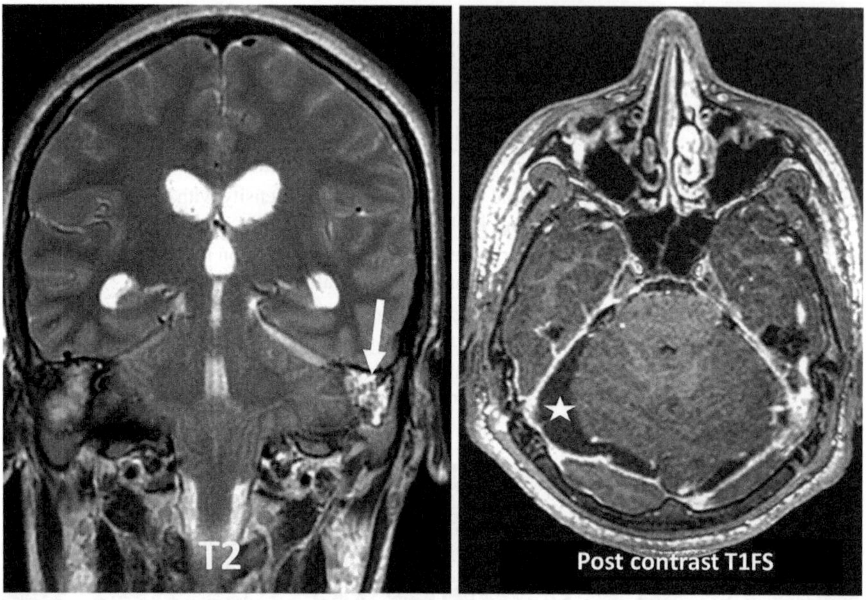

Fig. 15.3 Coronal T2-weighted image showing fluid signal in the left mastoid. Axial post-contrast image showing fluid collection along the tentorium cerebelli with peripheral enhancement

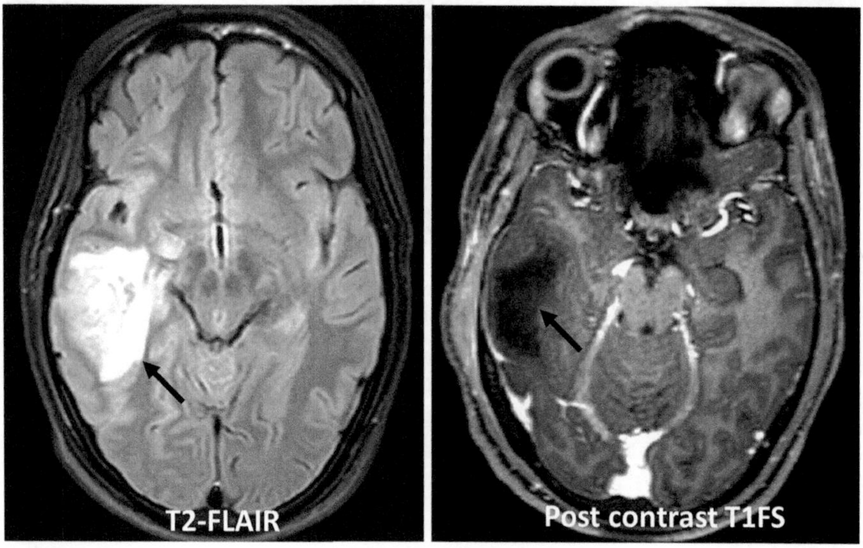

Fig. 15.4 Axial T2-FLAIR image showing focal edema in the right temporal lobe with faint enhancement on the post-contrast image

References

1. Penido ND, Chandrasekhar SS, Borin A, Maranhão AS, Testa JR. Complications of otitis media – a potentially lethal problem still present. Braz J Otorhinolaryngol. 2015;82(3):253–62.
2. Duarte MJ, Kozin ED, Barshak MB, Reinshagen K, Knoll RM, Abdullah KG, et al. Otogenic brain abscesses: a systematic review. Laryngoscope Investig Otolaryngol. 2018;3(3):198–208.

Chapter 16
Infections and Inflammatory Disease of Temporal Bone: Otomastoiditis with Labyrinthine Fistula

Rishabh Vaid and Aparna Irodi

Clinical Data A 60-year-old male with history of left ear discharge for 10 years with decreased hearing and on and off tinnitus.

Supplementary Information The online version contains supplementary material available at https://doi.org/10.1007/978-981-95-6132-2_16.

R. Vaid · A. Irodi (✉)
Department of Radiology, Christian Medical College, Vellore, India

H. Mahalingam (ed.), *Temporal Bone Imaging*,
https://doi.org/10.1007/978-981-95-6132-2_16

Radiological Findings (Fig. 16.1)

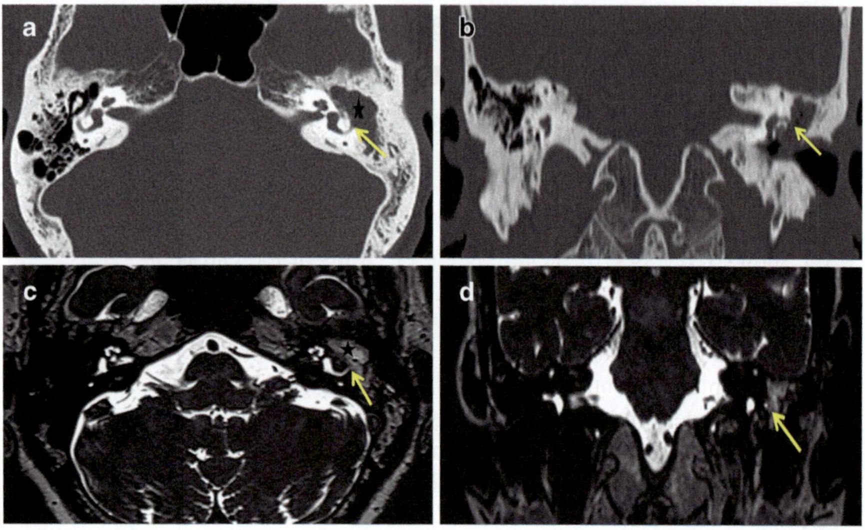

Fig. 16.1 (**a**, **b**) Axial and coronal images of HRCT temporal bone. (**c**, **d**) Axial and coronal images of heavily T2-weighted MRI; show erosion of the wall of the lateral semicircular canal suggesting labyrinthine fistula formation (yellow arrows in **a**, **b**, **c**, and **d**) between the lateral semicircular canal and the middle ear cavity. Compare with the normal bone overlying the lateral semicircular canal on the right side

Note also the complete opacification of the middle ear cavity with ossicular erosions (black star in a and c) as compared to the normal middle ear cavity on the right side. The opacification showed diffusion restriction (not shown) suggestive of a cholesteatoma. The rest of the inner ear structures appear normal.

Diagnosis Left-sided chronic otitis media with cholesteatoma; lateral semicircular canal erosion with labyrinthine fistula

Differential diagnosis Other middle ear lesions like squamous cell carcinoma in the middle ear cavity causing labyrinthine fistula

Clinical differential Other third window syndromes such as superior semicircular canal dehiscence

Discussion

Labyrinthine fistula or perilymphatic fistula refers to an abnormal direct communication between the fluid-filled inner ear and its surrounding structures, most classically with the air-filled middle ear through a defect. The symptoms usually include persistent tinnitus, hearing impairment, vertigo, and imbalance which may be isolated findings or associated with previously known ear pathologies [1].

Table 16.1 Etiologies for labyrinthine fistula

Congenital perilymph fistula	Associated with inner ear anomalies
Acquired perilymph fistula	Idiopathic (secondary to increased intracranial pressure such as labor, coughing, sneezing, diving, and flying barotrauma) Trauma Iatrogenic (stapes surgery) Cholesteatoma

Labyrinthine fistulas could be congenital or acquired (Table 16.1). Congenital fistulas are often associated with other inner ear anomalies, more frequently common cavity deformity and incomplete partition type II (Figs. 16.2 and 16.3). Oval or round window are the most common sites of congenital fistulous communication. Other sites include promontory, Hyrtl's fissure, anterior to semicircular canals, or roof of Eustachian tube. These patients with congenital fistulas often present with history of recurrent meningitis.

Traumatic perilymph fistula secondary to head injury is an important cause of post-traumatic hearing loss and giddiness. Iatrogenic fistula formation secondary to stapes surgery is also known. A majority of cases may also be idiopathic with the likely cause being secondary to increased intracranial pressure such as labor, coughing, sneezing, diving, and flying barotrauma [2].

Acquired perilymphatic fistulas are known to occur in cholesteatomas classically involving the lateral semicircular canal. However, the other semicircular canals may be involved as well. The reported incidence of cholesteatoma-induced perilymphatic fistula varies from 4% to 15%.

High-resolution computed tomography (HRCT) and thin section heavily T2W MRI sections such as CISS/FIESTA/DRIVE are reliable for the diagnosis of labyrinthine fistulas preoperatively. Air within the labyrinth (i.e., pneumolabyrinth) if seen can help in confirming the diagnosis. However, this may be missed if small. Other CT findings include fluid effusion of the window niches and a disturbed orientation of the stapes footplate. Heavily T2-weighted sequences are helpful in identifying fluid signal intensity in the middle ear and also to look for associated congenital ear anomalies which may be associated with fistula formation [3, 4].

Imaging Pitfalls

- False-positive cases secondary to motion artifacts, volume averaging, or normal hypodensities in the cochlea on CT. Fluid effusion in the middle ear can also be mistaken for perilymph leak but is less likely to be isointense to CSF.
- False-negative cases secondary to poor imaging resolution or due to intermittent nature of perilymph leak.
- Other third window pathologies such as a superior or posterior canal dehiscence and enlarged vestibular or cochlear aqueduct can present as perilymphatic fistula.

Definitive diagnosis can sometimes only be achieved with an exploratory tympanotomy.

Treatment

While there is currently no consensus on the management of labyrinthine fistulas, conservative management is preferred initially, and if symptoms persist or are recurrent, exploratory tympanotomy is the next step [5].

Additional Images

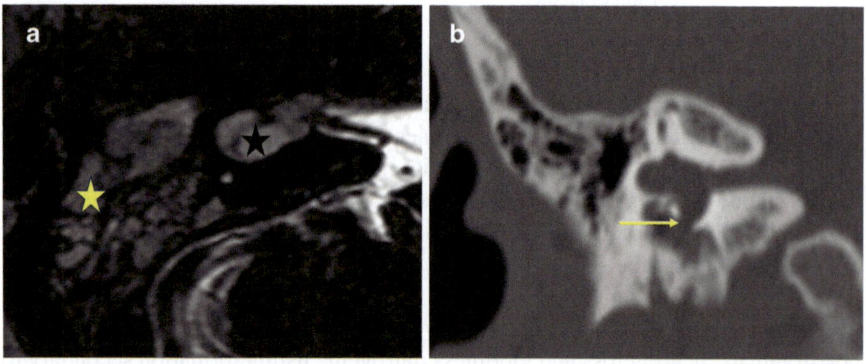

Fig. 16.2 (**a, b**) Axial DRIVE MRI and coronal HRCT temporal bone images in a case of cystic cochleovestibular anomaly (black star in **a**) demonstrating an enlarged round window with opacification suggestive of a perilymphatic fistula (yellow arrow in **b**). Also note the similar fluid signal intensity between the inner ear and middle ear (black and yellow stars) suggesting a fistulous communication

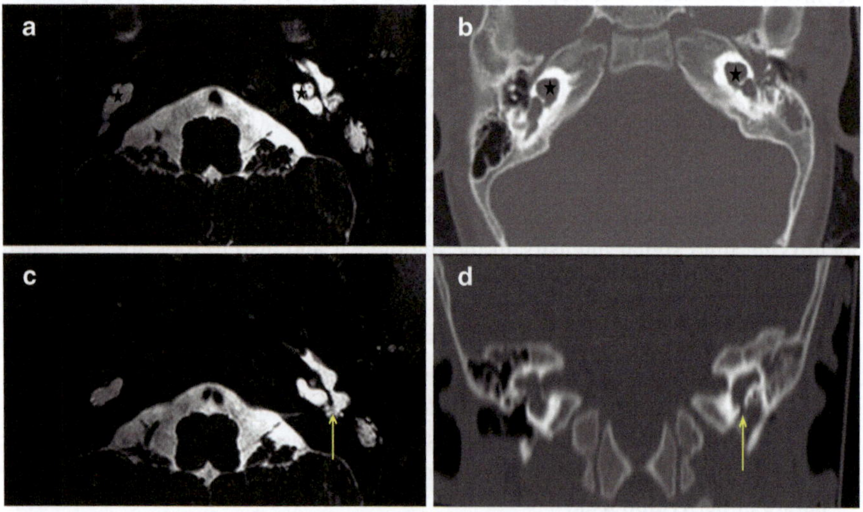

Fig. 16.3 (**a, b**) Axial DRIVE MRI and coronal HRCT temporal bone images in a 1-year-old child with severe hearing loss demonstrate bilateral cochlear anomalies (type 1 incomplete partition) (black stars). (**c, d**) Axial DRIVE MRI and coronal HRCT images in the same patient clearly demonstrate pathological fistulous communication between the inner ear and middle ear at the round window (yellow arrows) showing similar fluid intensity

References

1. Furhad S, Bokhari AA. Peri lymphatic fistula. [Updated 2023 Jul 19]. In: StatPearls [Internet]. Treasure Island: StatPearls Publishing; 2024.
2. Kurihara YY, Fujikawa A, Tachizawa N, Takaya M, Ikeda H, Starkey J. Temporal bone trauma: typical CT and MRI appearances and important points for evaluation. Radiographics. 2020;40(4):1148–62.
3. Venkatasamy A, Al Ohraini Z, Karol A, Karch-Georges A, Riehm S, Rohmer D, Charpiot A, Veillon F. CT and MRI for the diagnosis of perilymphatic fistula: a study of 17 surgically confirmed patients. Eur Arch Otorrinolaringol. 2020;277(4):1045–51. https://doi.org/10.1007/s00405-020-05820-3. Epub 2020 Feb 10.
4. Brooke S, Mehdi A, Catherine M, Shahrnaz J, Tina S, Djalilian Hamid R. Perilymphatic fistula: a review of classification, etiology, diagnosis, and treatment. Front Neurol. 2020;11:1046. https://doi.org/10.3389/fneur.2020.01046.
5. Geerse S, de Wolf MJF, Ebbens FA, van Spronsen E. Management of labyrinthine fistula: hearing preservation versus prevention of residual disease. Eur Arch Otorhinolaryngol. 2017;274(10):3605–12.

Chapter 17
Infections and Inflammatory Disease of Temporal Bone: Skull Base Osteomyelitis

Harshavardhan Mahalingam

Clinical Data A 66-year-old male with headache for 4 months, bilateral ear pain, and fever on and off. Patient is a known diabetic with a Hba1c level of 9.4%.

Radiological Findings (Fig. 17.1)

Diagnosis Skull base osteomyelitis

Differential diagnosis (if applicable) Nasopharyngeal carcinoma with skull base invasion, skull base malignancies (clival chordoma, metastasis, lymphoma/leukemia/myeloma), and inflammatory pseudotumor.

Discussion

Skull base osteomyelitis (SBO) can occur as a complication of a otogenic or sinonasal infection. It is more commonly encountered in the elderly and in immunocompromised patients. Clinical symptoms such as headache, facial pain, and otalgia, are non-specific and hence, diagnosis is often delayed.

It can be broadly divided into typical SBO (developing as complication of necrotizing otitis externa in diabetics) and atypical or central SBO (idiopathic or secondary to facial, sinus, or oral infections). Typical SBO is usually lateralized to one side while atypical SBO is central. Pseudomonas aeruginosa and Staphylococcus aureus are the most common causative agents of the typical and atypical forms, respectively [1].

Supplementary Information The online version contains supplementary material available at https://doi.org/10.1007/978-981-95-6132-2_17.

H. Mahalingam (✉)
Department of Radiology, SRIHER, Chennai, India

H. Mahalingam (ed.), *Temporal Bone Imaging*,
https://doi.org/10.1007/978-981-95-6132-2_17

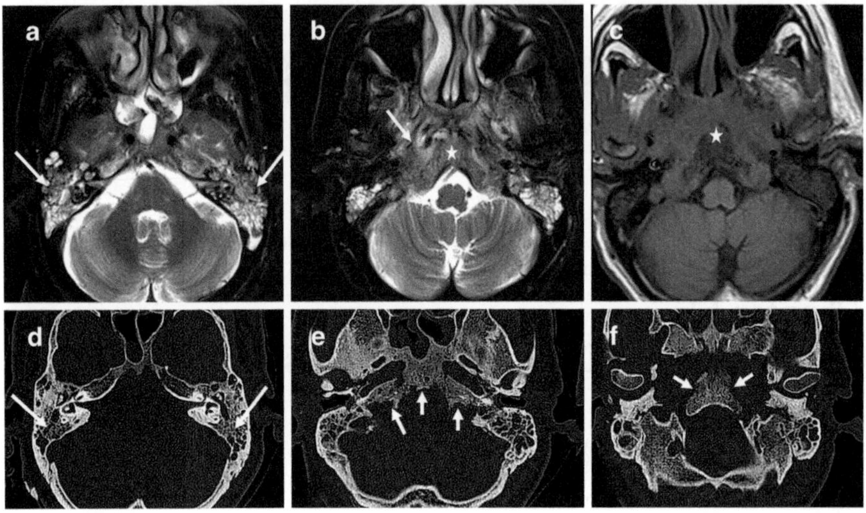

Fig. 17.1 (**a**) Axial T2-weighted image showing fluid signal within the bilateral middle ear and mastoid (arrows). (**b**) Axial T2-weighted image showing marrow edema in the clivus (star) with adjacent soft tissue edema (arrow). (**c**) Axial T1-weighted image shows loss of normal marrow fat signal—normal marrow T1 hyperintense signal is lost (star). (**d**–**f**) Axial HRCT temporal bone images showing bilateral otomastoiditis with multiple erosions in both petrous temporal bones and in the clivus (arrows)

Imaging findings on CT can be subtle, especially in early stages. These include cortical erosion and trabecular rarefaction in the skull base. Associated findings of fluid density in the middle ear/mastoid and in the paranasal sinuses may be present. Important areas to evaluate on HRCT include the bony external auditory canal, petrous apex, anterior clival margin, foramen lacerum, and jugular foramen. Contrast-enhanced CT can show enhancing soft tissue thickening in the infratemporal fossa and nasopharynx. Presence of abscesses can provide a clue to differential diagnosis from tumors.

MRI performs better than CT in evaluating the marrow and soft tissue involvement in SBO. Fat-suppressed T2-weighted images, non-fat-suppressed T1-weighted images, and fat suppressed post-gadolinium T1-weighted images are the most informative sequences for establishing the diagnosis. Diffusion-weighted imaging can help in identifying the presence of abscesses.

Nuclear medicine imaging techniques like Gallium-67 scintigraphy and FDG-PET play a complimentary problem-solving role in establishing the diagnosis [2].

Complications of SBO include cranial nerve palsies, internal carotid artery occlusion/pseudoaneurysm and internal jugular vein thrombosis.

Imaging Pearls

- Fat-saturated T2-weighted images are essential to identify skull base marrow edema.

- Loss of marrow T1 hyperintensity is an important clue to identify presence of disease.
- Careful attention to the cortical outline of skull base on CT is essential to detect subtle erosions.
- Identification of abscess formation can help in differentiating SBO from malignancies.

Imaging Pitfalls

- HRCT temporal bone is often the initial investigation done in suspected skull base osteomyelitis, and review of soft tissue window images is essential to pick up soft tissue swelling which may be the only finding on CT in early SBO.
- Skull base malignancies (especially nasopharyngeal carcinoma) can mimic SBO on imaging. Biopsy is often needed to differentiate these entities.

References

1. Chapman PR, Choudhary G, Singhal A. Skull base osteomyelitis: a comprehensive imaging review. AJNR Am J Neuroradiol. 2021;42(3):404–13.
2. Álvarez Jáñez F, Barriga LQ, Iñigo TR, Roldán LF. Diagnosis of skull base osteomyelitis. Radiographics. 2021;41(1):156–74.

Chapter 18
Infections and Inflammatory Disease of Temporal Bone: Otomastoiditis with Sinus Thrombosis

Harshavardhan Mahalingam and Karthik Kulanthaivelu

Clinical Data A 30-year-old male with history of headache for 2 days with blurring of vision.

Radiological Findings (Fig. 18.1)

Diagnosis Venous sinus thrombosis with raised intracranial tension – likely developing as a complication of right otomastoiditis.

Differential Diagnosis (If Applicable) Nil

Discussion

Venous sinus thrombosis can occur as a complication of acute or chronic otomastoiditis – either as a result of a defect in the sigmoid dural plate with resultant inflammation of sinus wall, or due to retrograde thrombophlebitis [1].

Diagnosis of sinus thrombosis on plain CT is sometimes possible due to the presence of a hyperdense clot within the sinus. This finding can be difficult to appreciate on HRCT sections and may require reconstruction of the CT images using a brain window with an appropriate reconstruction filter. Plain MRI can also provide clues, such as loss of the normal flow void of the venous sinuses; however, slow flow or hypoplastic sinuses may produce similar findings. Time-of-flight (TOF) MR

Supplementary Information The online version contains supplementary material available at https://doi.org/10.1007/978-981-95-6132-2_18.

H. Mahalingam (✉)
Department of Radiology, SRIHER, Chennai, India

K. Kulanthaivelu
Department of Neuroradiology, SRIHER, Chennai, India

H. Mahalingam (ed.), *Temporal Bone Imaging*,
https://doi.org/10.1007/978-981-95-6132-2_18

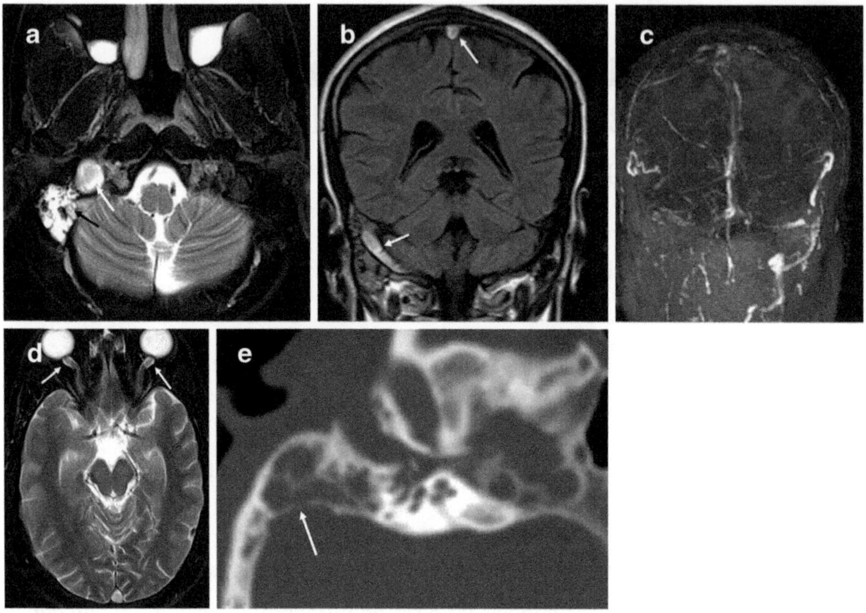

Fig. 18.1 (**a**) Axial fat-saturated T2-weighted image showing a dilated right IJV with loss of flow void (white arrow). Also note the fluid signal in the right mastoid (black arrow). (**b**) Coronal T2-FLAIR image showing loss of flow void in right transverse and superior sagittal sinuses. (**c**) Time of flight MR venogram shows no flow-related signal in the superior sagittal, right transverse, right sigmoid sinuses, and right internal jugular vein suggestive of extensive venous thrombosis. (**d**) Axial fat-saturated T2-weighted image showing prominent optic nerve sheaths with posterior scleral bulge (arrows) suggesting raised intracranial tension. (**e**) Axial HRCT section showing fluid density in the right mastoid with erosion of the sigmoid plate (arrow).

venogram can aid in diagnosis but is haunted by several pitfalls like slow flow, in-plane signal loss, and T1 shine through.

Definitive diagnosis of venous sinus thrombosis requires contrast-enhanced CT or MRI . On contrast enhanced imaging, an acute thrombus is seen as a complete or central filling defect within the venous sinus. Venous sinus thrombosis can further be complicated by development of venous infarcts and increased intracranial tension due to impaired intracranial venous drainage [2].

References

1. Zanoletti E, Cazzador D, Faccioli C, Sari M, Bovo R, Martini A. Intracranial venous sinus thrombosis as a complication of otitis media in children: critical review of diagnosis and management. Int J Pediatr Otorhinolaryngol. 2015;79(12):2398–403.
2. Canedo-Antelo M, Baleato-González S, Mosqueira AJ, Casas-Martínez J, Oleaga L, Vilanova JC, et al. Radiologic clues to cerebral venous thrombosis. RadioGraphics. 2019;39(6):1611–28.

Chapter 19
Temporal Bone in Head Trauma: Otic Capsule Sparing Temporal Bone Fractures

Jeffrey Skaria Joseph

Clinical Data A 40-year-old lady with history of high-impact motor vehicle accident-related trauma.

Radiological Findings (Fig. 19.1)

Supplementary Information The online version contains supplementary material available at https://doi.org/10.1007/978-981-95-6132-2_19.

J. S. Joseph (✉)
Department of Radiology, Chettinad Hospital and Research Institute,
Kelambakkam, Tamil Nadu, India

H. Mahalingam (ed.), *Temporal Bone Imaging*,
https://doi.org/10.1007/978-981-95-6132-2_19

Diagnosis Right longitudinal otic capsule sparing temporal bone fracture

Differential Diagnosis Pseudofractures

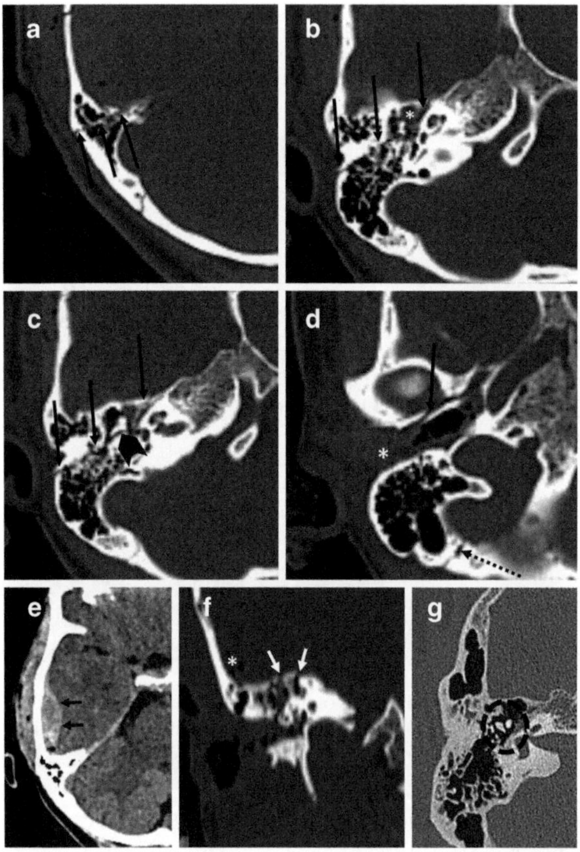

Fig. 19.1 Axial temporal bone CT images show a typical longitudinal (extralabyrinthine) otic capsule sparing right temporal bone fracture (black arrows, image **a–c**), running parallel to petrous pyramid, extending from the right mastoid into the middle ear cavity and reaching up to the groove for greater superficial petrosal nerve. Associated hemotympanum (white asterisk, image **b**) is seen, but the ossicular chain appears intact (black arrowhead, image **c**). Image **d** shows fracture of the anterior wall of the external auditory canal (black arrow) with associated blood in the EAC (white asterisk). Dotted black arrow represents occipitomastoid suture ("pseudofracture"). Axial CT brain image (image e) of the same patient shows associated epidural hematoma (EDH) in the right temporal region (black arrows). EDH is common in otic sparing fractures. Coronal reconstructed CT temporal bone (image f) shows fracture extending to the right tegmen, with multiple bone defects (white arrows) which are potential sites for CSF leaks. Pockets of pneumocephalus (white asterisk) are a secondary sign of temporal bone fracture. (Image courtesy Dr. Vinith. R) Axial HRCT temporal bone (image g) in another patient with prior history of trauma and persisting conductive hearing loss shows the "broken heart" sign (black circle) indicative of incudomalleolar joint separation.

19.1 Discussion

The temporal bone is prone to injury from high-impact trauma including road traffic accidents, assaults, falls, and sports injuries.

CT is the first-line imaging technique in head and neck trauma. In a setting of trauma, effusion/opacification in the mastoid or middle ear should raise suspicion for a temporal bone fracture and a dedicated high-resolution temporal bone CT with very thin slices (less than 1 mm) and small field of view should then be considered, subject to the patient's clinical status. Multiplanar reconstruction in coronal plane, Pöschl view, and Stenvers view is able to identify subtle fractures and contributes to a more complete assessment of fracture course [1].

Other *secondary* signs that should prompt a careful search for temporal bone fracture include external auditory canal opacification, air within the temporomandibular joint, pockets of pneumocephalus adjacent to the temporal bone, and pneumolabyrinth.

Traditionally, temporal bone fractures were classified (based on fracture line orientation to the long axis of the petrous part of temporal bone), into the more common longitudinal fracture (70%–90%), running lengthwise parallel to the petrous pyramid and the less common transverse fracture (10%–30%), running perpendicular to the petrous ridge (Fig. 19.2). A mixed or oblique subtype is a combination of both longitudinal and transverse fractures.

The limitation of this popular fracture classification system is its poor correlation with clinical outcomes and potential short-/long-term complications. As a result, other classification systems have been proposed.

One such system (Kelly and Tami 1994) classifies temporal bone fractures as otic capsule sparing (OCS, more common, 94%–97%) and otic capsule violating fractures (OCV, 3%–6%).

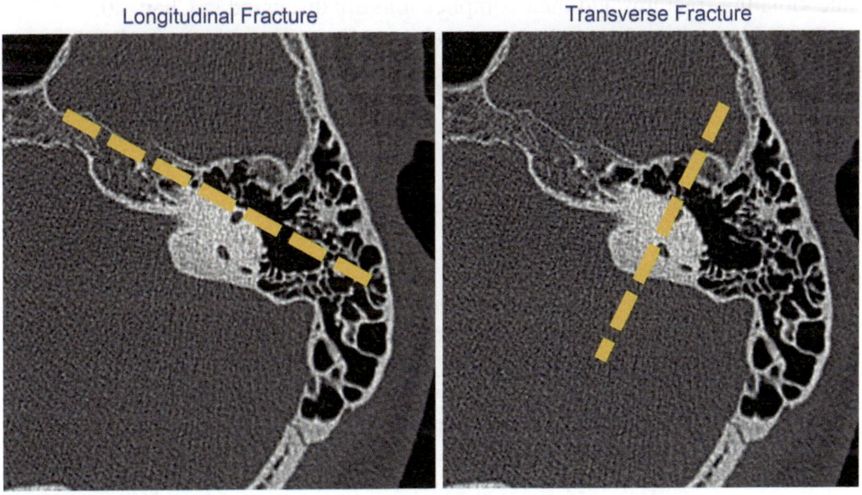

Fig. 19.2 Traditional temporal bone fracture classification according to fracture line orientation

Otic capsule sparing fractures result from a temporoparietal blow, usually involving the squamous temporal bone with fracture line extending to involve the posterosuperior external auditory canal, mastoid air cells, and traversing the middle ear, tegmen tympani, and tegmen mastoideum. They typically result in conductive hearing loss (CHL) due to ossicular injury. Other causes of transient traumatic CHL include hemotympanum and tympanic membrane perforation, which are usually managed conservatively; however, persisting CHL (diagnosed by a reassessment at 6 weeks) due to perforation may require interventions like tympanoplasty. Subarachnoid hemorrhage and epidural hematomas may also be associated with OCS fractures [2].

Injury to the ossicles manifests as ossicular fractures, ossicular subluxation, or dislocation, where there is frank disruption of the ossicular chain. Incus, being the largest ossicle with poor ligamentous support, is most frequently affected. Incudostapedial and incudomalleolar are the most common dislocations. Incudomalleolar joint dislocation results in loss of its typical ice-cream cone configuration. A "broken heart" or "Y sign" usually seen on coronal slices has been used sometimes to describe the slight lateral displacement of incus in incudomalleolar injury [3].

Potential difficulty in identifying incudostapedial separation in an acute setting is due to hemotympanum and its small anatomical structure.

Persistent CHL for >6 months is concerning and surgery for ossicular reconstruction may be indicated.

Ossicular fractures are uncommon, seen as subtle lucent lines through the ossicles or as displaced bone fragments. Stapes footplate fractures are attributed to transverse fractures extending through the oval window. Perilymphatic fistula, although more common in OCV fracture, is also a potential complication of transverse fractures traversing the footplate.

The bony labyrinth is rather strong compared to other temporal bone segments, requiring a greater impact to be fractured. So fractures through the bony labyrinth (also called otic capsule) are associated with more severe complications. Otic capsule violating fractures and their complications are discussed in Chap. 20.

Possible pitfall in diagnosing temporal bone fracture are the "pseudofractures," which are normal linear anatomical structures that complicate the identification of true fractures (Table 19.1 and Fig. 19.3).

Table 19.1 Temporal bone fracture mimics

S. no	Category	Examples
1	Aqueducts	Cochlear aqueduct, vestibular aqueduct
2	Canaliculi	Subarcuate canal, singular canal, inferior tympanic canaliculus, mastoid canaliculus, canal for chorda tympani, hiatus of facial canal
3	Grooves	Groove for greater petrosal nerve
4	Extrinsic fissures	Petrosphenoidal fissure, sphenosquamosal fissure, petro-occipital fissure, occipitomastoid suture
5	Intrinsic fissures	Tympanosquamosal fissure, petrosquamous fissure, petrotympanic fissure, tympanomastoid fissure

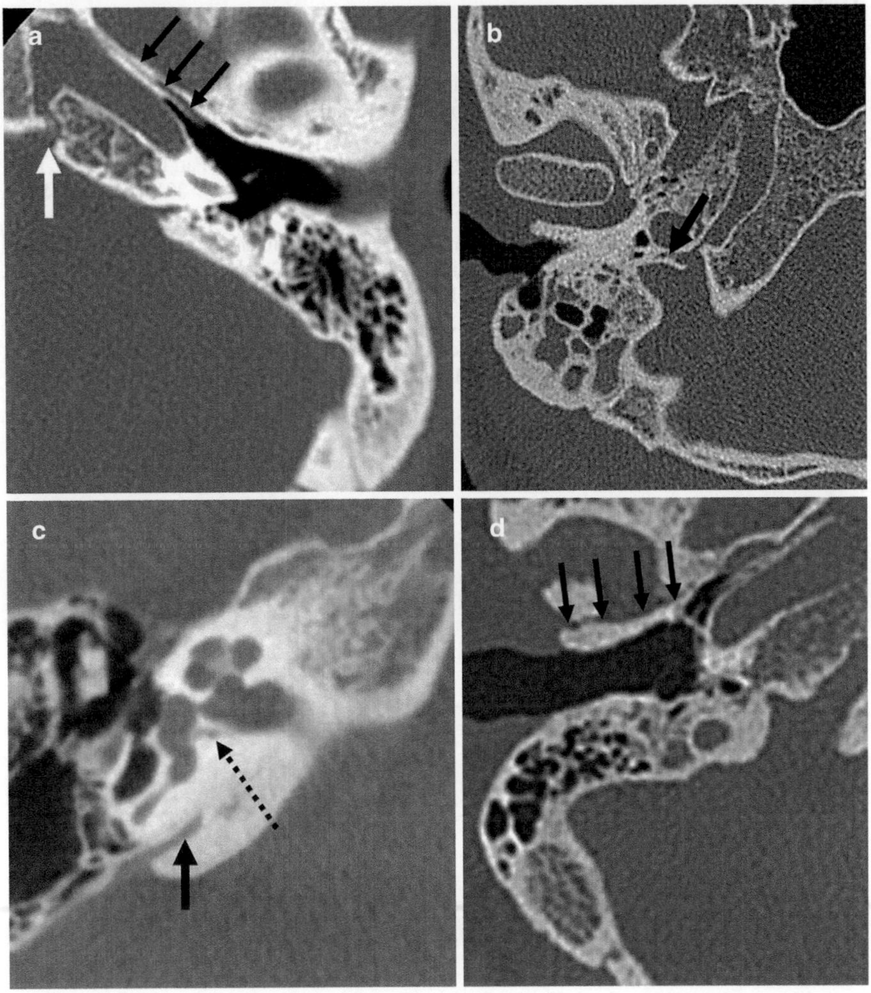

Fig. 19.3 Fracture mimics. (**a**) Petrosphenoidal fissure (black arrows) and petro-occipital fissure (white arrow), (**b**) inferior tympanic canaliculus (black arrow) (contains the Jacobson nerve), (**c**) vestibular aqueduct (black arrow) and singular canal (dotted black arrow), and (**d**) tympanosquamous fissure (black arrows)

Intrinsic fissures are those that form between the five native segments of the temporal bone. Extrinsic fissures separate the temporal bone from adjacent bones of the skull. Fissures can be differentiated by their corticated, sclerotic margins. Awareness of these normal linear structures is essential to avoid misinterpreting them as fracture lines [4].

When in doubt, compare with normal side and look for symmetry, as normal structures are typically symmetrical.

References

1. Kennedy TA, Avey GD, Gentry LR. Imaging of temporal bone trauma. Neuroimaging Clin N Am. 2014;24(3):467–86, viii. https://doi.org/10.1016/j.nic.2014.03.003. Epub 2014 May 21. PMID: 25086807
2. Juliano AF, Ginat DT, Moonis G. Imaging review of the temporal bone: Part II. Traumatic, postoperative, and noninflammatory nonneoplastic conditions. Radiology. 2015;276(3):655–72. https://doi.org/10.1148/radiol.2015140800. PMID: 26302389
3. Lantos JE, Leeman K, Weidman EK, Dean KE, Peng T, Pearlman AN. Imaging of temporal bone trauma: A clinicoradiologic perspective. Neuroimaging Clin N Am. 2019;29(1):129–43. https://doi.org/10.1016/j.nic.2018.08.005. Epub 2018 Oct 31. PMID: 30466637
4. Kurihara YY, Fujikawa A, Tachizawa N, Takaya M, Ikeda H, Starkey J. Temporal bone trauma: typical CT and MRI appearances and important points for evaluation. Radiographics. 2020;40(4):1148–62. https://doi.org/10.1148/rg.2020190023. Epub 2020 May 22. PMID: 32442046

Chapter 20
Temporal Bone in Head Trauma: Otic Capsule Violating Temporal Bone Fractures

Jeffrey Skaria Joseph

Clinical Data A 36-year-old male presenting to the ER with motor vehicle accident-related head injury.

Radiological Findings (Fig 20.1)

Diagnosis Left transverse otic capsule violating petrous temporal bone fracture

Differential Diagnosis Pseudofractures

20.1 Discussion

Otic capsule violating (OCV) fractures are less common than otic capsule sparing (OCS) fractures, occurring in about 3% to 6% of temporal bone fractures. They result from an occipital traumatic impact with fracture line extending from the foramen magnum through the petrous pyramid into the otic capsule, often involving the jugular foramen, foramen lacerum, and internal auditory canal. Axial CT sections are best to look for otic capsule violations, seen as fracture lines through the cochlea, vestibule, or semicircular canals.

OCV fractures are frequently associated with complications like profound sensorineural hearing loss (SNHL), cerebrospinal fluid leaks, and facial nerve injury.

Supplementary Information The online version contains supplementary material available at https://doi.org/10.1007/978-981-95-6132-2_20.

J. S. Joseph (✉)
Department of Radiology, Chettinad Hospital and Research Institute, Kelambakkam, Tamil Nadu, India

H. Mahalingam (ed.), *Temporal Bone Imaging*,
https://doi.org/10.1007/978-981-95-6132-2_20

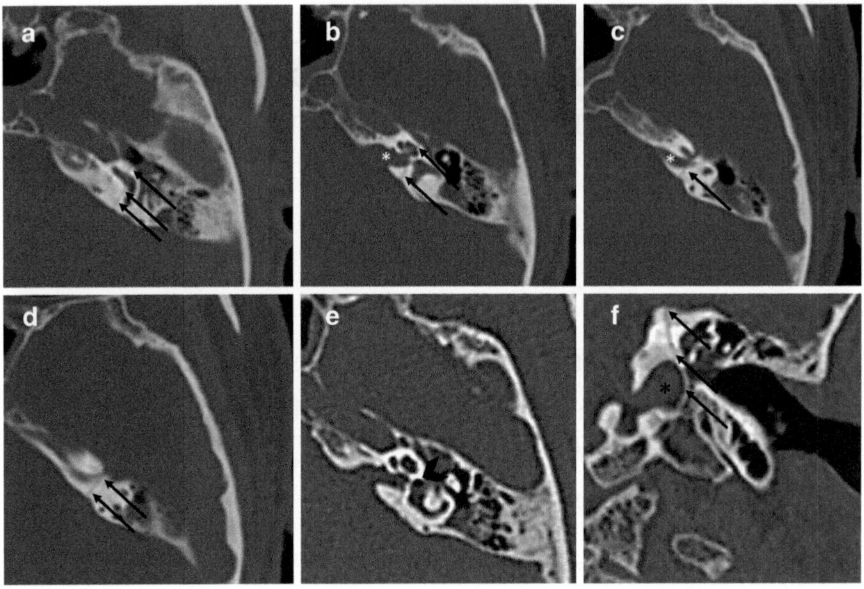

Fig. 20.1 Axial temporal bone CT images (**a–e**) show a typical transverse otic capsule violating left petrous temporal bone fracture (black arrows). The subtle fracture is seen coursing through the basal turn of the cochlea, propagating through the fundus of the internal auditory canal, traversing the apical cochlear turn, and reaching up to the tympanic segment of the facial nerve canal. Pneumolabyrinth, seen as a pocket of air in the vestibule (image e, black arrowhead), is an indirect sign that the otic capsule is breached. Coronal CT reconstruction (**f**) in the same patient shows, in addition, the fracture extending into the jugular foramen.

Patients may present clinically with SNHL post trauma, if the fracture crosses the labyrinth or internal auditory canal, injuring the cochlear nerve. Isolated post-traumatic intralabyrinthine hemorrhage without fractures may also present with SNHL, best seen on MRI as T1 hyperintensity in the vestibulocochlear apparatus [1].

Pneumolabyrinth (seen as air bubbles in the cochlea, vestibule, or semicircular canals) is a telltale sign of otic capsule violation, when the fracture is not immediately apparent. Fracture or contusion of the vestibule, semicircular canals, vestibular aqueduct, or vestibular nerve results in posttraumatic vertigo, but the symptoms usually resolve spontaneously over a year.

Posttraumatic perilymphatic fistula (abnormal communication between the fluid-filled inner ear and aerated middle ear, due to disruption at the oval/round window) is a difficult to diagnose complication in the absence of fracture, but to be suspected in a patient presenting acutely with fluctuating sensorineural hearing loss, persistent vertigo, and imaging showing middle ear effusion, opacification of the round window, and pneumolabyrinth.

A potential late complication of otic capsule violating fractures is the development of labyrinthitis ossificans. Earlier fibrous stage can be detected on high-resolution steady-state T2 MRI sequences, showing loss of normal fluid signal in the inner ear. Eventually, they progress to end-stage bone formation seen as osseous attenuation on CT [2].

Posttraumatic cerebrospinal fluid (CSF) leaks occur in about 13%–45% of patients with temporal bone fractures with its incidence at least 4 times more likely in otic capsule violating fractures than otic capsule sparing fractures. They are usually a result of direct tears to the dura by bone fractures and 7% of patients are at serious risk of developing meningitis, particularly those with persistent CSF leaks for >7 days. Patients may present either with otorrhea if the tympanic membrane is perforated or with CSF rhinorrhea through eustachian tube drainage, if the tympanic membrane is intact. Beta-2 transferrin testing can confirm suspected CSF leak, with beta-trace protein being more sensitive and specific for CSF [3].

A careful assessment of the integrity of tegmen using HRCT, including in coronal and sagittal reconstructions, is done to look for defects/potential sites of leak. It is essential to describe the location and size of the defect, the presence of displaced fracture fragment, and the presence of encephalocele – info that helps surgical decision-making. MR imaging is complementary, helping to distinguish fluid/blood or meningoencephalocele and detect associated focal meningitis.

The facial nerve is more commonly injured in otic capsule violating fractures (Fig. 20.2) and the geniculate ganglion region is most prone for injury. Scrutiny of the entire course of facial nerve is possible on CT. In patients with immediate posttraumatic paresis, disruption or displacement of the facial nerve canal or bony fragments along the nerve course may infer neural transection or compression by osseous fragment and is often an indication for surgical decompression. Delayed-onset facial palsy can be due to development of edema or expanding perineural hematoma causing neural compression of an intact nerve.

Vascular injuries can complicate temporal bone fractures when fracture lines traverse through the carotid canal or through the distal transverse and sigmoid sinuses. Injuries to the internal carotid artery are best evaluated by CT/MR angiography. Occlusion, dissection, pseudoaneurysm, and arteriovenous fistula are complications to be ruled out, especially if there is distraction of the carotid canal [4]. A checklist for reporting temporal bone fractures is presented in Table 20.1 [1].

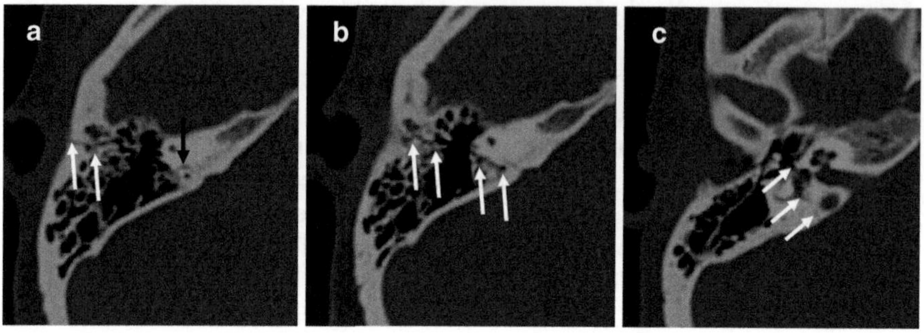

Fig. 20.2 Axial sections of HRCT temporal bone showing a posttraumatic transverse otic capsule violating temporal bone fracture, coursing through the right mastoid antrum (white arrows in image **a, b**), across the semicircular canal and vestibule to involve the tympanic segment of facial nerve canal (white arrows in image **c**). Note the curvilinear petromastoid canal/subarcuate canaliculus (black arrow in image **a**) seen between the limbs of the superior semicircular canal is a potential fracture mimic.

Table 20.1 Summary and checklist for reporting temporal bone fractures

Indirect signs of fracture	Look out for external auditory canal opacification, air within TM joint, pneumocephalus adjacent to temporal bone, pneumolabyrinth, middle ear opacification, mastoid air cell opacification, sphenoid sinus air fluid levels, and extra axial collections adjacent to the temporal bone.
Fracture location and direction	Trace entire fracture line (longitudinal/transverse/mixed oblique), petrous or nonpetrous location.
Otic capsule involvement	Is there violation of the cochlea, vestibule, vestibular aqueduct, or semicircular canals? Is the internal auditory canal involved? Presence of pneumolabyrinth
Ossicular chain integrity	Check malleus, incus, stapes, and ossicular joints for alignment/fracture/dislocation. Compare with normal side.
Facial nerve canal involvement	Trace the entire course of the nerve (internal auditory canal, fallopian canal, geniculate fossa, tympanic, mastoid). Is there need for surgical decompression (bone fragment indenting on nerve/disruption of facial canal borders)?
External auditory canal	Comment on fractures in this region (if ignored, can potentially complicate with stenosis).
Tegmen integrity	Assess tegmen tympani and mastoideum. Identify defect. Comment on location/size of defect, presence and orientation of distracted fracture fragment, and presence of encephalocele.
Vascular	Does the fracture line traverse the carotid canal (petrous/cavernous segments) or venous sinuses. Decide on CT angiography/venography to look for dissection, occlusion, pseudoaneurysm, or venous sinus thrombosis.

References

1. Kennedy TA, Avey GD, Gentry LR. Imaging of temporal bone trauma. Neuroimaging Clin N Am. 2014;24(3):467–86, viii. https://doi.org/10.1016/j.nic.2014.03.003. Epub 2014 May 21. PMID: 25086807
2. Juliano AF, Ginat DT, Moonis G. Imaging review of the temporal bone: Part II. Traumatic, postoperative, and noninflammatory nonneoplastic conditions. Radiology. 2015;276(3):655–72. https://doi.org/10.1148/radiol.2015140800. PMID: 26302389
3. Lantos JE, Leeman K, Weidman EK, Dean KE, Peng T, Pearlman AN. Imaging of temporal bone trauma: a clinicoradiologic perspective. Neuroimaging Clin N Am. 2019;29(1):129–43. https://doi.org/10.1016/j.nic.2018.08.005. Epub 2018 Oct 31. PMID: 30466637
4. Kurihara YY, Fujikawa A, Tachizawa N, Takaya M, Ikeda H, Starkey J. Temporal bone trauma: typical CT and MRI appearances and important points for evaluation. Radiographics. 2020;40(4):1148–62. https://doi.org/10.1148/rg.2020190023. Epub 2020 May 22. PMID: 32442046

References

Chapter 21
Temporal Bone in Head Trauma: Ossicular Disruption

Harshavardhan Mahalingam

Clinical Data A 16-year-old male involved in a road traffic accident presented with left ear bleed.

Radiological Findings (Fig. 21.1)

Diagnosis Comminuted, longitudinally oriented, otic capsule sparing fracture of petrous temporal bone (anterior subtype) with ossicular chain disruption

Differential Diagnosis (If Applicable) Transverse fracture

21.1 Discussion

In the context of head trauma, ossicular chain disruption can occur along with a temporal bone fracture or in isolation. It is more commonly associated with longitudinal fractures of petrous temporal bone than with transverse fractures. Post-traumatic conductive hearing loss is the usual clinical presentation [1].

With the malleus and stapes being well supported by ligaments, the incus is the ossicle most commonly involved in fractures and dislocations. Common patterns include incudostapedial subluxation (the most common), malleoincudal subluxation, incus dislocation, and stapes fracture and dislocation.

Supplementary Information The online version contains supplementary material available at https://doi.org/10.1007/978-981-95-6132-2_21.

H. Mahalingam (✉)
Department of Radiology, SRIHER, Chennai, India

H. Mahalingam (ed.), *Temporal Bone Imaging*,
https://doi.org/10.1007/978-981-95-6132-2_21

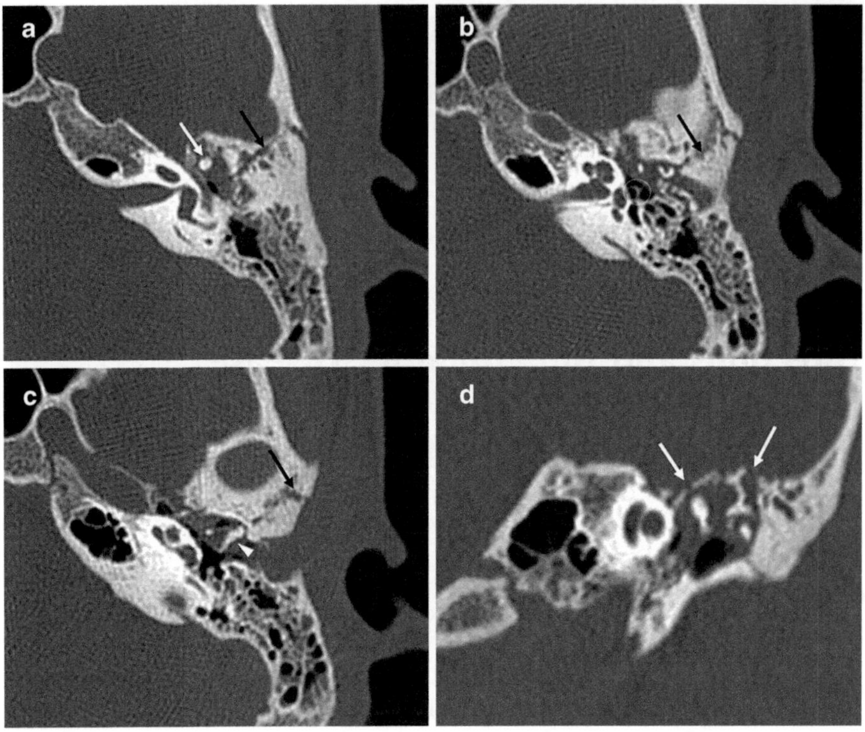

Fig. 21.1 (**a**, **b**, **c**) Axial sections of the left temporal bone from superior to inferior show a longitudinally oriented fracture of the petrous temporal bone (black arrows) with complete dislocation of the malleus and incus. The malleus (white arrow) is displaced anteriorly while the incus (arrowhead) is rotated transversely and lying inferior to the malleus. The stapes was normal (dotted circle). (**d**) Coronal section of the left temporal bone shows disruption of the tegmen tympani with comminution (arrows).

The axial plane is best suited for assessment of these subluxations. There can be anterior or posterior displacement of the lenticular process of incus in relation to the head of stapes in incudostapedial subluxation. In malleoincudal subluxation, there is separation of the "ice cream" from the "cone". Complete incus dislocation may also be encountered, in which the incus is displaced into the attic or even into the external auditory canal. Injury of the stapes should be suspected if the stapes superstructure is not visualized properly on axial images [2]. Recently, a grading system based on distance between the malleus and incus axes measured on HRCT, along with presence or absence of ossicular subluxation, has been shown to predict hearing outcomes [3].

References

1. Kurihara YY, Fujikawa A, Tachizawa N, Takaya M, Ikeda H, Starkey J. Temporal bone trauma: typical CT and MRI appearances and important points for evaluation. Radio Graphics. 2020 Jul;40(4):1148–62.
2. Maillot O, Attyé A, Boyer E, Heck O, Kastler A, Grand S, et al. Post traumatic deafness: a pictorial review of CT and MRI findings. Insights Imaging. 2016;7(3):341–50.
3. Mantokoudis G, Schläpfer N, Kellinghaus M, Hakim A, von Werdt M, Caversaccio MD, et al. Traumatic dislocation of middle ear ossicles: a new computed tomography classification predicting hearing outcome. PLoS One. 2021;16(2):e0245796.

Chapter 22
Neoplastic Diseases of Temporal Bone: External/Middle Ear Squamous Cell Carcinoma

Harshavardhan Mahalingam

Clinical Data A 60-year-old female with complaints of foul smelling discharge from the right ear for 2 months.

Radiological Findings (Fig. 22.1)
Otoscopic examination revealed nodular reddish soft tissue thickening in external auditory canal which on biopsy was diagnosed as squamous cell carcinoma.

Diagnosis External ear squamous cell carcinoma

Differential Diagnosis (If Applicable)
Otitis externa

22.1 Discussion

Malignancies of the external, middle and inner ear are rare. Squamous cell carcinoma (SCC) is the most common malignancy of temporal bone. Most of these lesions arise from the pinna with contiguous extension to the temporal bone. SCCs can also arise primarily from the EAC and rarely the middle or inner ear. The diagnosis of external auditory canal SCCs is often delayed, as they mimic otitis externa/media and cholesteatoma clinically, presenting with pain and otorrhea [1].

Supplementary Information The online version contains supplementary material available at https://doi.org/10.1007/978-981-95-6132-2_22.

H. Mahalingam (✉)
Department of Radiology, SRIHER, Chennai, India

H. Mahalingam (ed.), *Temporal Bone Imaging*,
https://doi.org/10.1007/978-981-95-6132-2_22

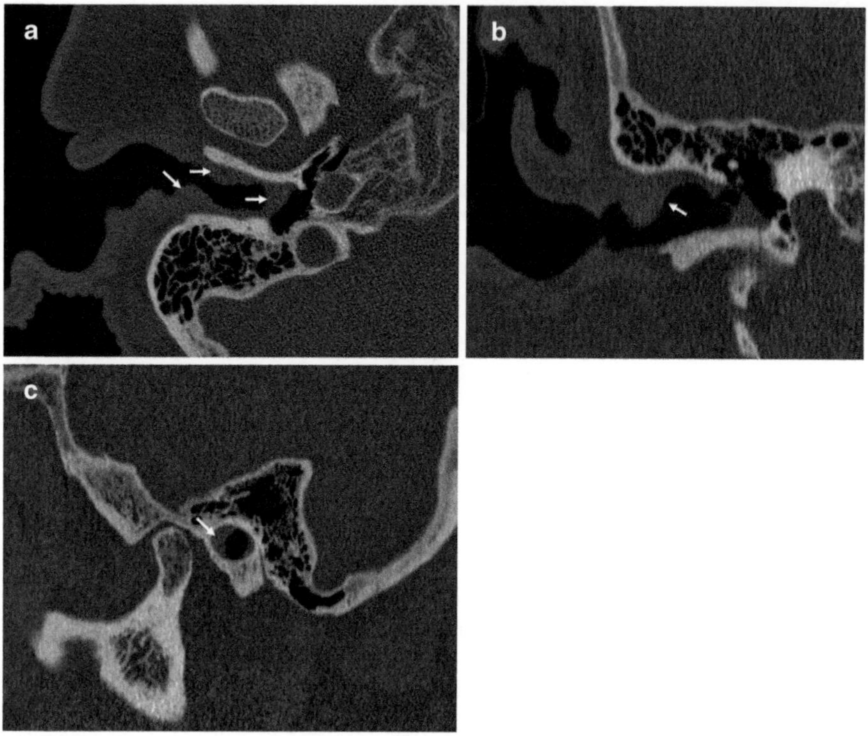

Fig. 22.1 (**a**, **b**, **c**) Axial, coronal, and sagittal reconstructed sections of the right temporal bone show asymmetric and nodular circumferential soft tissue thickening in the cartilaginous and bony parts of the right external auditory canal and involving the tympanic membrane (arrows). No bone erosions were seen.

CT is useful in identifying bone erosions in the EAC. MRI is especially useful in identifying local spread to the temporomandibular joint, parotid gland, and infratemporal fossa. Perineural spread along facial nerve course can be seen as enhancement and thickening of facial nerve on post-gadolinium images. MRI can also help in differentiating SCC from cholesteatoma (which can also show bone erosions), as SCC typically enhances brightly on post-gadolinium images while cholesteatoma does not show any enhancement. Local lymph nodal involvement (parotid, perimastoid, and level II cervical) also needs to be assessed [2].

Differentiation of SCC from necrotizing otitis externa may be difficult on imaging as both conditions can show soft tissue thickening, enhancement, and bone erosions in the EAC. Correlation with clinical findings and biopsy are essential to differentiate these entities.

Local staging of external ear and temporal bone SCC is presented in Table 22.1.

Table 22.1 T staging of external ear and temporal bone SCC according to modified Pittsburgh and modified Stell systems

Stage	Modified Pittsburgh	Modified Stell
T1	Tumor limited to EAC with no bone erosion or soft tissue extension	Tumor limited to EAC with no bone erosion or facial paresis
T2	Limited EAC bone erosion; limited (<0.5 cm) soft tissue involvement	Facial paresis or bone destruction without extension beyond organ of origin
T3	Full-thickness EAC bone erosion. Limited (<0.5 cm) soft tissue involvement. Extension to middle ear or mastoid	Extratemporal extension into parotid, TM joint, and skin
T4	Involves medial wall of middle ear, cochlea, carotid canal, jugular fossa, dura, TM joint, styloid process, and facial paresis	Extratemporal extension into dura and skull base

References

1. Allanson BM, Low TH, Clark JR, Gupta R. Squamous cell carcinoma of the external auditory canal and temporal bone: an update. Head Neck Pathol. 2018;12(3):407–18.
2. Tsuno NSG, Tsuno MY, Coelho Neto CAF, Noujaim SE, Decnop M, Pacheco FT, et al. Imaging the external ear: practical approach to normal and pathologic conditions. RadioGraphics. 2022;42(2):522–40.

Chapter 23
Neoplastic Diseases of Temporal Bone: Glomus Tympanicum

Madhavi Kandagaddala and Aparna Irodi

Clinical Data A 30-year-old man with a ringing sensation and progressive hearing loss.

Supplementary Information The online version contains supplementary material available at https://doi.org/10.1007/978-981-95-6132-2_23.

M. Kandagaddala (✉) · A. Irodi
Dept of Diagnostic Radiology, Division of Clinical Radiology, Christian Medical College & Hospital, Vellore, India

H. Mahalingam (ed.), *Temporal Bone Imaging*,
https://doi.org/10.1007/978-981-95-6132-2_23

Radiological Findings (Fig. 23.1)

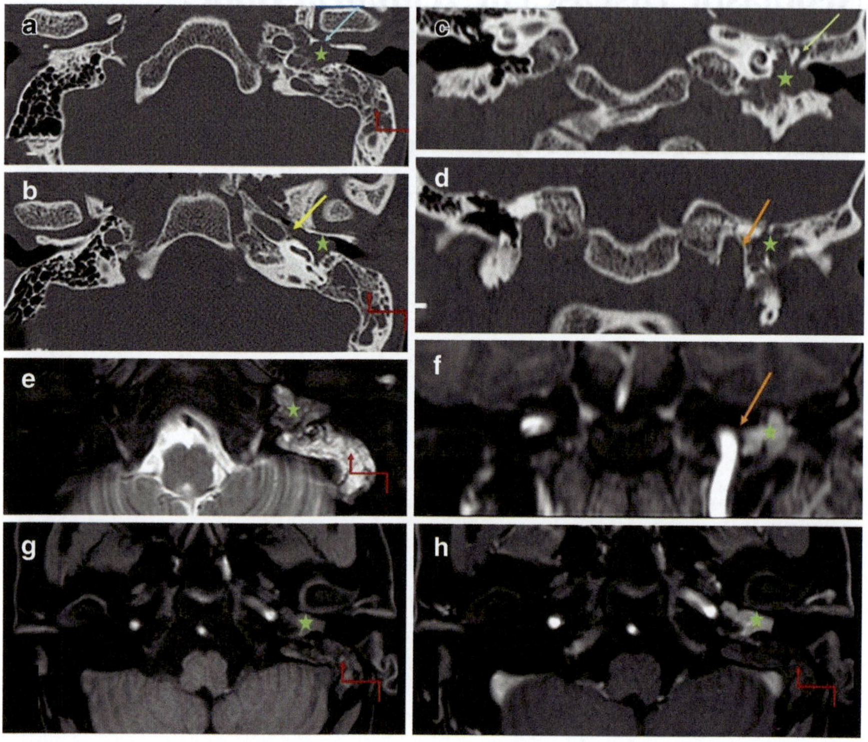

Fig. 23.1 (**a**, **b**): HRCT temporal bone axial images show a polypoidal lesion in the middle ear [green asterisk] with a base toward the promontory. There is focal erosion of the anterior wall of the external auditory canal [blue arrow] and extension into the eustachian tube [yellow arrow]. (**c**, **d**): HRCT temporal bone coronal images show encasement of the ossicles [green arrow] and extension into the hypotympanum. (**e**, **f**): MR images. The lesion appears hyperintense on T2-weighted images (**e**) with intense enhancement in the post-gadolinium image (**f**). The bone between the jugular bulb/fossa and middle ear mass is intact (orange arrow). (**g**, **h**): MR images. The lesion appears isointense to muscle on fat-suppressed T1-weighted images (**g**) with intense enhancement in the fat-suppressed post-gadolinium image (**h**). Also note the non-enhancing opacification of the mastoid air cells (red arrows in **a**, **b**, **f**, **g**, **h**) due to serous otitis media related to the glomus tympanicum extending into and obstructing the eustachian tube (see image **b**).

Diagnosis Glomus tympanicum

Differential Diagnosis
1. Glomus jugulare: Involves the jugular foramen and often presents with a dehiscent jugular bulb. However, in glomus tympanicum, the bone between the lesion in the middle ear and the jugular bulb or fossa is intact.
2. Aberrant internal carotid artery: It is imperative to distinguish glomus tympanicum from an aberrant internal carotid artery, as the latter manifests as a tubular structure traversing the middle ear cavity. The aberrant artery is typically associated with an absent or underdeveloped vertical segment of the carotid canal within the petrous bone, which may distort the inferior tympanic canaliculus.

23.1 Discussion

Glomus tympanicum tumors originate from paraganglia cells of neural crest origin in the tympanic plexus in the middle ear. These anatomical structures are located in proximity to Jacobson's nerve, a branch of cranial nerve IX, and Arnold's nerve, the auricular branch of cranial nerve X.

The primary symptoms of glomus tympanicum tumors consist of pulsatile tinnitus, with or without associated hearing loss. An otoscopic examination typically reveals a red, pulsating mass located behind an intact tympanic membrane; however, this examination does not provide information regarding the entire extent of the tumor.

Imaging is a critical component in the diagnosis of glomus tumors as it accurately assesses size and extent, which aids in deciding on a management strategy and surgical approach. Moreover, imaging aids in distinguishing conditions that may clinically mimic glomus tumors, such as an aberrant internal carotid artery or a high jugular bulb. The preferred imaging modalities include high-resolution computed tomography (HRCT) and high-resolution fat-suppressed contrast-enhanced magnetic resonance imaging (MRI).

High-resolution CT scans are particularly effective in evaluating the margins of the jugular fossa and the bony crest delineating the carotid artery from the jugular fossa. Conversely, contrast-enhanced MRI excels in delineating the tumor margins and assessing its intracranial extent. This imaging also helps in evaluating the tumor's relationship with adjacent anatomical structures, such as the jugular vein, carotid artery, membranous labyrinth, and any intracranial extension. The key imaging feature of a glomus tumor is an intensely enhancing mass located in the middle ear, characterized by a flat base oriented towards the cochlear promontory [1].

The commonly used classification systems for glomus tympanicum include the "Glasscock and Jackson" system, which is based on the location and extent of the tumor (Table 23.1). Another well-known system is the "Fisch" classification, which also categorizes tumors according to their location and extent, but it encompasses both the glomus tympanicum and glomus jugular [2].

Table 23.1 Glasscock and Jackson classification for glomus tumors

Type	Feature (location/extent)
Type I	Small mass limited to the promontory (Fig. 23.2)
Type II	Tumor completely filling middle ear space
Type III	Tumor filling the middle ear and extending into the mastoid
Type IV	Tumor filling middle ear, mastoid or external auditory canal, or intracranial extension

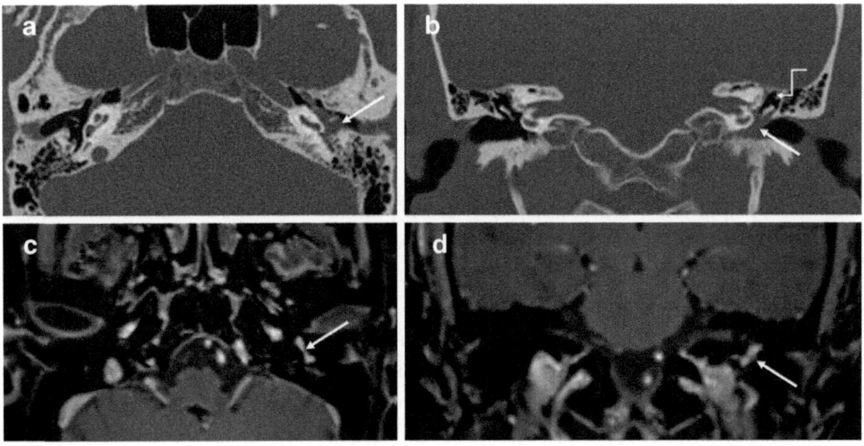

Fig. 23.2 a, b: HRCT temporal bone axial (**a**) and coronal (**b**) images show a polypoidal lesion in the middle ear [straight arrow] with a base toward the promontory. Lesion is in the meso- and hypotympanum with sparing of the epitympanum (elbow arrow in b).c, d: Fat-suppressed post-gadolinium MR – axial (**c**) and coronal (**d**) images show intense enhancement of the lesion seen overlying the promontory on the CT

Management: Surgical resection is the preferred treatment for glomus tympanicum tumors due to its relatively low risk and favorable long-term outcomes [1].

References

1. Sweeney AD, Carlson ML, Wanna GB, Bennett ML. Glomus tympanicum tumors. Otolaryngol Clin North Am. 2015;48(2):293–304. https://doi.org/10.1016/j.otc.2014.12.004. Epub 2015 Feb 4. PMID: 25659513
2. Tuan AS, Chen JY, Mafee MF. Glomus tympanica and other intratympanic masses: role of imaging. Oper. Tech. Otolaryngol Head Neck Surg. 2014;25:49–57.

Chapter 24
Neoplastic Diseases of Temporal Bone: Petrous Apex Lesions

Harshavardhan Mahalingam and Karthik Kulanthaivelu

Clinical Data A 31-year-old male with history of right-sided facial pain.

Supplementary Information The online version contains supplementary material available at https://doi.org/10.1007/978-981-95-6132-2_24.

H. Mahalingam (✉)
Department of Radiology, SRIHER, Chennai, India

K. Kulanthaivelu
Department of Neuroradiology, SRIHER, Chennai, India

H. Mahalingam (ed.), *Temporal Bone Imaging*,
https://doi.org/10.1007/978-981-95-6132-2_24

Radiological Findings (Fig. 24.1)

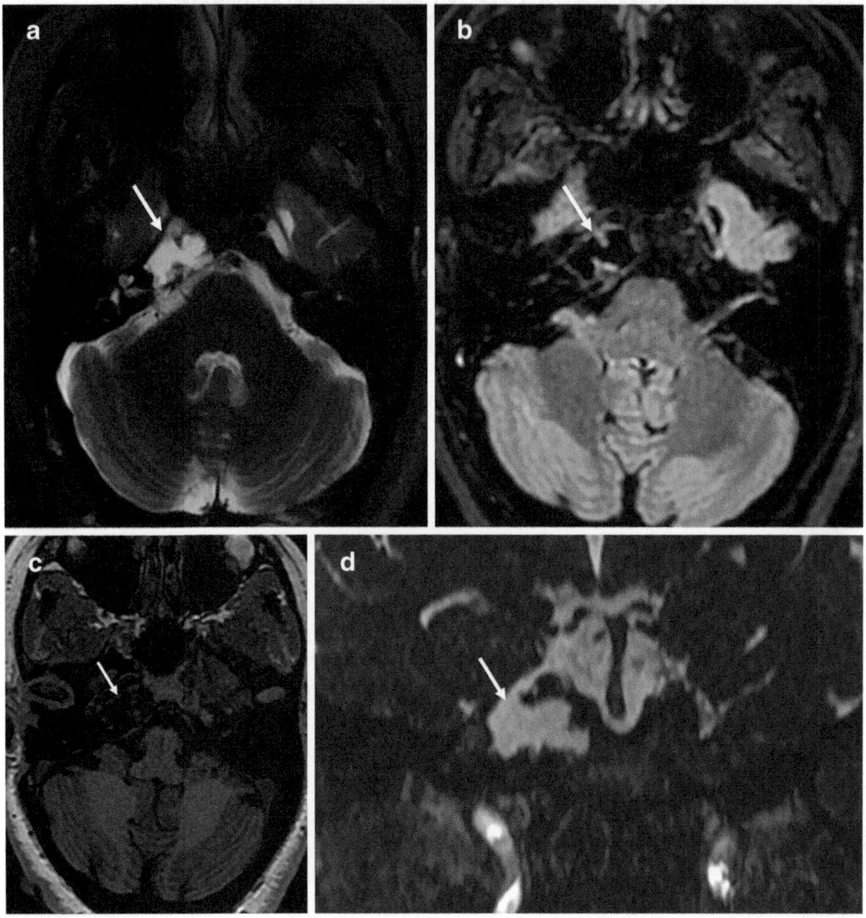

Fig. 24.1 (**a**) T2-weighted axial image shows a CSF signal intensity lesion in the right petrous apex (arrow). (**b**) T2-FLAIR image showing complete suppression of the fluid signal within the lesion. (**c**) T1-weighted axial image showing T1 hypointense nature of the lesion. (**d**) Coronal reformatted 3D heavily T2-weighted image shows communication of the lesion with CSF space (arrow). Trigeminal nerve branches were seen entering the lesion

Diagnosis Petrous apex cephalocele

Differential Diagnosis (If Applicable) Petrous apex effusion, cholesterol granuloma, mucocele

24.1 Discussion

Petrous apex cephaloceles are herniations of the meninges from the Meckel's cave into the petrous apex. These are postulated to occur due to chronic raised intracranial pressure transmitted to Meckel's cave and are often bilateral. These are often incidentally detected; however, they can present with headache and CSF otorrhea.

On CT, a smooth marginated lytic area is seen in the petrous apex. The lesion follows the signal of CSF on all sequences on MRI. Communication with the subarachnoid space can be demonstrated on thin section heavily T2-weighted images [1].

Clinical Data A 6-year-old boy with an incidental lesion on MRI brain.

Radiological Findings (Fig. 24.2)

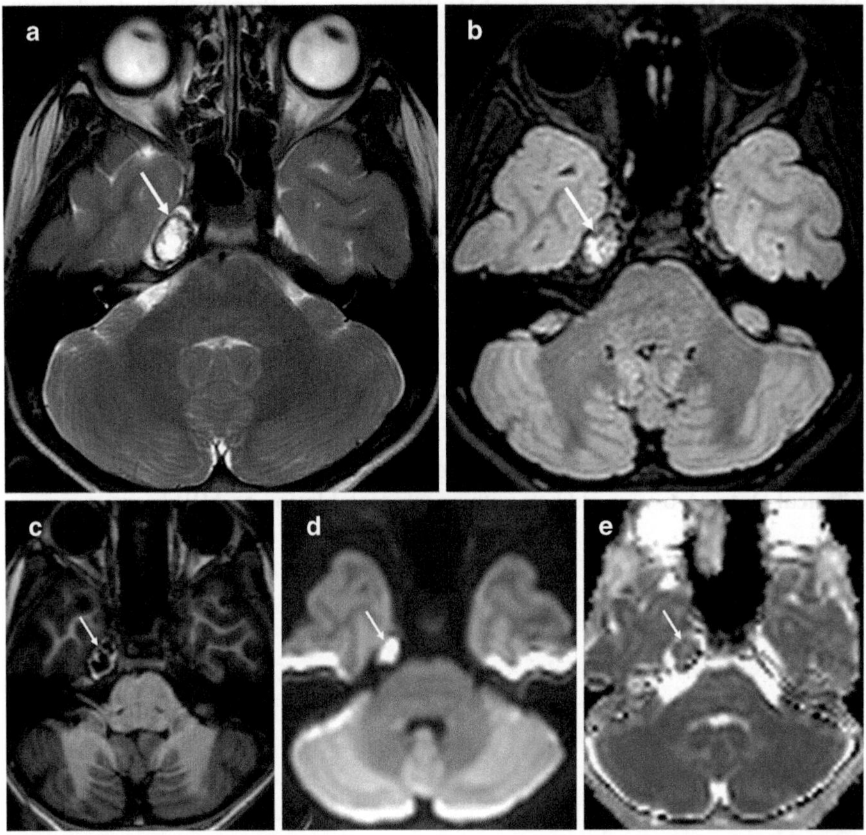

Fig. 24.2 (**a**) T2-weighted axial image showing a T2 hyperintense lesion in the right petrous apex having signal similar to CSF and a peripheral T2 hypointense wall (arrow). (**b**) T2-FLAIR image showing no suppression of signal within. (**c**) T1-weighted axial image showing T1 hypointense content with T1 hyperintense wall. (**d**, **e**) Diffusion-weighted image and apparent diffusion coefficient map showing diffusion restriction within the lesion (arrows)

Diagnosis Petrous apex cholesteatoma

Differential Diagnosis (If Applicable) Petrous apex effusion, cholesterol granuloma, mucocele

24.2 Discussion

Petrous apex cholesteatomas, or epidermoids, are cystic lesions lined by squamous epithelium and filled with keratinaceous debris. They are typically seen in children and young adults. They can be congenital, arising from ectopic rests of ectoderm trapped in the petrous apex during embryogenesis, or acquired as a result of repeated infections of the petrous apex. the congenital type is thought to be more common.

On CT, these present as an expansile lytic lesion in the petrous apex with or without associated bone destruction. On MRI, these lesions have high signal on T2 and FLAIR images and low signal on T1-weighted images. The characteristic feature of this lesion is presence of diffusion restriction with lack of enhancement on post-gadolinium images [2].

Clinical Data An 18-year-old female with incidentally detected lesion in the petrous temporal bone on CT done for evaluation of trauma

Radiological Findings (Fig. 24.3)

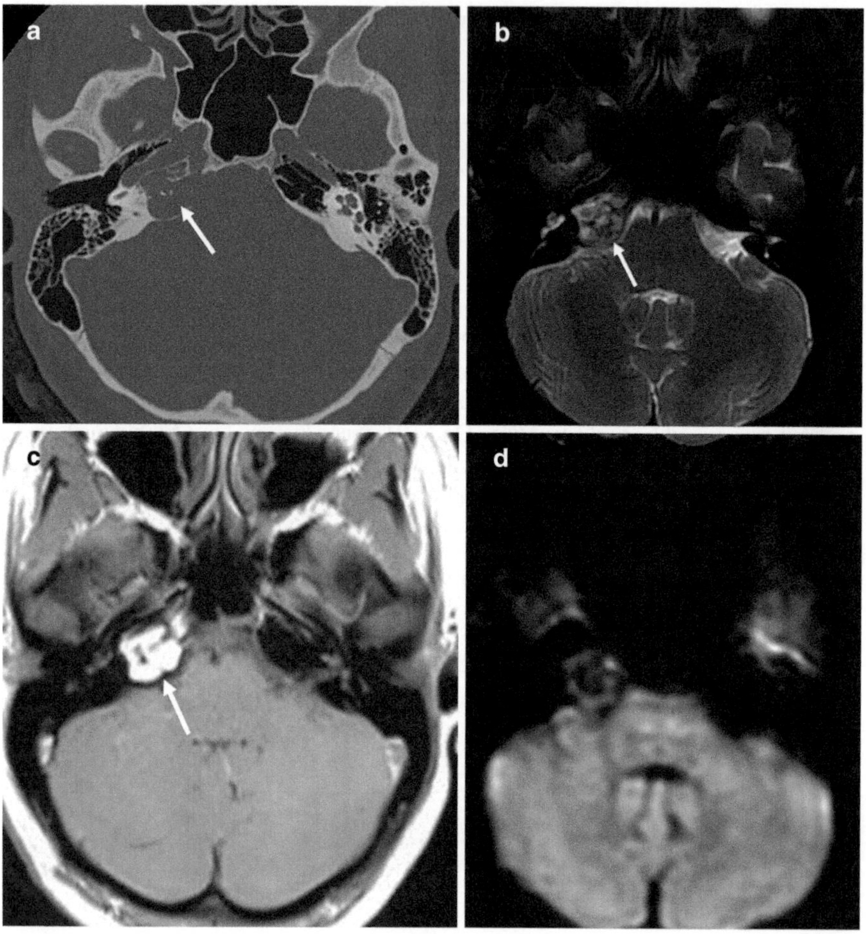

Fig. 24.3 (**a**) Axial section of HRCT temporal bone shows a mildly expansile lytic lesion in the right petrous apex (arrow). (**b**) Fat-saturated T2-weighted MR image shows predominantly T2 hyperintense signal within the lesion in the right petrous apex. (**c**) T1-weighted image shows intensely bright appearance of the lesion (arrow). (**d**) Diffusion-weighted MR image shows no diffusion restriction within the lesion

Diagnosis Petrous apex cholesterol granuloma

Differential Diagnosis (If Applicable) Petrous apex cholesteatoma, petrous apex effusion

24.3 Discussion

A wide spectrum of lesions can occur in the petrous apex with cholesterol granuloma being the most common. Cholesterol granulomas are cystic lesions with gelatinous fluid, hemorrhage, and cholesterol crystals as content with a fibrous capsule. It is postulated to arise due to either inadequate ventilation of air cells in the petrous apex or spontaneous hemorrhage into pneumatized petrous apex from the adjacent marrow.

On CT, these lesions typically present as unilocular lytic expansile lesions. MRI clinches the diagnosis due to presence of high T1 signal within (ascribed to cholesterol crystals and hemorrhage). Typically, this high signal is not suppressed on T1 fat-saturated images. A peripheral T2 hypointense rim may be seen. They do not show any diffusion restriction or post-gadolinium enhancement. Asymptomatic lesions are usually treated conservatively. Larger lesions with mass effect might require surgical resection or decompression [3].

Diagnostic Pitfall When there is asymmetric pneumatization of petrous apices, the non-pneumatized petrous apex will have high T1 signal due to marrow fat. This can mimic high T1 signal from cholesterol granuloma. However, the normal marrow fat will lack a well-defined margin and thus can be differentiated from cholesterol granuloma.

Common lesions of petrous apex lesions and some diagnostic clues are presented in Table 24.1.

A detailed discussion on imaging of petrous apex lesions is presented in Chap. 37.

Table 24.1 Differential diagnosis of petrous apex lesions based on imaging

Lesion	Diagnostic clues
Cholesterol granuloma	T1 and T2 hyperintensity with no diffusion restriction
Cholesteatoma	Diffusion restriction; no post-gadolinium enhancement
Cephalocele	Follows CSF signal on all MRI sequences; communication with subarachnoid space
Petrous apicitis	Fluid signal with post-gadolinium enhancement, usually associated with otomastoiditis
Schwannoma	Ovoid/dumbbell shaped with continuity with trigeminal nerve
Chondrosarcoma	Chondroid matrix calcifications on CT; T2 bright enhancing lesion
Metastasis/myeloma/lymphoma	Aggressive bone destruction and enhancement
ICA aneurysm	Rounded shape; continuity with ICA
Pseudolesion	On MRI – due to asymmetric pneumatization

References

1. Razek AA, Huang BY. Lesions of the petrous apex: classification and findings at CT and MR imaging. RadioGraphics. 2012;32(1):151–73.
2. Mafee MF, Kumar A, Heffner DK. Epidermoid cyst (cholesteatoma) and cholesterol granuloma of the temporal bone and epidermoid cysts affecting the brain. Neuroimaging Clin N Am. 1994;4(3):561–78.
3. Isaacson B, Kutz JW, Roland PS. Lesions of the petrous apex: diagnosis and management. Otolaryngol Clin North Am. 2007;40(3):479–519, viii.

Chapter 25
Neoplastic Diseases of Temporal Bone: Jugular Foramen Tumor

Harshavardhan Mahalingam and Karthik Kulanthaivelu

Clinical Data A 61-year-old female with history of headache, dysphagia, and hoarseness of voice for 4 months.

Supplementary Information The online version contains supplementary material available at https://doi.org/10.1007/978-981-95-6132-2_25.

H. Mahalingam (✉)
Department of Radiology, SRIHER, Chennai, India

K. Kulanthaivelu
Department of Neuroradiology, SRIHER, Chennai, India

H. Mahalingam (ed.), *Temporal Bone Imaging*,
https://doi.org/10.1007/978-981-95-6132-2_25

Radiological Findings (Fig. 25.1)

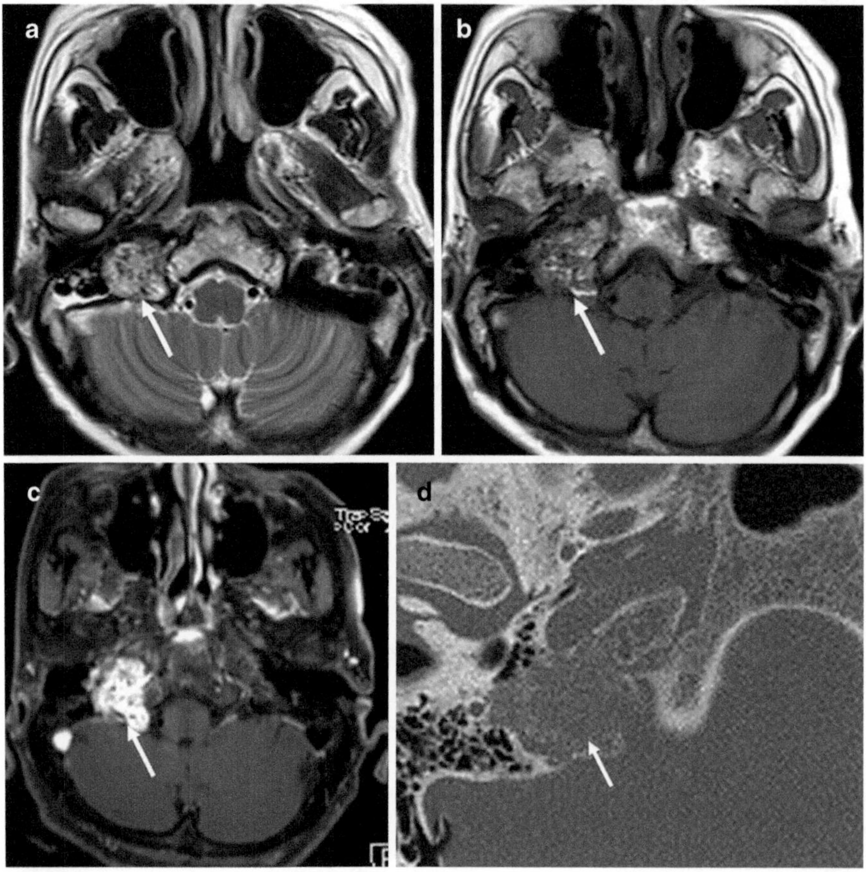

Fig. 25.1 (**a**) T2-weighted axial image at the level of the jugular foramen shows a predominantly T2 hyperintense mass lesion in the right jugular foramen with multiple T2 hypointense foci within. (**b**) T1-weighted axial image shows mixed T1 hyperintense and hypointense areas within the mass (salt-and-pepper appearance). (**c**) Axial post-gadolinium fat-saturated image shows intense enhancement of the mass lesion with multiple small dark flow voids within. (**d**) Axial HRCT section showing permeative lytic destructive lesion in the jugular foramen

Diagnosis Glomus jugulare/jugular foramen paraganglioma

Differential Diagnosis (If Applicable) Jugular foramen nerve sheath tumor, metastasis, meningioma, plasmacytoma

25.1 Discussion

The jugular foramen is located on the inferomedial surface of the petrous pyramid and is oriented anterolaterally coursing superior to inferior. It is divided into two compartments – anteriorly placed pars nervosa (containing the glossopharyngeal nerve and inferior petrosal sinus) and posteriorly placed pars vasculosa (containing the internal jugular vein, vagus, and spinal accessory nerve). The jugular foramen is separated superiorly from the middle ear cavity by a bony septum. The carotico-jugular spine separates it from the carotid canal and jugular tubercle separates it from the hypoglossal canal [1]. Refer to Fig. 1.4 in Chap. 1.

Jugular foramen lesions classically present with triad of loss of taste in posterior tongue, dysphagia/vocal cord paralysis, and sternocleidomastoid/trapezius weakness. This combination of symptoms is called Vernet syndrome. Other symptoms include tinnitus, headache, and hearing loss.

A wide spectrum of pathologies can occur in the jugular foramen and are listed in Table 25.1.

Jugular paragangliomas are the most common primary mass lesion of the jugular foramen. They arise from paraganglia located along the walls of jugular bulb and along the cranial nerves at site of superior vagal ganglion. They belong to the wider group of paragangliomas/chemodectomas which can secrete vasoactive substances. They typically present in 5th and 6th decades of life. These lesions are usually benign but locally aggressive [2].

On CT, these lesions typically show permeative or moth-eaten pattern of bone erosion. The floor of the middle ear cavity, caroticojugular spine, and jugular tubercle are common sites of erosion. Large lesions can erode the bony labyrinth. Intense enhancement is seen on post-contrast images [3].

Table 25.1 Etiological classification of spectrum of pathologies which occur in the jugular foramen

Jugular foramen pathologies		
Vascular	Infections	Neoplasms
High-riding jugular bulb	Abscess	Glomus/paraganglioma
Asymmetry (pseudolesion)		Nerve sheath tumors
IJV thrombosis	Cholesteatoma	Metastasis
Arteriovenous malformation		Meningioma
Jugular diverticulum		Plasmacytoma
		Chondrosarcoma

On MRI, these lesions show variegated signal intensity on T1- and T2-weighted images which has been called as a salt-and-pepper appearance. This is due to presence of flow voids, slow flow, and hemorrhages within the lesion. Post-gadolinium sequences show intense enhancement within these lesions. Presence of intradural extension and indistinct medial border of the lesion suggests possible cranial nerve encasement/infiltration [4].

References

1. Caldemeyer KS, Mathews VP, Azzarelli B, Smith RR. The jugular foramen: a review of anatomy, masses, and imaging characteristics. RadioGraphics. 1997;17(5):1123–39.
2. Vogl TJ, Bisdas S. Differential diagnosis of jugular foramen lesions. Skull Base. 2009;19(1):3–16.
3. Valavanis A, Schubiger O, Oguz M. High-resolution CT investigation of nonchromaffin paragangliomas of the temporal bone. AJNR Am J Neuroradiol. 1983;4(3):516–9.
4. Robertson JH, Gardner G, Cocke EW. Glomus jugulare tumors. Clin Neurosurg. 1994;41:39–61.

Chapter 26
Neoplastic Diseases of Temporal Bone: Cerebellopontine Angle Tumors

Amrutha Ranganath and Aparna Irodi

Clinical Data A 48-year-old female with reduced hearing on the right side for 2 years, giddiness, and imbalance while walking for 4 months prior to admission.

Supplementary Information The online version contains supplementary material available at https://doi.org/10.1007/978-981-95-6132-2_26.

A. Ranganath
Department of Radiology, Christian Medical College, Vellore, India

A. Irodi (✉)
Department of Radiology, Christian Medical College, Vellore, India

H. Mahalingam (ed.), *Temporal Bone Imaging*,
https://doi.org/10.1007/978-981-95-6132-2_26

Radiological Findings (Fig. 26.1)

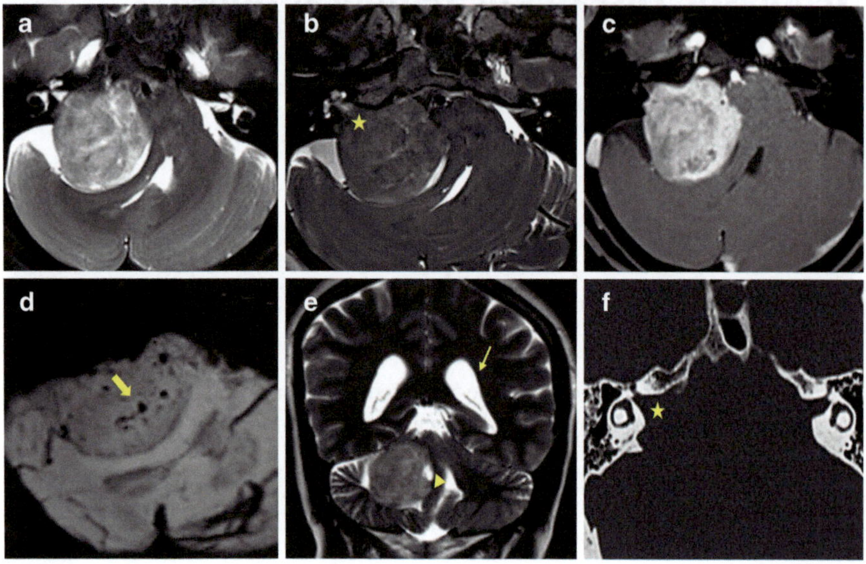

Fig. 26.1 (**a**) T2 axial, (**b**) FLAIR axial, (**c**) T1FS post-contrast axial, (**d**) SWI axial, and (**e**) T2 coronal sections of MRI brain show a large predominantly solid, intensely enhancing (image **c**) extra axial cerebellopontine angle lesion, extending to the internal auditory canal with widening of porus acusticus (marked by yellow asterisk in images **b** and **f**), intralesional hemorrhage (thick yellow arrow shows blooming foci on SWI in image **d**), and mass effect on middle cerebellar peduncle and fourth ventricle (yellow arrowhead in image **e**) with resultant dilated third (not shown in images) and lateral ventricles (thin yellow arrow shown in image **e**). Image **f**, axial section HRCT temporal bone shows widening of IAC on the right and no bone erosions

Diagnosis Right cerebellopontine angle vestibular schwannoma with mild hydrocephalus

Differential Diagnosis Cerebellopontine angle meningioma, CP angle epidermoid

26.1 Discussion

Large number of neoplastic and non neoplastic lesions can present as cerebellopontine angle masses. The key factors to be kept in mind while approaching any cerebellopontine angle mass is to identify its site of origin and distinctive signal characteristics. Most common of these lesions in order of their frequency of occurrence include vestibular Schwannoma, meningioma, and epidermoid cyst.

Vestibular schwannomas are the most common (75–90%), benign WHO grade 1 tumor arising from Schwann cells in association with vestibulocochlear nerve (95% from inferior division of vestibular component). Most of them are sporadic and unilateral. Presence of bilateral lesions is highly suggestive of neurofibromatosis type 2 (NF2). Median age of presentation is usually in 4th–5th decade of life [1].

Characteristically, they are solid and intensely enhancing intracanalicular lesions widening the porus acusticus and extending into the CP angle, with the larger lesions demonstrating cystic areas, intralesional hemorrhage, and mass effect on the cerebellar hemisphere, adjacent brainstem, and fourth ventricle, causing upstream hydrocephalus. On MRI, they are T1 hypo to isointense with variable T2 signal and enhancement pattern based on the consistency of the lesion. Computed tomography better delineates the widening of the porus acusticus [2, 3].

Koos classification system is used to grade the lesions based on their location (Fig. 26.2).

Differentials

- *CP angle meningiomas* present as intensely enhancing lesions with its broad base to the petrous temporal bone with or without bony hyperostosis. IAC most often remains intact (Fig. 26.3).
- *CP angle epidermoids* are typically non-enhancing lesions with diffusion restriction, insinuating into the potential spaces around CP angle (Fig. 26.4).

Key points in differentiating the abovementioned CP angle lesions are as shown in Table 26.1.

Broad overview on imaging differentials for cerebellopontine angle lesions is shown in Fig. 26.5.

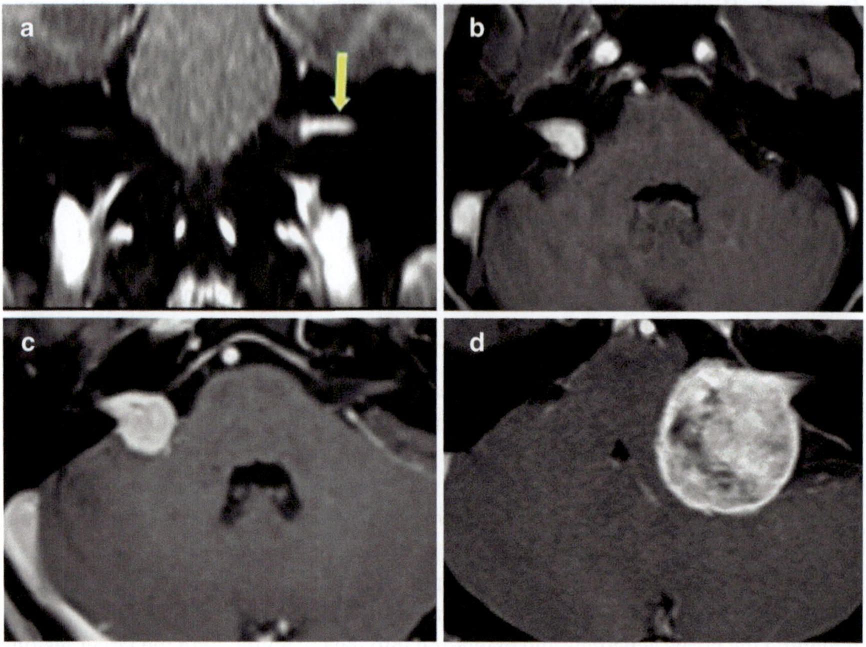

Fig. 26.2 Koos classification for CP angle schwannoma. Image (**a**): Grade1 – predominantly intracanalicular lesion with no CP angle extensions (marked as yellow arrow). Image (**b**): Grade 2 – includes those lesions arising from internal auditory canal extending into the CP angle and shows no contact with cerebellum or brainstem. Image (**c**): Grade 3 – refers to a larger CP angle lesion in contact with brainstem without causing any mass effect. Image (**d**): Grade 4 – includes large CP angle lesions in contact with brainstem and cerebellum, causing mass effect and usually associated with hydrocephalus

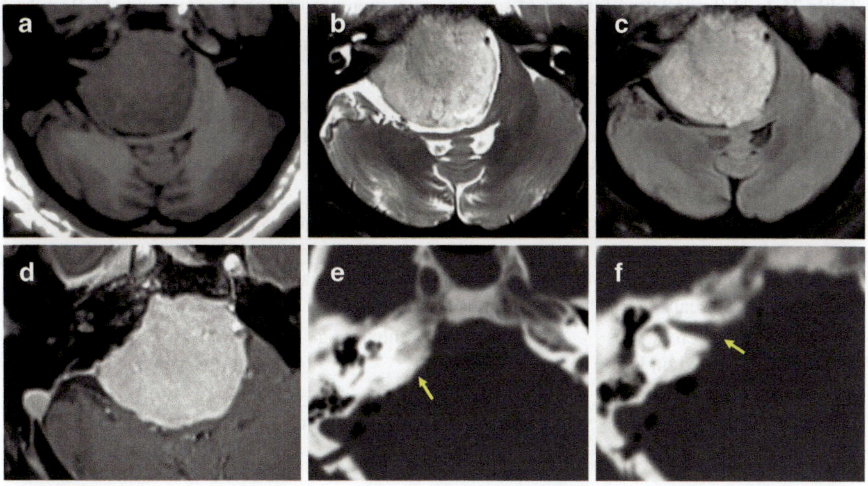

Fig. 26.3 Right cerebellopontine angle meningioma: Image (**a**): T1 axial image shows well-defined T1 hypointense extra axial lesion in the right CP angle with broad base to the petrous temporal bone. Image (**b**, **c**): T2/FLAIR axial images demonstrate the hyperintense signal of lesion and mass effect on brainstem, fourth ventricle, and adjacent right cerebellar hemisphere. Image (**d**) shows the intense and homogenous post-contrast enhancement on T1FS post-contrast sequence. Images (**e**, **f**) are CT images demonstrating the hyperostotic right petrous temporal bone (image e) and a normal internal auditory canal (image **f**), both marked with yellow arrows

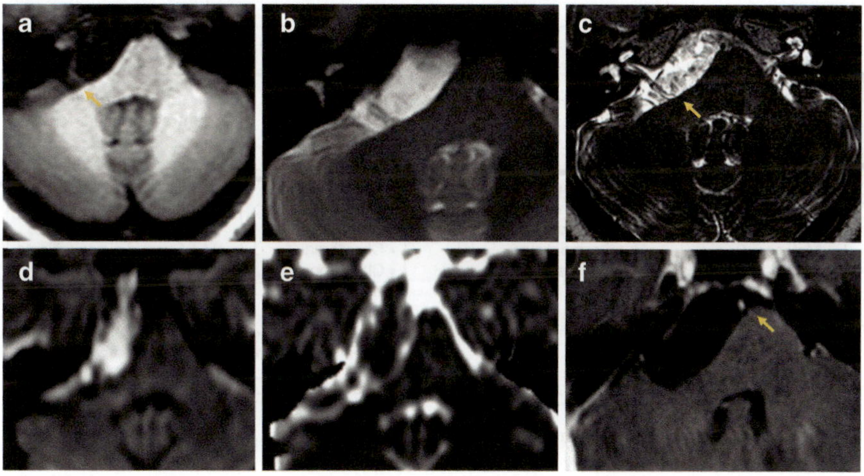

Fig. 26.4 Right cerebellopontine angle epidermoid cyst. A series of axial MRI brain images show a well marginated (**a**) T1 hypointense, (**b**, **c**) T2/DRIVE hyperintense lesion in the right CP angle, without encasing the right 7th/8th nerve complex (seen separately from the lesion represented with yellow arrow in image **c**) (**d**, **e**) with diffusion restriction on DWI/ADC and (**f**) no post-contrast enhancement on T1 post-contrast sequence. Also note mild extension into the prepontine cistern, insinuating around the basilar artery (enhancing dot in the image marked by yellow arrow in image **f**) with mass effect on the pons and right middle cerebellar peduncle

Table 26.1 Differentiating features of schwannoma, meningioma, and epidermoid at CP angle

CP angle schwannoma	CP angle meningioma	CP angle epidermoid
Most common CP angle lesion	Second most common – 5–10% of CP angle lesions	Third most common CP angle lesion
Present as globular masses, commonly extending from the internal auditory canal	Present with a broad base to petrous bone	Well-marginated lesions demonstrating plasticity
Intratumoral calcifications are less common (+)	Intratumoral calcifications are more common (+++)	No intratumoral calcifications (−)
Associated with widening of the internal auditory canal	Internal auditory canal is mostly normal.	Internal auditory canal is normal.
Moderate and heterogenous enhancement based on lesion composition	Intensely enhancing lesions	No post-contrast enhancement
Absence of dural tail sign	Dural tailing is commonly seen	Absence of dural tail sign

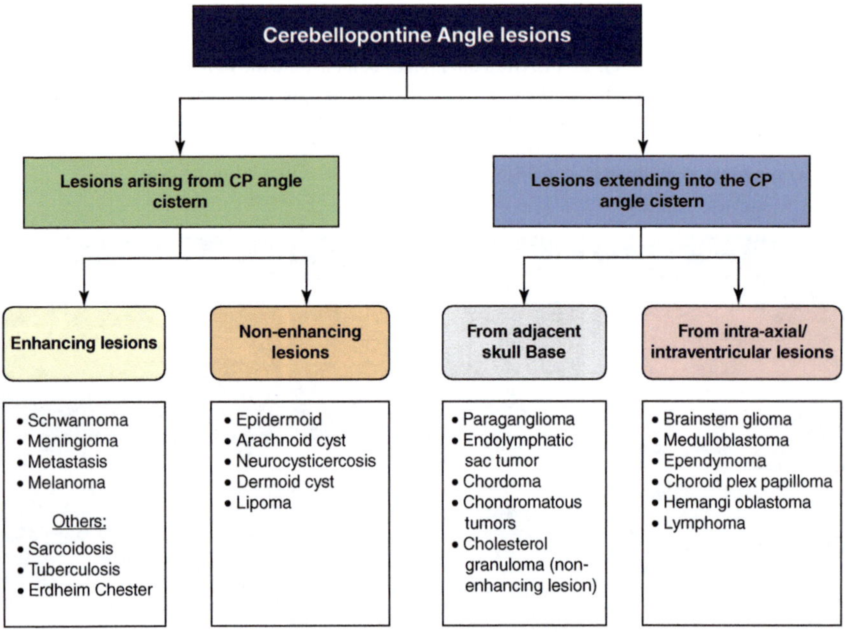

Fig. 26.5 Imaging-based differential diagnosis of cerebellopontine angle lesions

References

1. Smirniotopoulos JG, Yue NC, Rushing EJ. Cerebellopontine angle masses: radiologic-pathologic correlation. Radiographics. 1993;13:1131–47.
2. Bonneville F, Sarrazin JL, Marsot-Dupuch K, Iffenecker C, Cordoliani YS, Doyon D, et al. Unusual lesions of the cerebellopontine angle: a segmental approach. Radiographics. 2001;21:419–38.
3. Fink JR. Imaging of cerebellopontine angle masses: self-assessment module. Am J of Roentgenol. 2010;195(3_supplement):S15–21.

Chapter 27
Miscellaneous Temporal Bone Pathologies: Otosclerosis – Fenestral and Retrofenestral

Aparna Irodi

Clinical Data A 40-year-old gentleman presented with bilateral hearing loss and tinnitus.

Supplementary Information The online version contains supplementary material available at https://doi.org/10.1007/978-981-95-6132-2_27.

A. Irodi (✉)
Department of Radiology, Christian Medical College, Vellore, India

H. Mahalingam (ed.), *Temporal Bone Imaging*,
https://doi.org/10.1007/978-981-95-6132-2_27

Radiological Findings (Fig. 27.1)

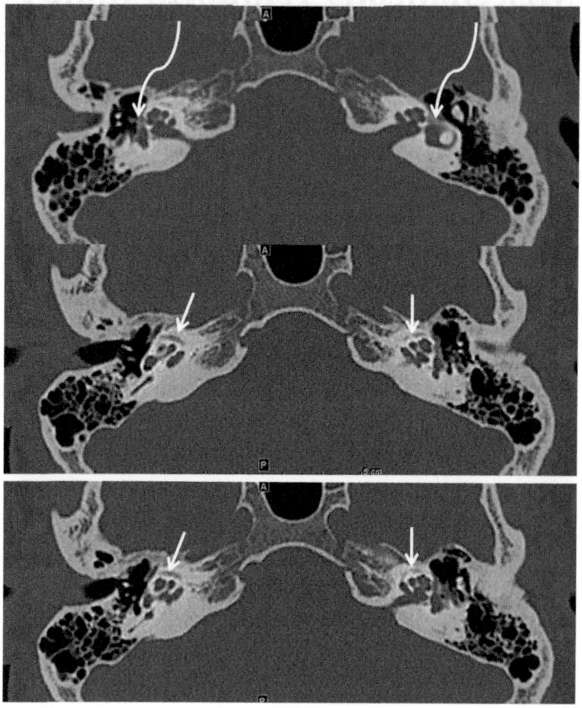

Fig. 27.1 Serial axial images of HRCT temporal bone show a small area of demineralization in the fissula ante fenestram (curved long arrows) and curvilinear lucency of demineralization around the cochlea (short straight arrows) on both sides, giving double ring sign. These findings are consistent with fenestral and retrofenestral (cochlear) otosclerosis.

Diagnosis Cochlear/retrofenestral otosclerosis

Differential Diagnosis Cochlear cleft

27.1 Discussion

Pathology in Otosclerosis The dense avascular endochondral bone (middle layer) of the otic capsule is replaced by vascular foci of immature bone tissue.

It occurs in two phases – active otospongiotic phase and inactive otosclerotic phase.

Clinical Presentation Progressive conductive or mixed hearing loss in adults (commonly 15–45 years). Tinnitus, vestibular symptoms, and paracusis may also be seen.

Examination
Otoscopy – Hyperemia on the cochlear promontory may be seen "Schwartze sign."

Audiogram Conductive or mixed hearing loss (initially at lower frequencies) with widened air-bone gap. Drop in bone conduction at around 2000 Hz frequency region (Carhart notch) is typically described in otosclerosis, but it is not pathognomonic.

HRCT Temporal Bone Findings depend on the stage of the disease and extent of involvement. Most common finding in the active otospongiotic phase is a focus of demineralization seen as a hypodense focus just anterior to the oval window (known as the fissula ante fenestram) seen in 80–90% of cases, and when only this area is involved, it is called as *fenestral otosclerosis* (Fig 27.2). Fissula ante fenestram is a groove between the oval window and the cochleariform process.

As it progresses, the hypodensity can extend to the pericochlear area (*retrofenestral or cochlear otosclerosis*), giving rise to a halo around the cochlea which is sometimes called as double ring of Valvassori (Fig. 27.1). In the inactive otosclerotic phase, the otic capsule can become more sclerotic and a thickness of >2.3 mm at the level of the cochleariform process on axial CT image can be a helpful pointer. Although the severity may vary, 80–85% of the cases are bilateral [1].

Rotteveel (Table 27.1) and Symons and Fanning (Table 27.2) are some of the grading systems which can be used to grade the extent of involvement in otosclerosis.

Reporting Checklist
- Size and location of otospongiotic and otosclerotic foci
- Narrowing of the oval or round window
- Findings that may affect surgery like course of facial nerve canal, high-riding jugular bulb, status of middle ear cavity, ossicles, and any inner ear anomalies

Table 27.1 Rotteveel grading of otosclerosis

Grade 1	Purely fenestral
Grade 2	2a – Double ring sign 2b – Narrowed basal turn of cochlea 2c – Double ring and narrowed basal turn of cochlea
Grade 3	Severe cochlear involvement with unrecognizable otic capsule

Table 27.2 Symons and Fanning grading of otosclerosis

Grade 1	Purely fenestral with thickened stapes footplate (Fig. 27.2)
Grade 2a	Hypodensity around posterior basal turn of cochlear and round window niche
Grade 2b	Hypodensity around apical and middle turns of cochlear
Grade 3	Diffuse, confluent involvement of the otic capsule (Fig. 27.3)

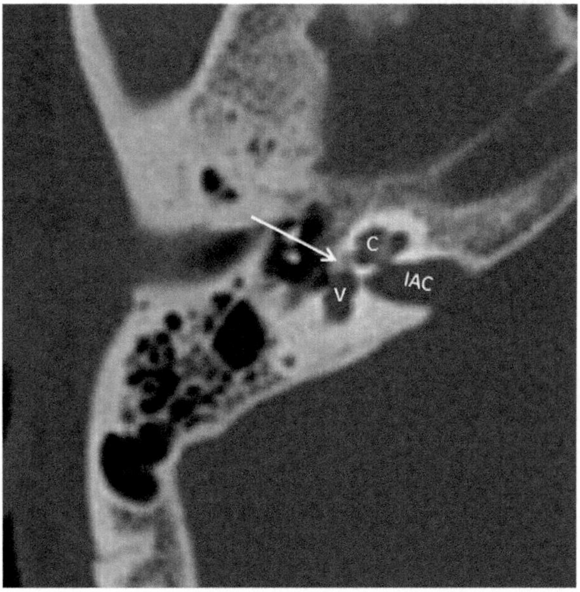

Fig. 27.2 Fenestral otosclerosis. Focused axial image of HRCT temporal bone showing a focus of demineralization in the fissula ante fenestram (arrow), suggestive of fenestral otosclerosis. C, cochlea, V, vestibulae, IAC, internal auditory canal

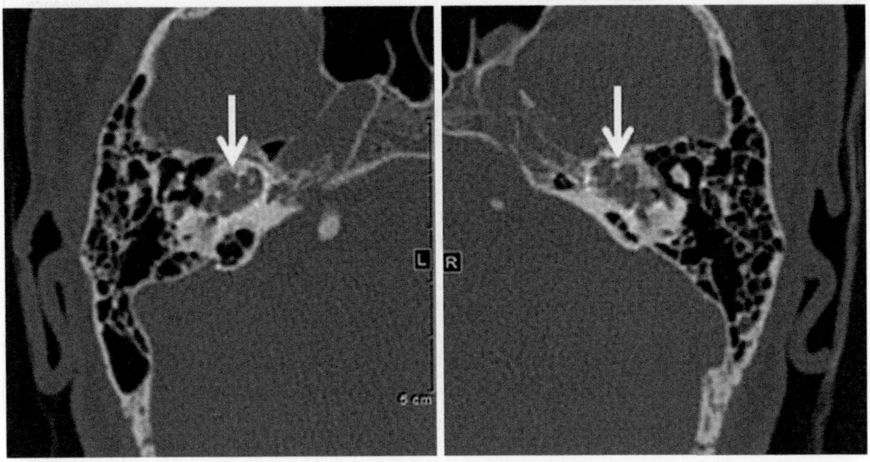

Fig. 27.3 Cochlear otosclerosis with diffuse involvement of the otic capsule on both sides (arrows), with extensive disease and unrecognizable normal structure of the cochlea

Fig. 27.4 Cochlear cleft. Focused axial HRCT of the temporal bone showing a curvilinear lucency (arrow) which is parallel and lateral to the basal turn of the cochlea

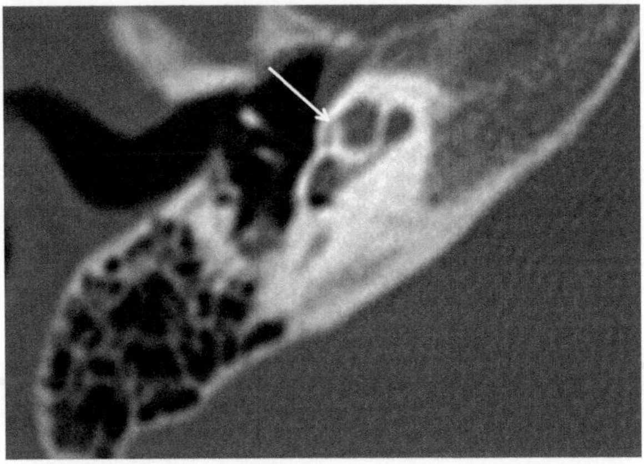

MRI Less often used in the diagnosis of otosclerosis, and if larger areas are involved, they may be seen as intermediate signal on T1W and high signal on T2W images and can show enhancement in the active phases

Imaging Pitfalls

Cochlear cleft (Fig. 27.4) is a normal variant seen as thin linear lucency around the cochlea due to incomplete endochondral ossification. It can be variable in size and can extend from fissula ante fenestram area toward the promontory. Cochlear cleft is more often seen in children and is not associated with any hearing impairment [2].

References

1. Mangia LRL, Coelho LOM, Carvalho B, de Oliveira AKP, Hamerschmidt R. Imaging studies in otosclerosis: an up-to-date comprehensive review. Int Arch Otorhinolaryngol. 2021;25(2):e318–27. https://doi.org/10.1055/s-0040-1715149. Epub 2020 Sep 24. PMID: 33968239; PMCID: PMC8096512
2. Sanverdi SE, Ozgen B, Dolgun A, Sarac S. Incomplete endochondral ossification of the otic capsule, a variation in children: evaluation of its prevalence and extent in children with and without sensorineural hearing loss. Am J Neuroradiol. 2015;36(1):171–5. https://doi.org/10.3174/ajnr.A4128.

Chapter 28
Miscellaneous Temporal Bone Pathologies: External Auditory Canal Osteoma

Jeffrey Skaria Joseph

Clinical Data A 39-year-old male presenting with reduced hearing in the left ear and otologic examination showing a hard oval mass in the external auditory canal.

Supplementary Information The online version contains supplementary material available at https://doi.org/10.1007/978-981-95-6132-2_28.

J. S. Joseph (✉)
Department of Radiology, Chettinad Hospital and Research Institute, Kelambakkam, Tamil Nadu, India

H. Mahalingam (ed.), *Temporal Bone Imaging*,
https://doi.org/10.1007/978-981-95-6132-2_28

Radiological Findings (Fig. 28.1)

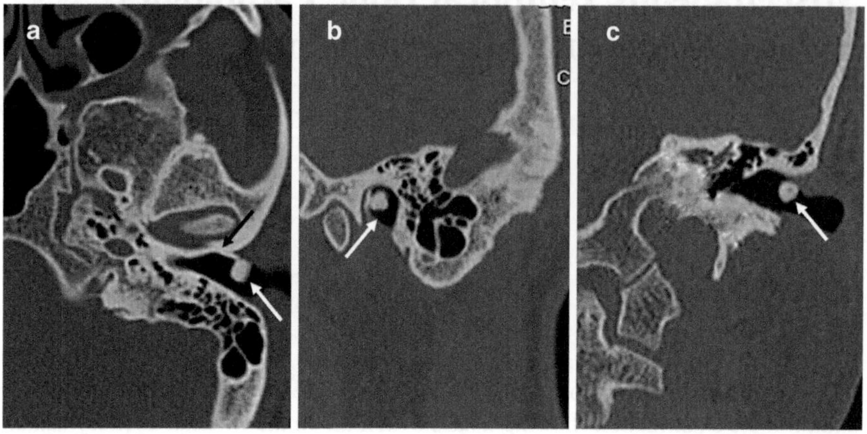

Fig. 28.1 HRCT of the temporal bone axial (**a**) with sagittal and coronal (**b**, **c**) reconstructions shows a well-defined solitary 4 × 4.5 mm pedunculated dense osseous lesion (white arrows), nestled along the anterior wall of the left external auditory canal and protruding into the lumen at the lateral tip of the isthmus. The lesion is closely associated with the tympanosquamous fissure (black arrow in Fig. a) (Image courtesy Dr. Einstein)

Diagnosis Left external auditory canal osteoma

Differential Diagnosis External auditory canal exostosis

28.1 Discussion

Osteomas are benign slow-growing tumors arising from the lamellar bone. They have a predilection for the facial bones, paranasal sinuses, external auditory canal (EAC), mandible, and mastoid cortex. In the temporal bone, EAC is the most common site of osteomas. They are rare (0.05% of total otologic surgeries), noninvasive, and indolent until they become large enough to cause mass effect, auditory canal obstruction (Fig. 28.2), or hearing loss (usually conductive hearing loss) [1].

Canal obstruction may lead to cerumen buildup and secondary infections, medial to the obstructing osteoma. Clinically, they may be seen as smooth pedunculated mass, often covered by apparently normal skin.

CT is the best modality to assess EAC osteomas. They are typically seen as a solitary, unilateral, well-defined, pedunculated hyperattenuating mass, arising lateral to the isthmus and protruding into the EAC. On occasion, they can appear as a lobulated bony mass. EAC osteomas are closely related to the tympanosquamous and tympanomastoid suture lines. MRI may show high signal on T1-weighted images, indicative of bone marrow within the lesion.

Identification of a single osteoma should prompt a search for other osteomas in the skull as multiple osteomas are associated with Gardner syndrome (a colonic polyposis syndrome).

The closest differential diagnosis for EAC osteoma is exostosis of the EAC (Surfer's ear), which are reactive osseous thickening typically in individuals with repetitive cold-water and wind exposure, seen on CT as bilateral broad-based bony outgrowths (Table 28.1).

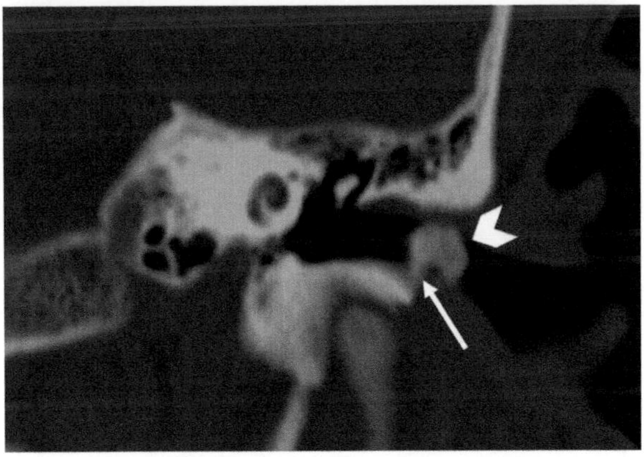

Fig. 28.2 Coronal section of HRCT of the temporal bone showing a pedunculated, lobulated osteoma (white arrowhead) with stalk (white arrow) in the lateral aspect of the left EAC and protruding into and occluding the canal lumen. (Image courtesy Dr. Madhavi K)

Table 28.1 External auditory canal osteoma vs exostoses

Osteoma	Exostoses
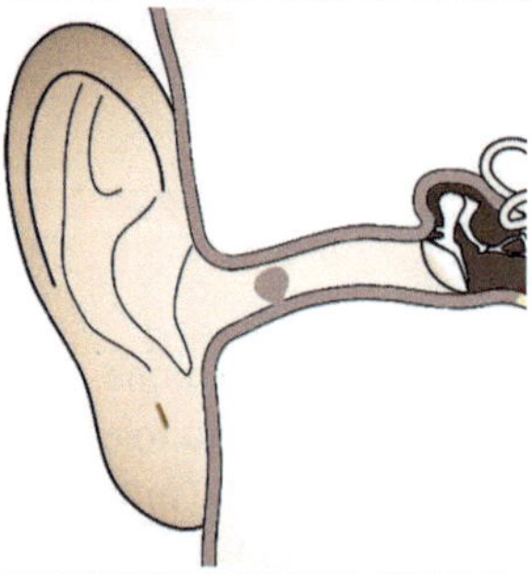	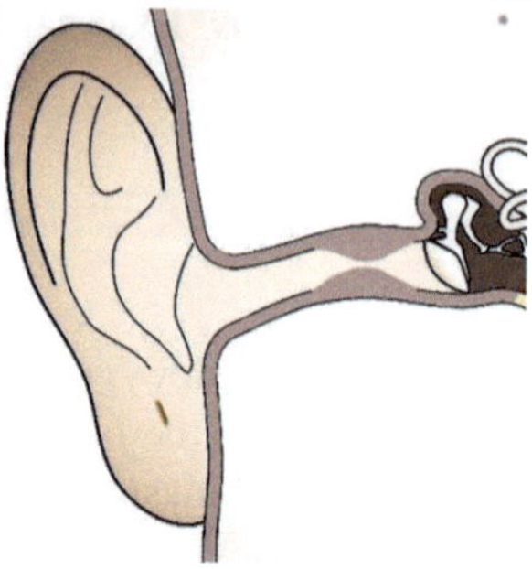
Benign neoplasm with uncertain etiology, often incidental	Reactive osseous change to repetitive cold-water exposure
Unilateral	Often bilateral
Usually solitary lesion, pedunculated	Sessile and broad-based bony overgrowth
Closely associated with suture lines (tympanosquamous, tympanomastoid)	Not related to sutures
Lateral to isthmus	Medial to isthmus

It may be difficult to distinguish osteomas from exostoses histopathologically. CT may be beneficial to differentiate the two, although management of these conditions remains the same. In symptomatic patients, surgical excision is the standard treatment, often with good prognosis [2].

References

1. Carbone PN, Nelson BL. External auditory osteoma. Head Neck Pathol. 2012;6(2):244–6. https://doi.org/10.1007/s12105-011-0314-7. Epub 2011 Dec 20. PMID: 22183765; PMCID: PMC3370017
2. Tsuno NSG, Tsuno MY, Coelho Neto CAF, Noujaim SE, Decnop M, Pacheco FT, Souza SA, Fonseca APA, Garcia MRT. Imaging the external ear: practical approach to normal and pathologic conditions. Radiographics. 2022;42(2):522–40. https://doi.org/10.1148/rg.210148. Epub 2022 Feb 4. PMID: 35119966

Chapter 29
Miscellaneous Temporal Bone Pathologies: Keratosis Obturans

Harshavardhan Mahalingam and Asthik Biswas

Clinical Data A 6-year-old girl with bilateral earache and reduced hearing noticed by parents.

Radiological Findings (Fig. 29.1)

Diagnosis Keratosis obturans

Differential Diagnosis (If Applicable) External ear cholesteatoma, medial canal fibrosis

29.1 Discussion

Keratosis obturans (KO) is characterized by accumulation of keratinaceous debris in the medial part of the external auditory canal (EAC) with surrounding granulation tissue. It is typically encountered in children and young adults. Patients usually present with pain as the primary complaint. Hearing impairment may be present. In

Supplementary Information The online version contains supplementary material available at https://doi.org/10.1007/978-981-95-6132-2_29.

H. Mahalingam (✉)
Department of Radiology, SRIHER, Chennai, India

A. Biswas
Department of Pediatric Neuroradiology, Great Ormond Street Hospital, NHS foundation trust, London, United Kingdom

H. Mahalingam (ed.), *Temporal Bone Imaging*,
https://doi.org/10.1007/978-981-95-6132-2_29

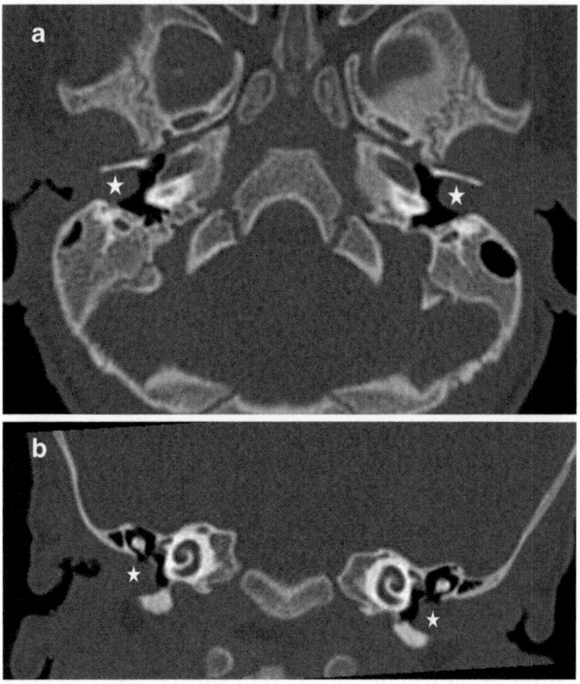

Fig. 29.1 (**a**, **b**) Axial and coronal HRCT images of the temporal bone show soft tissue density filling and occluding the lumen of the bony part of the bilateral external auditory canal (star). No bone erosions are seen. The soft tissue is reaching medially up to the level of the tympanic membrane.

children, KO can be bilateral and can be associated with bronchiectasis and sinusitis [1].

Diagnosis of KO is usually apparent on otoscopic examination, which shows keratinaceous debris within the EAC with a silvery matrix and surrounding granulation tissue. The keratinaceous debris of KO is usually difficult to remove. On CT, KO manifests as a soft tissue plug in the EAC, with or without associated circumferential bone rarefaction. However, no focal bone erosions are present, which differentiates this condition from EAC cholesteatoma [2]. KO is managed conservatively with multiple sessions of aural toileting.

References

1. Chong AW, Raman R. Keratosis obturans: a disease of the tropics? Indian J Otolaryngol Head Neck Surg. 2017;69(3):291–5.
2. Tsuno NSG, Tsuno MY, Coelho Neto CAF, Noujaim SE, Decnop M, Pacheco FT, et al. Imaging the external ear: practical approach to normal and pathologic conditions. RadioGraphics. 2022;42(2):522–40.

Chapter 30
Miscellaneous Temporal Bone Pathologies: Osteopetrosis

Harshavardhan Mahalingam and Asthik Biswas

Clinical Data An 8-year-old girl with known skeletal dysplasia referred for reduced hearing.

Supplementary Information The online version contains supplementary material available at https://doi.org/10.1007/978-981-95-6132-2_30.

H. Mahalingam (✉)
Department of Radiology, SRIHER, Chennai, India

A. Biswas
Department of Pediatric Neuroradiology, Great Ormond Street Hospital, NHS foundation trust, London, United Kingdom

H. Mahalingam (ed.), *Temporal Bone Imaging*,
https://doi.org/10.1007/978-981-95-6132-2_30

Radiological Findings (Fig. 30.1)

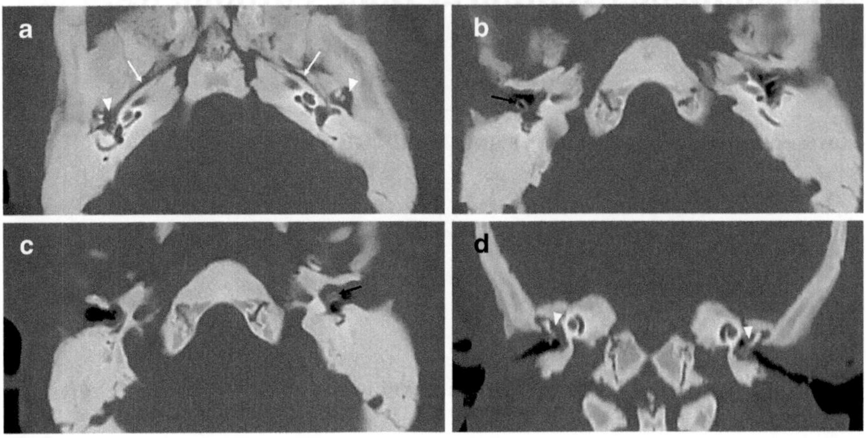

Fig. 30.1 (**a**) Axial HRCT section of the temporal bones shows diffuse thickening and sclerosis of the skull and facial bones. Soft tissue density is seen completely filling the bilateral middle ear cavities (arrowheads). Also note the severely narrowed bony part of the Eustachian tubes on both sides (white arrows). (**b**, **c**) Axial HRCT sections of the temporal bones show soft tissue density filling the bilateral middle ear cavities with tympanostomy tubes in situ (black arrows). (**d**) Coronal HRCT section shows similar findings of diffuse skull thickening and sclerosis with soft tissue density (arrowheads) in bilateral middle ear cavities

Diagnosis Osteopetrosis with bilateral otitis media

Differential Diagnosis (If Applicable) Nil

30.1 Discussion

Osteopetrosis is an inherited sclerosing bone dysplasia caused by subnormal osteoclast function. Two forms of this disease have been described – autosomal dominant (usually manifests in early adulthood and has benign course) and autosomal recessive (manifests in neonatal period or in infancy and is associated with multiple serious complications like bone marrow failure, neurological deficits, and fractures). The latter is also called "malignant osteopetrosis" due to a rapid debilitating course and early death. Multiple genes have been implicated in this disorder [1].

Decreased hearing is one of the common manifestations of autosomal recessive osteopetrosis during the first year of life. The most common cause of reduced hearing in these patients is otitis media with effusion due to severe stenosis of Eustachian tubes. These patients are also prone to repeated infections (including acute otitis media) due to bone marrow failure. Hearing loss can also occur due to other causes like stenosis of the EAC, poorly pneumatized mastoids, ossicular ankylosis, and fixation of stapes. Stenosis of internal auditory canal can cause compression of the vestibulocochlear and facial nerves resulting in sensorineural hearing loss and facial palsy [2].

References

1. Penna S, Villa A, Capo V. Autosomal recessive osteopetrosis: mechanisms and treatments. Dis Model Mech. 2021;14(5):dmm048940.
2. Dozier TS, Duncan IM, Klein AJ, Lambert PR, Key LL. Otologic manifestations of malignant osteopetrosis. Otol Neurotol Off Publ Am Otol Soc Am Neurotol Soc Eur Acad Otol Neurotol. 2005;26(4):762–6.

Chapter 31
Miscellaneous Temporal Bone Pathologies: Fibrous Dysplasia

Harshavardhan Mahalingam and Asthik Biswas

Clinical Data A 14-year-old girl with skull deformity and reduced hearing in right ear.

Radiological Findings (Fig. 31.1)

Diagnosis Fibrous dysplasia

Differential diagnosis (if applicable) Paget's disease, hyperparathyroidism, sclerosteosis, osteopetrosis

Discussion

Fibrous dysplasia (FD) is a benign but progressive bone disease characterized by replacement of normal bone by fibrous tissue. It can be monostotic or polyostotic. The polyostotic form can have syndromic associations (e.g., McCune-Albright syndrome). Patients with FD usually present with deformities, pathological fractures, and nerve compression due to bone expansion.

FD can affect any bone in the body. Involvement of the temporal bone in FD is less common and is usually seen in the polyostotic form as a part of generalized craniofacial involvement. Isolated FD of the temporal bone is exceedingly rare. Temporal bone involvement in FD can cause symptoms due to EAC stenosis (typically at the junction of bony and cartilaginous parts), Eustachian tube narrowing/occlusion leading to otitis media, EAC cholesteatoma, and middle ear

H. Mahalingam (✉)
Department of Radiology, SRIHER, Chennai, India

A. Biswas
Department of Pediatric Neuroradiology, Great Ormond Street Hospital, NHS Foundation Trust, London, UK

H. Mahalingam (ed.), *Temporal Bone Imaging*,
https://doi.org/10.1007/978-981-95-6132-2_31

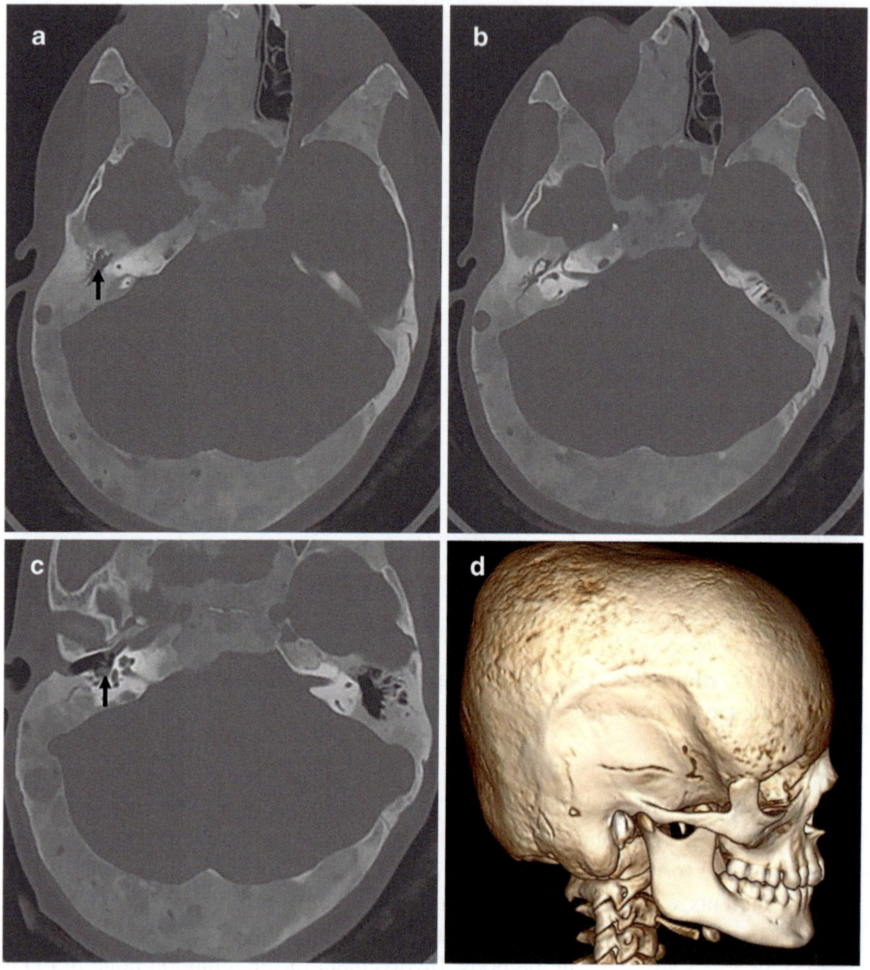

Fig. 31.1 (**a**–**c**) Serial axial section of HRCT of the temporal bone shows multifocal areas of bone expansion with ground-glass matrix involving the calvarium, skull base, and facial skeleton. Also note the soft tissue density in the right middle ear and mastoid (arrow) s/o otitis media. (**d**) Volume-rendered image of the head shows deformity of the skull with multiple areas of bone expansion

cholesteatoma. Less commonly, it causes sensorineural hearing loss due to involvement of the inner ear structures or internal auditory canal narrowing [1].

On CT, FD usually shows expansion of the bone with cortical thinning and radiolucent areas with loss of trabecular architecture called ground-glass appearance. FD can have three patterns—pagetoid (mixed dense and lucent areas), sclerotic, and cystic. On MRI, the lesions tend to be hypointense on T1-weighted images and of varying signal on T2-weighted images due to admixture of fibrosis with cysts. Blood-fluid levels can also be seen within the lesions [2].

Paget's disease is an enigmatic systemic disorder of the elderly population involving the bone with a wide spectrum of clinical manifestation ranging from asymptomatic incidentally detected lesions on imaging to life-threatening complications. It can involve the skull base and temporal bone with resultant hearing loss, tinnitus, and vertigo. It manifests on CT as areas of mixed lysis and sclerosis with cortical thickening and bone expansion. Involvement of the temporal bone often begins at the petrous apex and advances laterally. Resorption of the otic capsule can occur. Stapes footplate fixation is common. Severe skull base involvement can lead to basilar invagination.

References

1. Mierzwiński J, Kosowska J, Tyra J, Haber K, Drela M, Paczkowski D, et al. Different clinical presentation and management of temporal bone fibrous dysplasia in children. World J Surg Oncol. 2018;16(1):5.
2. Zhang K, Qu P, Wang B, Zhang E, Chen B. Management of the temporal bone fibrous dysplasia with external auditory canal stenosis and secondary cholesteatoma in an Asian population: a 11-case series. Ear Nose Throat J. 2021;100(10):NP469–74.

Part III
Topographic Approach to Differential Diagnosis

Chapter 32
Topographic Approach to Differential Diagnosis: Approach to External Ear Pathologies

Harshavardhan Mahalingam

The conditions affecting the external ear can be broadly divided into those primarily affecting the pinna and those primarily affecting the EAC, although some conditions can affect both regions of the external ear.

32.1 Conditions Affecting the Pinna

The pinna is easily amenable to clinical examination and hence, imaging plays a minor role in differential diagnosis. Imaging may be necessary to assess the deeper extent of lesions or to assess associated abnormalities in the middle ear, skull base, and mastoid. HRCT of the temporal bone is usually the first-line imaging investigation. A separate soft tissue reconstruction of the temporal bone scan (in addition to the high-resolution bone algorithm reconstruction) is essential for imaging assessment of external ear. A 3D volume-rendered reconstruction of the pinna is also useful. MRI can be useful in certain situations as a problem-solving tool.

The conditions affecting the pinna which are referred for imaging can be divided into congenital malformations and mass lesions.

32.1.1 Microtia/Anotia

Microtia refers to a small and usually deformed pinna. Anotia refers to completely absent pinna. Severity can be graded according to the Marx classification (Table 32.1)

H. Mahalingam (✉)
Department of Radiology, SRIHER, Chennai, India

H. Mahalingam (ed.), *Temporal Bone Imaging*,
https://doi.org/10.1007/978-981-95-6132-2_32

Table 32.1 Marx classification of microtia severity [1]

Grades	Clinical features
1	Small pinna with normal morphology
2	Rudimentary, malformed, but retains few normal features
3	Severely attenuated, lump of deformed tissue (peanut ear)
4	Anotia

Microtia is usually unilateral. Microtia is usually accompanied by anomalies of the EAC, such as stenosis and atresia, and middle ear anomalies, such as dysplastic ossicles and falls under the spectrum of congenital aural dysplasia. The severity of microtia has a direct correlation with the severity of EAC and middle ear anomalies. Inner ear anomalies may also coexist but are not necessarily correlated to the severity of the microtia [2]. Many syndromes can be associated with microtia, including Goldenhar syndrome, Treacher Collins syndrome, CHARGE syndrome, Crouzon syndrome, Pierre Robin sequence, and Down syndrome [1].

32.1.2 Preauricular Sinus

It is seen as a dimple in the skin close to the crus helix of the pinna. Rarely, it can be located near the tragus. It occurs due to incomplete fusion of the auricular hillocks resulting in a blind-ending, epithelium-lined tract. It is usually a benign clinical finding and is often asymptomatic. Superadded infection can result in discharge from the sinus and ulceration. The sinus is almost always attached to the perichondrium of the auricular cartilage. These sinuses are usually posterosuperior to the parotid gland and facial nerve, although extension into the parotid has been described. High-resolution ultrasound can be useful in demonstrating the course of the sinus in relation to the parotid gland and to look for underlying cystic component or abscess. CT and MRI have limited utility in this clinical setting. Syndromes associated with preauricular sinus are Beckwith-Wiedemann syndrome and Melnick-Fraser syndrome [3, 4].

32.1.3 First Branchial Cleft Anomalies

They account for less than one-tenth of all branchial cleft anomalies (note that the 2nd branchial cleft anomalies are much more common). First branchial cleft anomalies can manifest as a cyst, sinus, or fistula near the EAC. They can be situated anterior or posterior to the pinna and can extend up to the angle of the mandible. Parotid gland may or may not be involved. These can be divided into two types. In type 1, the cyst or sinus is located in the preauricular region, is parallel to the EAC

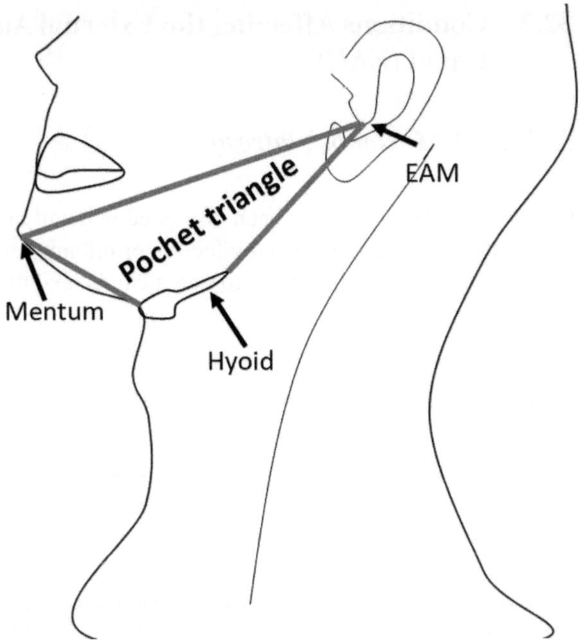

Fig. 32.1 Schematic representation of the Pochet triangle

within parotid gland, and is lateral to facial nerve. In type 2, the tract extends to the angle of the mandible with tract closely related to the facial nerve branches [5]. Clinical presentation can be in the form of recurrent periauricular swelling or a mass, sinus opening, or discharge from the external ear or angle of mandible. First branchial cleft anomalies are usually encountered in a triangular region anterior to the sternocleidomastoid called the Pochet triangle bounded by EAC, mentum, and hyoid bone (Fig. 32.1)

32.1.4 *Mass Lesions in the Pinna*

A wide variety of mass lesions can occur in the pinna, with the most common being skin/adnexal lesions. Benign lesions include epidermal cyst, nevus, hypertrophic scar, keloid, vascular malformations, and hemangioma. Hematomas and pseudocyst can also be encountered. Malignant lesions include squamous cell carcinoma and basal cell carcinoma [6].

32.1.5 Calcification of the Elastic Cartilage of the Pinna

Differential diagnosis for calcification of the pinna includes diabetes mellitus, relapsing polychondritis, gout, ochronosis, and post-traumatic calcification.

32.2 Conditions Affecting the External Auditory Canal (EAC)

32.2.1 EAC stenosis/atresia

Congenital EAC atresia has been discussed in detail in Chap. 4. Acquired EAC stenosis can occur due to repeated infection or inflammation, or due to trauma. This is described in the subsequent section on medial canal fibrosis.

32.2.2 Diffuse wall thickening in the EAC

Circumferential diffuse wall thickening in the EAC is most commonly due to infective and inflammatory causes. These include otitis externa (OE), necrotizing otitis externa (NOE), herpes zoster oticus, and relapsing polychondritis. NOE is discussed in Chap. 10.

Herpes zoster oticus (Ramsay Hunt syndrome) is characterized by auricular herpes zoster vesicles, otalgia, and facial nerve palsy. MRI can show hyperenhancement in the facial nerve and occasionally in the vestibulocochlear nerve compared to the opposite side. Note that the normal facial nerve can show enhancement on post-gadolinium images at the 1st genu and in tympanic and mastoid segments. However, any enhancement in cisternal, canalicular, and proximal labyrinthine segments is abnormal.

Relapsing polychondritis is an autoimmune condition characterized by recurrent inflammation of cartilages in the ear, nose, and tracheobronchial tree. HRCT of the temporal bone can show diffuse thickening of the cartilaginous part of the EAC and also of the pinna with or without calcifications.

Rarely, squamous cell carcinoma of the EAC can present with diffuse wall thickening. Squamous cell carcinoma of EAC is discussed in Chap. 22.

HRCT helps in identifying the extent of thickening, associated bone erosions, and extension into adjacent structures. Sagittal reconstruction of the EAC is especially helpful in accurately assessing these features.

32.2.3 Focal Soft Tissue Thickening or Mass Lesion in EAC

A focal soft tissue thickening or mass in the EAC is a commonly encountered situation when interpreting HRCT temporal bone exams. It has a wide differential diagnosis, the most important of which are discussed below. Table 32.2 provides the salient imaging features for differentiating these pathologies.

Table 32.2 Differential diagnosis of focal soft tissue thickening in EAC

Diagnosis	Imaging clues to differential diagnosis
Cerumen	Peripheral rim of air surrounding the soft tissue
Medial canal fibrosis	Crescentic-shape soft tissue density with no bone erosion
Cholesteatoma	Focal bone destruction—especially along posteroinferior part of bony EAC. Diffusion restriction on MRI
Keratosis obturans	Expansion of bony EAC with circumferential bone thinning
Cholesterol granuloma	T1 and T2 hyperintensity on MRI

Earwax or cerumen—Earwax is produced by ceruminous glands in the EAC. It is incidentally noted on many HRCT temporal bone examinations and needs to be differentiated from more sinister pathologies. The diagnostic clues to identify cerumen are a peripheral rim of air surrounding the soft tissue within the EAC and a change in appearance on follow-up examinations. Impacted cerumen may completely obstruct the EAC, but it does not show any expansion of the canal or any bone erosion.

Medial canal fibrosis—It is otherwise called acquired atresia or stenosis of the EAC. It is characterized by crescent-shaped soft tissue density occluding the medial part of the EAC abutting the tympanic membrane. No bone erosions are seen. Almost half of these patients have bilateral involvement. It usually occurs due to development of a fibrous tissue plug in the EAC following repeated infections, radiotherapy, or trauma [7].

Cholesteatoma— The external ear is an uncommon site of cholesteatoma with most of these lesions occurring in the middle ear. Both congenital and acquired cholesteatomas can occur in the EAC. EAC cholesteatoma can also occur due to preexisting EAC stenosis. Most cases, are however, are idiopathic with the posteroinferior aspect of the bony EAC being most commonly affected. HRCT shows a soft tissue density mass with bone erosions and intralesional bone fragments. The lesion can erode into the middle ear, mastoid, and facial nerve canal. Intense diffusion restriction on MRI is a helpful clue to diagnosis. Keratosis obturans (KO) is a close differential diagnosis on imaging. Compared to KO, cholesteatoma usually affects older individuals, is usually unilateral, and has more of eccentric bone destruction.

Keratosis obturans has been discussed in Chap. 29.

Cholesterol granuloma—The most common site of cholesterol granuloma is the petrous apex with EAC being a rare site of involvement. The CT appearance is nonspecific, showing a soft tissue density lesion with or without bone thinning. MRI is more helpful as it shows T1 and T2 hyperintensity with peripheral T2 hypointense rim.

EAC osteoma has been discussed in Chap. 28.

A wide variety of skin/adnexal lesions can manifest as masses within the EAC. In addition to common skin lesions like nevi and papillomas, benign neoplasms arising from the ceruminous glands like ceruminous adenoma and ceruminous pleomorphic adenoma can also be encountered in the EAC. HRCT appearance is nonspecific with a nodular soft tissue density in EAC.

Skin malignancies like basal cell carcinoma and squamous cell carcinoma can also manifest as a mass within the EAC [8]. Squamous cell carcinoma of EAC is discussed in Chap. 22.

32.2.4 Foreign Body in EAC

Foreign bodiesin the EAC are commonly encountered in the pediatric age group. Hyperdense foreign bodies like metal, stone, and glass can be readily apparent on HRCT while organic materials like wood, cotton, fabric and plastic buds may mimic other soft tissue lesions on imaging.

32.2.5 Fractures of EAC

Fractures of EAC can occur due to extension from other parts of the temporal bone or due to impaction of the mandibular condyle. Fractures of EAC can be longitudinal or transverse. The Poschl view shows EAC fractures more conspicuously. Potential pitfalls in diagnosing EAC fractures include a persistent foramen tympanicum, tympanosquamous, and tympanomastoid sutures [9].

References

1. Zhang TY, Bulstrode N, Chang KW, Cho YS, Frenzel H, Jiang D, et al. International consensus recommendations on microtia, aural atresia and functional ear reconstruction. J Int Adv Otol. 2019;15(2):204–8.
2. Calzolari F, Garani G, Sensi A, Martini A. Clinical and radiological evaluation in children with microtia. Br J Audiol. 1999;33(5):303–12.
3. Matev B, Lyutfi E, Stoyanov GS, Sapundzhiev NR. Preauricular sinus: a tale of forgetful rediscovery. Cureus. 2020;12(6):e8885.
4. Scheinfeld NS, Silverberg NB, Weinberg JM, Nozad V. The preauricular sinus: a review of its clinical presentation, treatment, and associations. Pediatr Dermatol. 2004;21(3):191–6.
5. Maithani T, Pandey A, Dey D, Bhardwaj A, Singh VP. First branchial cleft anomaly: clinical insight into its relevance in otolaryngology with pediatric considerations. Indian J Otolaryngol Head Neck Surg. 2014;66(Suppl 1):271–6.
6. Jung SY, Kim MG, Boo SH, Yeo EK, Kwon C, Lee SK, et al. Clinical analysis of auricular benign masses. Korean J Audiol. 2012;16(1):10–3.
7. Luong A, Roland PS. Acquired external auditory canal stenosis: assessment and management. Curr Opin Otolaryngol Head Neck Surg. 2005;13(5):273–6.
8. Tsuno NSG, Tsuno MY, Coelho Neto CAF, Noujaim SE, Decnop M, Pacheco FT, et al. Imaging the external ear: practical approach to normal and pathologic conditions. Radiographics. 2022;42(2):522–40.
9. Wood CP, Hunt CH, Bergen DC, Carlson ML, Diehn FE, Schwartz KM, et al. Tympanic plate fractures in temporal bone trauma: prevalence and associated injuries. Am J Neuroradiol. 2014;35(1):186–90.

Chapter 33
Topographic Approach to Differential Diagnosis: Approach to Middle Ear and Mastoid Pathologies

Harshavardhan Mahalingam

The normal middle ear and mastoid are air-filled structures. Opacification of middle ear and mastoid can occur due to a variety of causes (Fig. 33.1).

The HRCT appearance of these various etiologies shows considerable overlap and requires correlation with clinical symptoms and signs to arrive at a proper diagnosis. Hence, reviewing the clinical notes and discussing with the referring physician are of paramount importance in arriving at a proper diagnosis. The role of HRCT is more oriented toward assessing the extent of the disease rather than providing a histological or etiological diagnosis.

By far the most common cause of opacification of the middle ear and/or mastoid on HRCT of the temporal bone is various types of otitis media. It is important to look for the imaging clues that suggest possibility of other diagnoses to avoid misdiagnosis as otitis media in such cases. The presence of serous otitis media in adults should prompt a search for a nasopharyngeal mass lesion. Some clues to differential diagnosis are presented in Table 33.1.

Imaging of otomastoiditis and cholesteatoma and their various complications are discussed in Chaps. 11, 12, 13, 14, 15, 16, 17, and 18.

Temporal bone trauma is discussed in Chaps. 19, 20, and 21.

Glomus tumors of the middle ear are discussed in Chap. 23.

Aberrant ICA, high-riding jugular bulb, and dehiscent jugular bulb are discussed in Chaps. 8 and 9.

H. Mahalingam (✉)
Department of Radiology, SRIHER, Chennai, India

H. Mahalingam (ed.), *Temporal Bone Imaging*,
https://doi.org/10.1007/978-981-95-6132-2_33

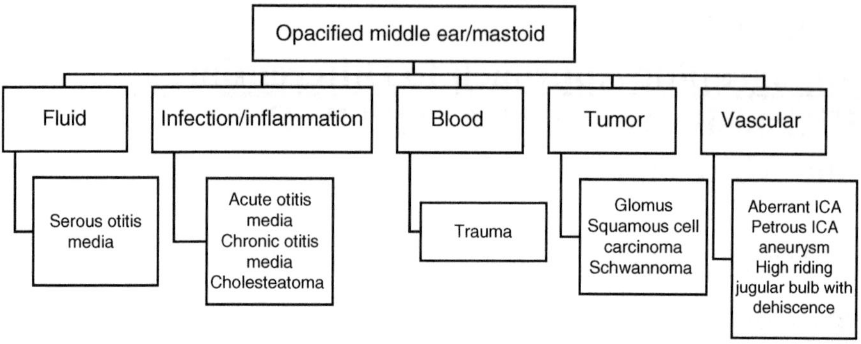

Fig. 33.1 Schematic representation of differential diagnosis of middle ear and mastoid opacification

Table 33.1 Causes of middle ear opacification other than otitis media

Differential diagnosis of the middle ear opacification	Imaging clues for diagnosis
Cholesteatoma	Most commonly located in epitympanum. Bone erosions especially in scutum and tegmen
Glomus tumor	Located in meso- or hypotympanum. Permeative pattern of bone destruction. Intense post-contrast enhancement
Facial nerve schwannoma	Expansion of the facial canal
Aberrant ICA	Tubular structure coursing across the cochlear promontory. Absent vertical segment of the carotid canal with dehiscence of carotid plate
Dehiscent jugular bulb	"Mass" located in the posteroinferior part of the middle ear cavity with defect in the floor of the middle ear cavity

Facial nerve schwannoma will be discussed in the following paragraphs.

Facial nerve schwannomas can arise anywhere along the course of the facial nerve from the cisternal segment to the intraparotid location. They can be sporadic or associated with type 2 neurofibromatosis. Most commonly, they present with facial palsy, twitching, or hemifacial spasm. Other symptoms include sensorineural/conductive hearing loss and vertigo.

The imaging morphology of the lesion depends on the site of origin. Tumors of CPA-IAC region show morphology indistinguishable on imaging from vestibular schwannoma. Tumors of the labyrinthine segment and geniculate ganglion show tubular morphology. Tumors of the tympanic segment protrude into the middle ear cavity and can present as a middle ear mass on clinical examination. Tumors of mastoid segment erode into the mastoid air cells and can mimic an aggressive lesion [1].

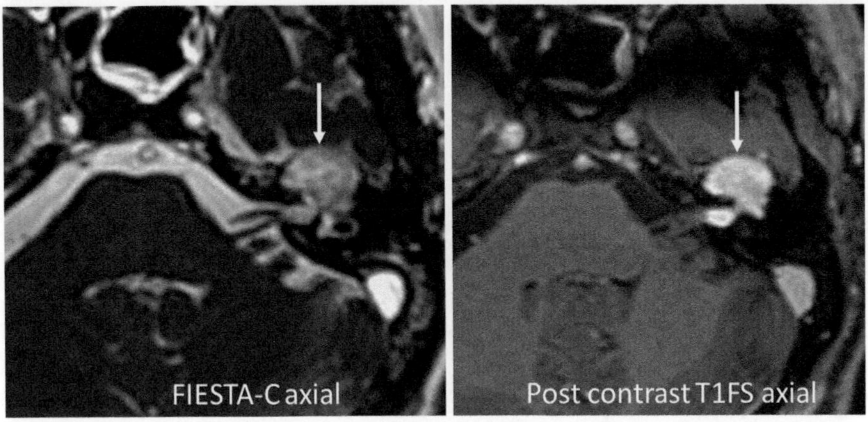

Fig. 33.2 Heavily T2-weighted thin section (FIESTA-C) axial image and post-contrast T1 fat-saturated image at the level of cerebellopontine angle showing a hyperintense, intensely enhancing mass lesion in the left temporal bone in the region of cochlea and 1st genu of the facial nerve

These tumors typically show facial canal expansion with smooth bone scalloping rather than bone erosion or destruction. On MRI, they appear T2 hyperintense and T1 iso- to hypointense to gray matter. Small lesions enhance homogeneously while larger lesions can have cystic and hemorrhagic areas within. MR imaging appearance of a facial nerve schwannoma centered at the geniculate ganglion is demonstrated in Fig. 33.2.

Reference

1. Wiggins RH, Harnsberger HR, Salzman KL, Shelton C, Kertesz TR, Glastonbury CM. The many faces of facial nerve schwannoma. AJNR Am J Neuroradiol. 2006;27(3):694–9.

Chapter 34
Topographic Approach to Differential Diagnosis: Approach to Inner Ear Pathologies

Harshavardhan Mahalingam

Diseases affecting the inner ear can be broadly divided into congenital malformations and acquired pathologies.

34.1 Congenital Inner Ear Malformations

Inner ear malformations (IEM) occur due to arrested development of the inner ear structures during the 1st and 2nd trimesters of fetal life. Sensorineural hearing loss (SNHL) is the primary manifestation of these conditions. SNHL is identified in the newborn period in most cases due to routine screening programs. IEMs can be idiopathic due to environmental agents like teratogens and congenital infections or could be due to inherited genetic syndromes (e.g., Pendred syndrome, CHARGE syndrome, X-linked deafness, etc.).

From an imaging standpoint, IEMs can be broadly divided into those that have no imaging abnormality (accounting for majority of cases, nearly 80%) and those that have manifest abnormalities on imaging.

The former group, which has no detectable abnormalities on imaging, are those that occur due to a developmental arrest a much later stage of development of inner ear in the 2nd trimester of fetal life. This manifests as abnormalities of the membranous labyrinth and of the sensory end organs with normal bony labyrinthine structure. Detection of abnormalities in the structures of the membranous labyrinth is beyond the maximum resolution possible with current clinical CT and MRI scanners.

H. Mahalingam (✉)
Department of Radiology, SRIHER, Chennai, India

H. Mahalingam (ed.), *Temporal Bone Imaging*,
https://doi.org/10.1007/978-981-95-6132-2_34

The latter group accounting for the remaining 20% of patients with IEMs have abnormalities in bony labyrinth which are readily identified with CT and MRI. Imaging plays an important role in this group of patients in deciding the mode of treatment and surgical technique. Factors which need to be addressed in management of IEMs are choosing cochlear implantation vs auditory brainstem implantation, choosing the surgical approach, choosing an appropriate electrode, risk of CSF gusher, meningitis, and anomalous course of facial nerve.

The IEMs with abnormalities of the bony labyrinth are classified into eight groups [1]. This classification is presented in Table 34.1. Some examples of congenital inner ear anomalies are presented in Chap. 6.

Complete labyrinthine aplasia (also called Michel deformity) is characterized by absence of recognizable inner ear structures with varying degrees of hypoplasia or aplasia of the petrous temporal bone and otic capsule. A rudimentary otocyst is characterized by a tiny cyst measuring a few millimeters in dimension with no IAC.

Cochlear aplasia can be of two types absent cochlea with normal vestibule and absent cochlea with dilated vestibule. Absent cochlea with dilated vestibule can appear similar to common cavity (CC) malformation. In CC, the IAC opens into the center of the cyst, whereas in absent cochlea with dilated vestibule, the cyst is posterior to the IAC fundus.

Common cavity malformation shows a single cystic chamber with the IAC opening into its center. Cochlear hypoplasia is characterized by a smaller than normal cochlea with a lesser number of turns. It is divided into four types—small bud-like cochlea, cystic hypoplastic cochlea with absent modiolus, cochlea with less than

Table 34.1 Classification of inner ear malformations

	Type	Imaging	CSF gusher	Facial nerve anomaly	Treatment
1	Complete labyrinthine aplasia	No bony inner ear structure	–	+	ABI
2	Rudimentary otocyst	Tiny remnant cystic structure	–	+	ABI
3	Cochlear aplasia	No cochlea	–	+	ABI
4	Common cavity	Single cyst in place of cochlea and vestibule	–	+	CI/ABI
5	Cochlear hypoplasia	Small-sized cochlea	Possible	+	HA/CI/ABI
6	IP1	Cystic cochlea	+	Possible	CI/ABI
	IP2	Cystic cochlear apex	Possible	–	HA/CI
	IP3	Absent modiolus	+	+	HA/CI
7	Enlarged VA	Normal cochlea, enlarged VA	Possible	–	HA/CI
8	Cochlear aperture abnormality	Small/absent cochlear aperture	–	–	CI/ABI

Adapted from Ref. [1]

ABI auditory brainstem implant, *CI* cochlear implant, *CSF* cerebrospinal fluid, *HA* hearing aid, *IP* incomplete partition, *VA* vestibular aqueduct two turns, and cochlea with hypoplastic middle and apical turns. Cochlear nerve deficiency is commonly seen in cochlear hypoplasia and hence needs to be carefully looked for.

Incomplete partition (IP) is a group of anomalies where there is a separate cochlea and vestibule with normal cochlear dimensions. However, the internal structure of cochlea is abnormal. IP-1 shows cystic cochlea with no modiolus or interscalar septa and dilated vestibule. IP-2 shows defective apical part of modiolus and corresponding interscalar septa giving rise to a cystic cochlear apex with normal basal turn. Triad of a cystic cochlear apex, mildly dilated vestibule, and dilated vestibular aqueduct is called Mondini deformity. IP-3 shows defective modiolus but interscalar septa are present. IP-3 defect is seen in patients with X-linked deafness.

Enlarged vestibular aqueduct (EVA) is defined as a midpoint vestibular aqueduct (VA) diameter greater than 1.5 mm. In EVA, the cochlea and vestibule are normal.

The cochlear aperture can be hypoplastic (width less than 1.4 mm) or aplastic (not visualized on mid-modiolar section). It can occur with a narrow IAC (width less than 2.5 mm). Cochlear aperture abnormalities are often accompanied by hypoplastic or absent cochlear nerve. The cochlear nerve is considered hypoplastic when its size is smaller than thc accompanying facial nerve on oblique sagittal cisternographic MR images.

34.2 Other Malformations

Isolated SCC dysplasia—Isolated abnormalities of the SCC can occur with normal cochlea. These anomalies do not directly fit into the classification system described above. It can have syndromic associations; for example, CHARGE syndrome has absent SCCs. Isolated absence of posterior SCC can be seen in Alagille syndrome.

Isolated lateral SCC abnormality—The lateral SCC is last to develop and hence is the one most commonly involved by malformations. Isolated lateral SCC dysplasia with other bony labyrinthine structures being normal is common. Bony island of the lateral SCC normally measures more than 2.6 mm in width. In isolated lateral SCC dysplasia, the bony island may be small or even absent.

Congenital fistulous communications involving inner and middle ear are discussed in Chap. 9. Inner ear involvement in osteopetrosis is discussed in Chap. 30.

34.3 Acquired Abnormalities of Inner Ear

Common acquired pathologies of the inner ear include labyrinthitis (discussed in Chap. 14), labyrinthine hemorrhage, labyrinthine fistula (discussed in Chap. 16), Meniere's disease, otosclerosis (discussed in Chap. 27), tumors of inner ear, and inner ear involvement in systemic osteodystrophies such as fibrous dysplasia and

Paget's disease (discussed in Chap. 31). Some of the pathologies which have not been presented elsewhere are discussed in the following paragraphs.

Labyrinthine hemorrhage—Hemorrhage can occur due to trauma or bleeding diatheses. Hemorrhage is seen on MRI as T1 hyperintensity and reduced signal of the intralabyrinthine fluid on fluid-sensitive sequences. CT can be useful in identifying associated fractures but is not sensitive in detecting labyrinthine hemorrhage.

Meniere's disease—It is a disease characterized by fluctuating sensorineural hearing loss, tinnitus, and vertigo or sensation of aural pressure most commonly presenting in the 5th or 6th decade of life. Symptoms are usually unilateral. It is thought to occur due to increased pressure of the endolymph (endolymphatic hydrops). Routine MRI usually does not demonstrate any abnormality in Meniere's disease. MRI demonstration of dilated endolymphatic structures depends on delayed post-contrast imaging after 24 hours of intratympanic or after 4 hours of intravenous administration of gadolinium-based contrast agents (GBCA). The GBCA is taken up selectively by the perilymph while the endolymph does not take up the contrast. A 3D FLAIR sequence can then be used to selectively null the endolymphatic fluid signal. Diagnostic criteria and grading systems have been proposed to diagnose and quantify endolymphatic hydrops [2].

Inner ear tumors—Primary tumors arising from the inner ear structures are rare. Intralabyrinthine schwannomas arise from the branches of the vestibulocochlear nerve within the inner ear structures and are much less common than the CP angle schwannomas. On MRI, these lesions appear as filling defects within the inner ear structures on fluid-sensitive sequences and show homogeneous enhancement on post-gadolinium images. Based on location, these tumors can be intracochlear, transmodiolar, intravestibular, vestibulocochlear, and transotic (extending to the middle ear) [3].

Endolymphatic sac tumor (ELST) is a neuroectodermal neoplasm arising from the endolymphatic sac/duct. It is a benign, but locally aggressive, neoplasm. Clues to diagnosis on imaging are its location in the posterior part of the petrous temporal bone with expansion/destruction of vestibular aqueduct, calcific foci within or along the rim of the lesion on CT, and T1 hyperintense areas with heterogeneous enhancement on MRI. Signal heterogeneity within the lesion is a hallmark feature of this tumor and is due to presence of calcifications and hemorrhages [4]. ELSTs have a strong association with von Hippel-Lindau syndrome.

References

1. Sennaroğlu L, Demir BM. Classification and current management of inner ear malformations. Balk Med J. 2017;34(5):397–411.
2. de Pont LMH, van Steekelenburg JM, Verbist BM, van Buchem MA, Blom HM, Hammer S. State of the art imaging in Menière's disease. Tips and tricks for protocol and interpretation. Curr Radiol Rep. 2020;8(11):25.

3. Salzman KL, Childs AM, Davidson HC, Kennedy RJ, Shelton C, Harnsberger HR. Intralabyrinthine schwannomas: imaging diagnosis and classification. Am J Neuroradiol. 2012;33(1):104–9.
4. Patel NP, Wiggins RH, Shelton C. The radiologic diagnosis of endolymphatic sac tumors. Laryngoscope. 2006;116(1):40–6.

Chapter 35
Topographic Approach to Differential Diagnosis: Approach to Cerebellopontine Angle and Internal Acoustic Canal Pathologies

Harshavardhan Mahalingam

The cerebellopontine angle (CPA) is a CSF-filled subarachnoid space that lies between the pons/middle cerebellar peduncle medially and dura covering the petrous temporal bone laterally. It is limited superiorly by the 5th cranial nerve and inferiorly by the 9th, 10th, and 11th cranial nerves. It is traversed by the VII and VIII cranial nerves and anterior inferior cerebellar artery (AICA). The flocculus of the cerebellum projects into the medial part of the CPA.

The CPA is laterally continuous with the internal auditory canal (IAC) which extends from the porus acusticus internus to the fundus adjacent to the bony labyrinth. Anatomy of the IAC is reviewed in Chap. 1.

The spectrum of lesions which can affect the CP angle and IAC are presented in Fig. 35.1.

By far, the most common mass lesion affecting the CPA/IAC is the vestibular schwannoma (accounting for nearly three-fourths or 75% of all such lesions). Meningioma and epidermoid are less common. Other mass lesions are exceedingly rare in this region.

Symptoms of CPA/IAC lesions are usually due to cranial nerve compression such as sensorineural hearing loss (SNHL), vertigo, and trigeminal neuralgia. Large lesions can compress the brainstem and/or cause hydrocephalus. Facial nerve palsy due to a CPA mass is uncommon.

CP angle/IAC schwannomas are discussed in Chap. 26.

The imaging features of other CPA mass lesions are presented in Table 35.1.

Petrous apex lesions are discussed separately in Chaps. 24 and 36.

H. Mahalingam (✉)
Department of Radiology, SRIHER, Chennai, India
e-mail: drharsha@sriramachandra.edu.in

H. Mahalingam (ed.), *Temporal Bone Imaging*,
https://doi.org/10.1007/978-981-95-6132-2_35

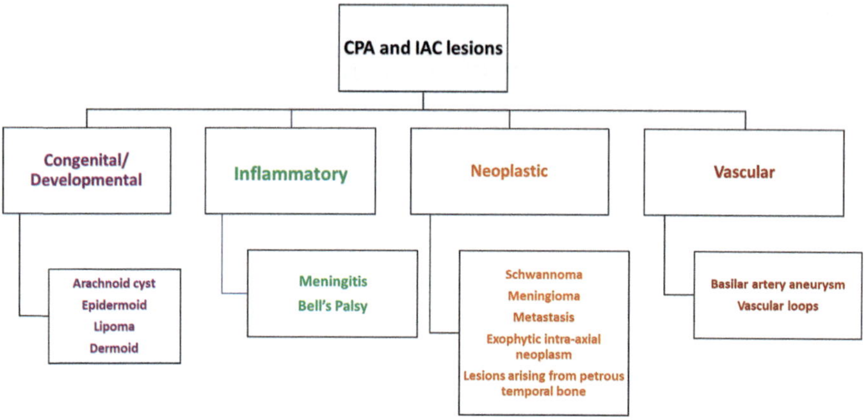

Fig. 35.1 Schematic representation of the classification of CP angle lesions

Table 35.1 Differential diagnosis of CPA and IAC lesions based on imaging features

	CPA/IAC lesion	Imaging features on CT	Imaging features on MRI
Congenital/ developmental	Epidermoid cyst (Fig. 35.2)	CSF density lesion expanding subarachnoid space	T2 hyperintense, T1 hypointense, partial suppression on FLAIR, diffusion restriction, minimal to absent enhancement
	Arachnoid cyst	CSF density lesion expanding subarachnoid space	T2 hyperintense, T1 hypointense, complete suppression on FLAIR, no diffusion restriction, absent enhancement (mirrors the signal of CSF in all sequences)
	Lipoma	Fat density lesion (around −100 HU)	T1 and T2 hyperintense with signal suppression on fat-saturated sequences

(continued)

Table 35.1 continued

	CPA/IAC lesion	Imaging features on CT	Imaging features on MRI
Neoplastic	Meningioma (Fig. 35.3)	Mildly hyperdense intensely enhancing lesion with broad base to dura. Adjacent bone may show hyperostosis.	T1 isointense, T2 hypo- to hyperintense intensely enhancing lesion with broad base to dura and dural tail
	Schwannoma	Isodense mass lesion in CP angle extending into IAC with IAC widening	Ice-cream cone appearance. Small lesions are homogeneous and enhance intensely. Larger lesions often show cystic and hemorrhagic areas within.
	Metastasis	Variable density. Aggressive features in form of bone destruction and disproportionate mass effect	Disproportionate vasogenic edema in adjacent brain parenchyma with mass effect. Leptomeningeal metastasis can manifest as smooth or nodular meningeal thickening within the IAC.
	Exophytic lesions from brain parenchyma[a] (Fig. 35.4)	Compress and narrow the CP angle cistern instead of widening it	Lack of CSF cleft around the lesion differentiates from extra-axial lesions (thin section FIESTA/T2-SPACE might be helpful).
Vascular	Basilar artery aneurysm	Isodense rounded mass on plain CT. CT angiography shows the vascular origin of the lesion.	May be T2 dark due to flow void. May show variable signal due to slow flow and/or thrombosis. Rounded shape is a diagnostic clue.

[a]Exophytic lesions from brain parenchyma—medulloblastoma, ependymoma, choroid plexus papilloma, glioma, and lymphoma

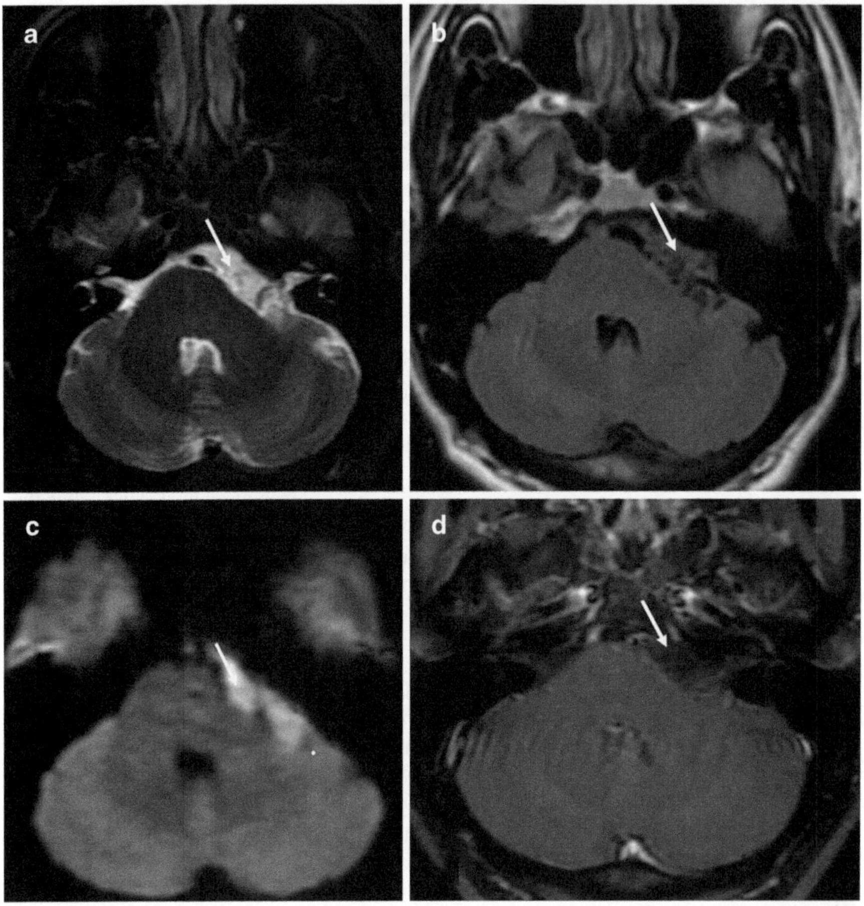

Fig. 35.2 Epidermoid cyst. (**a**) Axial T2-weighted image showing expansion of the left CP angle cistern (arrow). (**b**) Axial T2-FLAIR-weighted image showing partial suppression of signal within the left CP angle cistern. (**c**) Diffusion-weighted image showing restriction diffusion within the lesion. (**d**) Post-gadolinium T1-weighted image shows no enhancement within the lesion

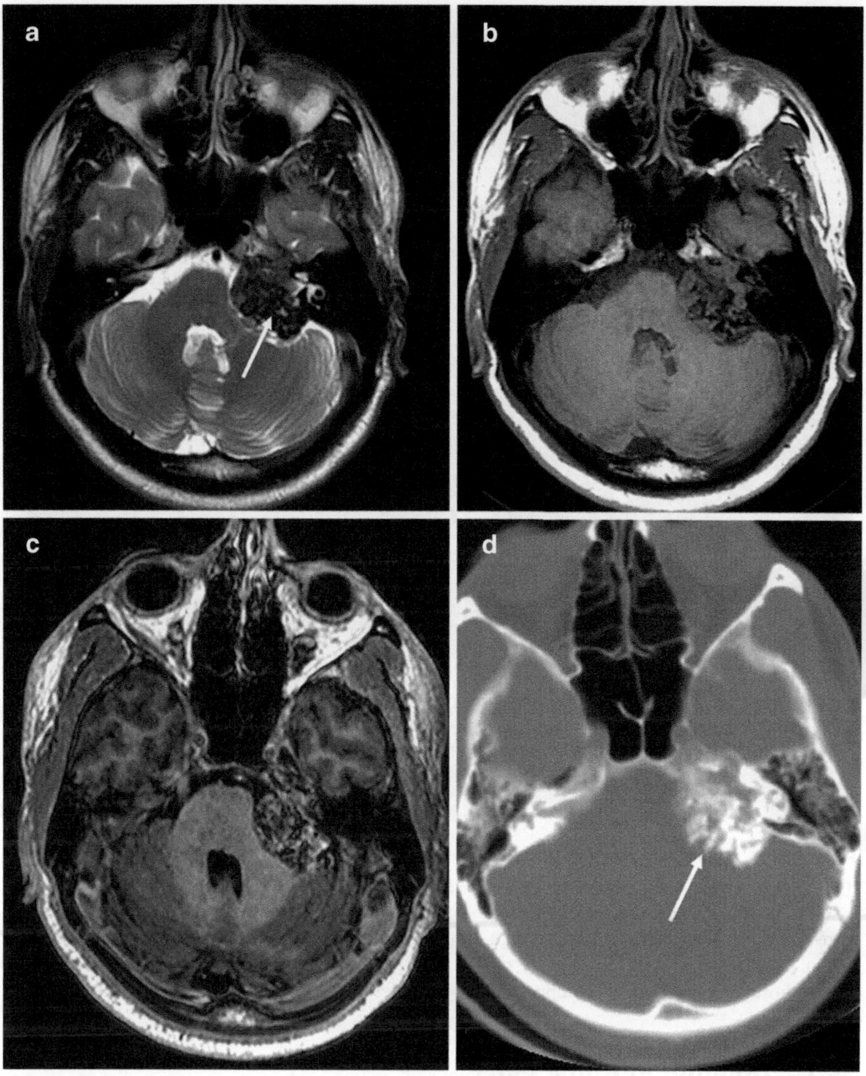

Fig. 35.3 Meningioma. (**a**) Axial T2-weighted image showing T2 hypointense extra-axial mass lesion in left CP angle with extension into the left IAC (arrow). (**b**) Axial T2-FLAIR-weighted image showing iso- to hypointense signal. (**c**) Axial T1-weighted image showing few T1 hyperintense areas within. (**d**) Axial HRCT image shows densely calcified nature of the lesion with involvement of the petrous temporal bone

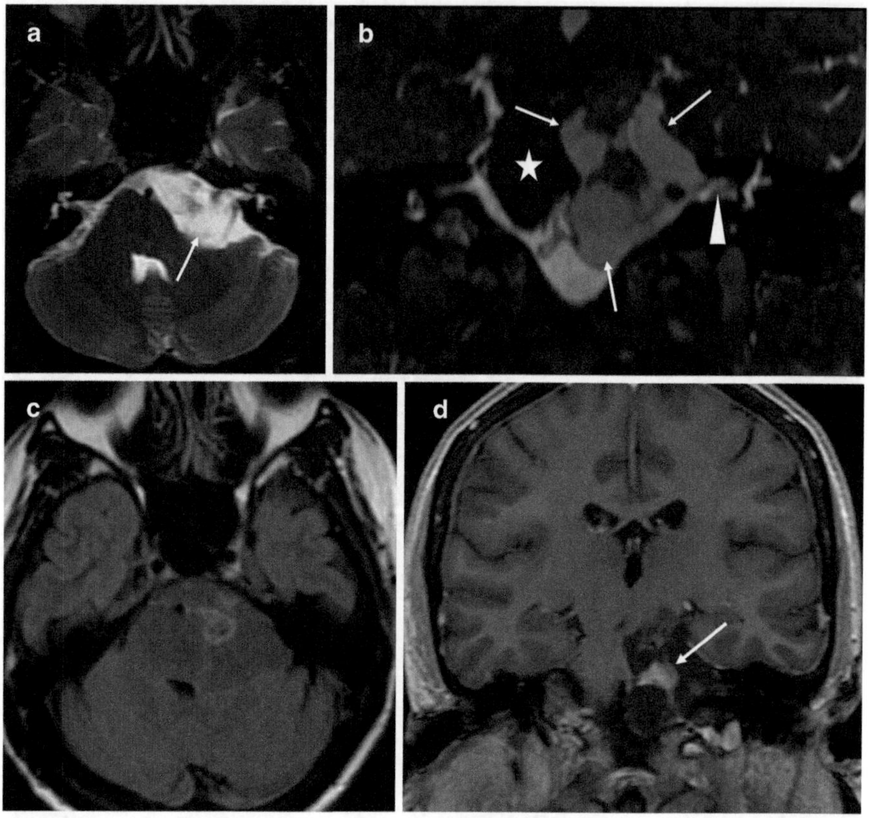

Fig. 35.4 Exophytic intra-axial lesion (glioma). (**a**) Axial T2-weighted image showing expansion of the left CP angle cistern (arrow) and left IAC. (**b**) Coronal heavily T2-weighted image showing a solid-cystic septated lesion pushing pons (star) to the right side and extending into left IAC (arrowhead). (**c**) Axial T2-FLAIR image shows few hyperintense solid components within the lesion. The lesion was infiltrating the pons and expanding it. (**d**) Post-gadolinium T1-weighted image shows enhancing solid component within the lesion

35.1 Imaging in Bell's Palsy

Bell's palsy is an idiopathic sudden-onset unilateral lower motor neuron palsy of the 7th cranial nerve. It is characterized by sudden-onset often reaching peak severity within 72 h from onset. Features of unilateral facial palsy (characteristically involving both upper and lower halves of the face) are often accompanied by auricular or postauricular pain, hyperacusis, altered facial sensation, and altered taste. The median age of affliction is 40 years.

It is a diagnosis of exclusion and imaging is not needed when the clinical presentation is classical. Imaging may be essential to rule out other causes of facial nerve palsy when the clinical presentation is atypical. Red flags which suggest an alternate diagnosis are slow progression with prolonged course, sudden complete palsy, bilateral involvement, recurrent disease, segmental facial involvement, history of recent trauma, presence of ear discharge, fever, difficulty hearing, and parotid mass on examination [1].

In patients with an atypical clinical presentation, HRCT of the temporal bone and contrast-enhanced MRI can be utilized for further evaluation depending on the clinical suspicion. Common differential diagnoses of unilateral facial palsy includes tumors of facial nerve (such as schwannoma), CP angle tumors, parotid tumors, and granulomatous diseases like sarcoidosis.

In Bell's palsy, HRCT of the temporal bone does not show any abnormality while contrast-enhanced MRI may show hyperenhancement of the intracanalicular and labyrinthine segments of the nerve, though not in all patients. It is pertinent to note that the geniculate ganglion and tympanomastoid segments of the facial nerve can normally show some enhancement [2].

35.2 Vascular Loops in IAC

The presence of a vascular loop in the CPA or IAC is a frequently encountered finding on imaging studies. Most of these loops arise from the anterior inferior cerebellar artery which normally courses through the CPA. Multiple studies have found no significant correlation between the presence of a vascular loop and any audiovestibular symptoms attributable to the neurovascular contact [3, 4].

References

1. Bell's palsy: aetiology, clinical features and multidisciplinary care. J Neurol Neurosurg Psychiatry [Internet]. [cited 2024 Jul 8]. Available from: https://jnnp.bmj.com/content/86/12/1356.long.
2. Seok JI, Park JH, Park JA, Do Y. Contrast-enhanced MRI findings of patients with acute bell palsy within 7 days of symptom onset: a retrospective study. Medicine (Baltimore). 2023;102(48):e36337.
3. Deep NL, Fletcher GP, Nelson KD, Patel AC, Barrs DM, Bendok BR, et al. Magnetic resonance imaging assessment of vascular contact of the facial nerve in the asymptomatic patient. J Neurol Surg B Skull Base. 2016;77:503–9.
4. Zidan MA, Almansor N. Presence of vascular loop in patients with audio-vestibular symptoms: is it a significant finding? Evaluation with 3-tesla MRI 3D constructive interference steady state (CISS) sequence. Egypt J Radiol Nucl Med. 2020;51(1):114.

Chapter 36
Topographic Approach to Differential Diagnosis: Approach to Petrous Apex Pathologies

Harshavardhan Mahalingam

The petrous apex is a pyramid-shaped structure formed by the medial part of the temporal bone. Margins of this region are formed by the bony labyrinth laterally and the petro-occipital suture medially. It is a region with multitude of important vascular and neural structures, either passing through it or and in close relation to it. This gives rise to a wide spectrum of possible pathologies [1].

The petrous apex is divided by the internal auditory canal (IAC) into a medial part that contains either bone marrow or is pneumatized, and a small lateral part formed by dense bone of the otic capsule. Imaging appearance of medial part of normal petrous apex, especially on MRI, is dependent on the extent of pneumatization. The non-pneumatized petrous apex has relatively a high signal in adults on both T1- and T2-weighted images due to fatty marrow while the pneumatized petrous apex has a low signal due to the presence of air. Occasionally, the medial part of the petrous apex may be sclerotic, showing low-signal intensity on all MRI sequences. The lateral part of the petrous apex always has low signal on all MRI sequences due to dense bone (Fig. 36.1).

Clinical presentation of petrous apex lesions can be variable, ranging from incidentally detected lesions (on scans done for other unrelated indications) to headache, ear pain, and cranial neuropathies. The V and VI cranial nerves are the most common cranial nerves affected by petrous apex lesions. MRI is more helpful in tissue characterization and, thus, is more useful for the differential diagnosis of petrous apex lesions in the majority of situations [2].

The spectrum of petrous apex lesions is represented in Fig. 36.2.

Some of the petrous apex lesions have already been presented in the case-based approach section in chapter 24. A short summary of diagnostic clues to individual lesions of petrous apex is presented in Table 36.1.

H. Mahalingam (✉)
Department of Radiology, SRIHER, Chennai, India
e-mail: harsha.mahalingam@gmail.com

H. Mahalingam (ed.), *Temporal Bone Imaging*,
https://doi.org/10.1007/978-981-95-6132-2_36

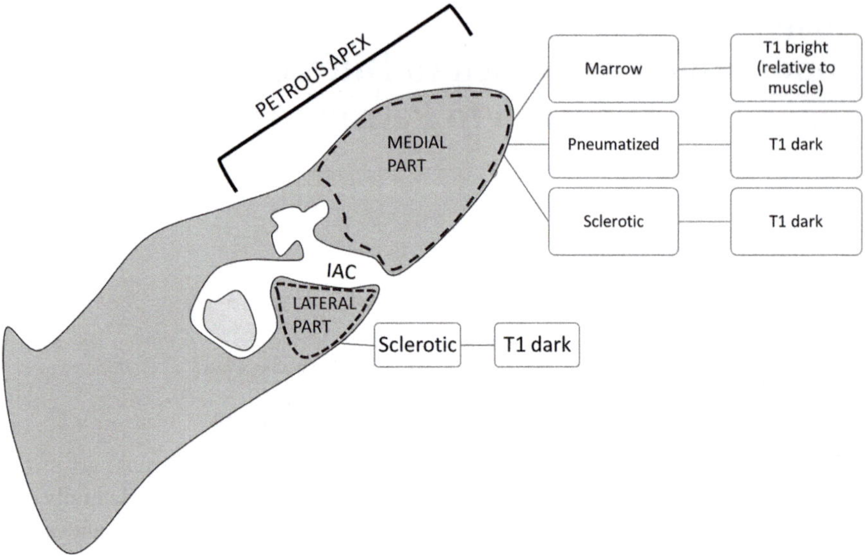

Fig. 36.1 Schematic representation of variable MRI signal of petrous apex

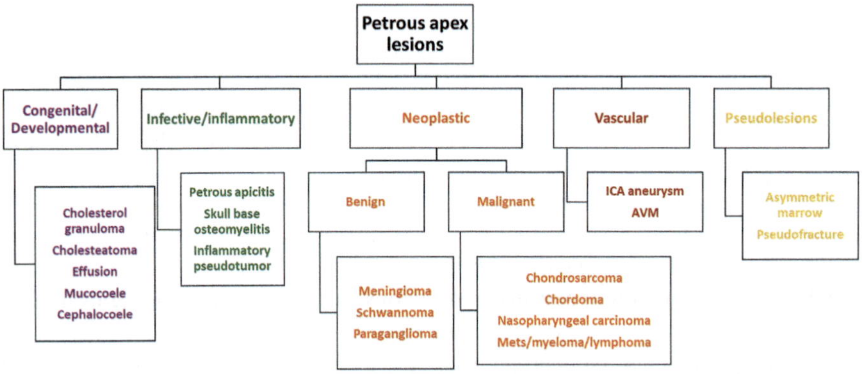

Fig. 36.2 Etiological classification of the petrous apex lesions

Table 36.1 Imaging clues to differential diagnosis of petrous apex lesions

	Petrous apex lesion	Imaging features on CT	Imaging features on MRI	Figures
	Pseudolesion—asymmetric petrous apex	Asymmetric pneumatization in up to 10%. Readily apparent on CT	The non-pneumatized petrous apex can be mistaken for a lesion (especially cholesterol granuloma) due to T1 hyperintense marrow	
Congenital/ developmental	Cholesteatoma	Expansile lytic lesion with variable bone erosion	T2 hyperintense, T1 hypointense, central diffusion restriction is key feature. Minimal to absent enhancement	Presented in Chap. 24
	Cholesterol granuloma[a]	Expansile lytic lesion. Long-standing large lesions can have bone gaps mimicking destruction.	T2 and T1 hyperintense, no diffusion restriction, not suppressed on fat-saturated images	Presented in Chap. 24
	Mucocele	Formed by obstruction of pneumatized petrous apex. Expansile lytic lesion	T2 hyperintense, low to intermediate signal on T1	
	Cephalocele	Erosion of petrous apex with scalloped margin	CSF signal intensity on all sequences Continuity with Meckel's cave on heavily T2-weighted 3D images	Presented in Chap. 24
Infective/ inflammatory	Petrous apicitis[b]	Opacification of petrous apex air cells with/without bone erosion	T2 hyperintense, T1 hypointense, post-gadolinium enhancement within the air cells with/without adjacent meningeal enhancement	Figure 36.3
	Osteomyelitis[c]	Erosion, fragmentation in acute stage, and irregular sclerosis in late stages	T2 hyperintense, T1 hypointense, post-gadolinium enhancement usually extends to infratemporal soft tissues.	Presented in Chap. 17
	Inflammatory pseudotumor	Bone erosion	Enhancing soft tissue replacing the bone—requires biopsy	

(continued)

Table 36.1 (continued)

	Petrous apex lesion	Imaging features on CT	Imaging features on MRI	Figures
Neoplastic	Meningioma	Mildly hyperdense to brain parenchyma, associated bone hyperostosis/sclerosis	Extra-axial dural-based intensely enhancing mass arising from CP angle/petroclival dura. Dural tail may be seen.	
	Schwannoma	Smooth marginated extra-axial lesions with bone scalloping	Extra-axial mass lesion arising from V, VII, or VIII cranial nerves, heterogeneous enhancement, may show cysts and fluid levels within	
	Paraganglioma	Secondary invasion from middle ear/ jugular foramen, moth-eaten appearance	Salt-and-pepper appearance, intense enhancement	
	Chondrosarcoma	Bone destruction with chondroid (punctate, ring, and arc calcifications) matrix	T2 very bright due to chondroid matrix (calcified regions can be hypointense), intense post-gadolinium enhancement	Figure 36.4
	Endolymphatic sac tumor	Located in the posterior midportion of the petrous temporal bone, permeative bone destruction, calcifications usually present	Heterogeneous signal on T1 and T2 due to intratumoral hemorrhage and calcifications	
	Nasopharyngeal carcinoma	Contiguous erosion of petrous apex	T2 hyperintense T1 hypointense infiltrative lesion, bulky cervical lymphadenopathy	
	Systemic malignancies (metastasis/myeloma/ lymphoma)	Aggressive bone destruction	Loss of normal marrow signal, infiltrative pattern, post-gadolinium enhancement	Figure 36.5
Vascular	ICA aneurysm	Expansion of carotid canal with scalloped bone margin	Variable signal intensity depending on variable flow patterns and possible thrombus within	

[a]Cholesterol granulomas are the most common lesions of the petrous apex seen on imaging
[b]Petrous apicitis occur due to extension of infection from otitis media to a pneumatized air cell in the petrous apex. Clinical presentation can be in form of ear pain, sixth cranial nerve palsy, and facial pain—Gradenigo triad
[c]Involvement of petrous apex by skull base osteomyelitis usually occurs secondary to necrotizing otitis externa in diabetics

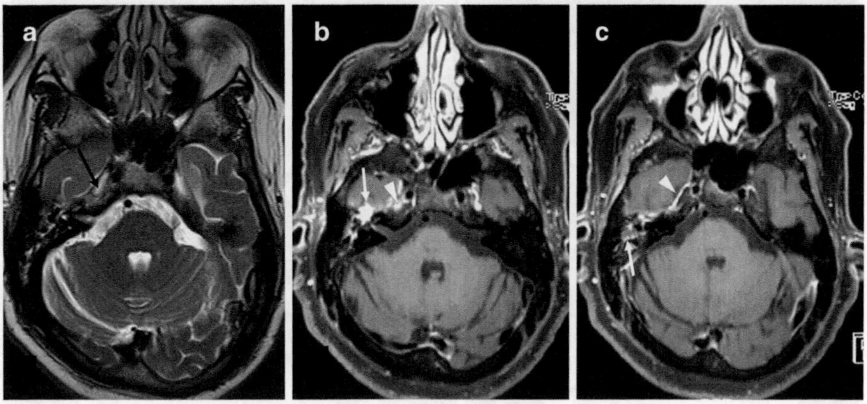

Fig. 36.3 Petrous apicitis. (**a**) T2-weighted axial image showing marrow edema in the right petrous apex (arrow). (**b**, **c**) Axial post-gadolinium T1-weighted fat-saturated images showing abnormal enhancement in the right middle ear, mastoid (white arrow), and petrous apex (arrowhead)

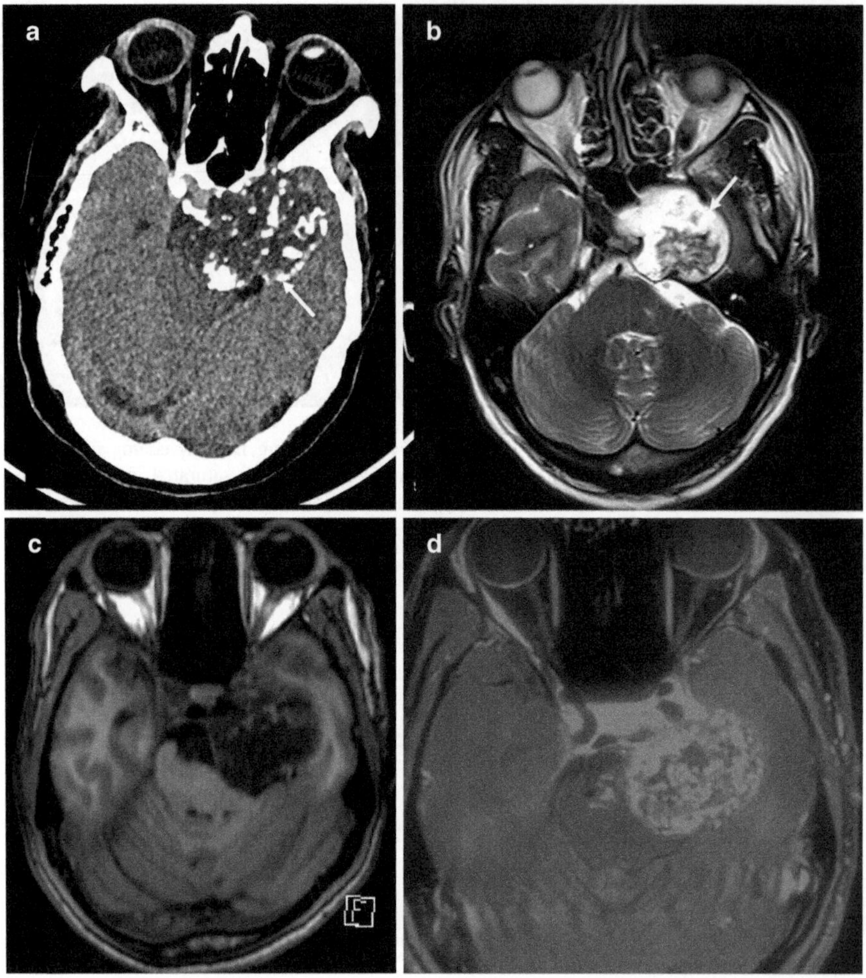

Fig. 36.4 Chondrosarcoma of petrous apex. (**a**) Axial CT section showing a large mass lesion in the region of left petrous apex with multiple calcific foci within (arrow). (**b**) T2-weighted axial image showing markedly T2 hyperintense mass with few T2 dark areas within. (**c**) T1-weighted axial image showing hypointense signal. (**d**) Axial post-gadolinium T1-weighted fat-saturated image showing intense enhancement of the mass

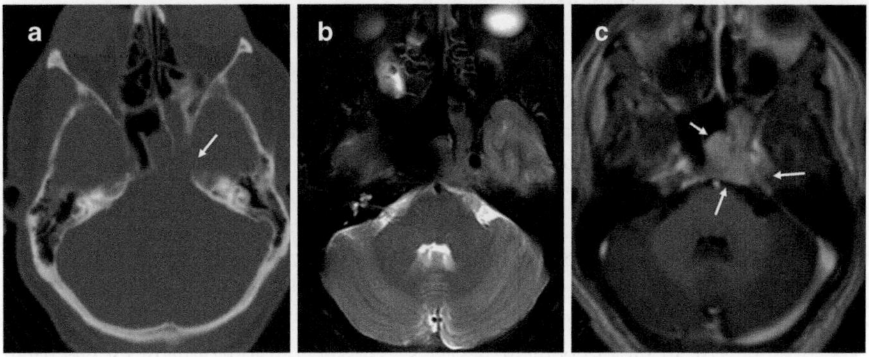

Fig. 36.5 Myeloma. (**a**) Axial HRCT section in bone window showing lytic destruction of the left petrous apex (arrow). (**b**) T2-weighted axial image showing infiltrative T2 hyperintense mass in the region of left petrous apex and left cavernous sinus. (**c**) Axial post-gadolinium T1-weighted fat-saturated image showing intensely enhancing mass involving the petrous apex and sphenoid sinus (arrow). Bone marrow biopsy was suggestive of myeloma

References

1. Razek AA, Huang BY. Lesions of the petrous apex: classification and findings at CT and MR imaging. Radiographics. 2012;32(1):151–73.
2. Isaacson B, Kutz JW, Roland PS. Lesions of the petrous apex: diagnosis and management. Otolaryngol Clin N Am. 2007;40(3):479–519, viii.

Part IV
Special Considerations in Temporal Bone

Chapter 37
Imaging in Cochlear Implantation

Shivaprakash B. Hiremath, Neetika Gupta, Andrea Para, Pejman Maralani, Pradeep Krishnan, and Elka Miller

37.1 Imaging in Cochlear Implantation

Sensorineural hearing loss (SNHL) results from disruption of the auditory pathway, including the organ of Corti, inner ear, cochlear nerve, and central auditory centers of the brain. It is characterized by impaired sound detection and localization, as well as reduced speech recognition and discrimination. According to WHO estimates, approximately 5% of the global population, more than 700 million individuals will suffer from disabling sensorineural hearing loss by 2050 [1]. Cochlear implantation is the standard of care for patients with severe to profound SNHL with limited or no benefit from auditory rehabilitation by hearing aids.

Magnetic resonance imaging (MRI) and computed tomography (CT) serve complementary roles in the presurgical evaluation for cochlear implantation [2–4]. A 3D T2 SPACE and oblique sagittal T2-weighted sequences enable a thorough

S. B. Hiremath (✉) · A. Para
Division of Neuroradiology, Joint Department of Medical Imaging, Toronto Western Hospital, Univeristy Health Network, University of Toronto, Toronto, ON, Canada

Department of Medical Imaging, University of Toronto, Toronto, ON, Canada

N. Gupta · P. Krishnan · E. Miller
Department of Medical Imaging, Children's Hospital of Eastern Ontario, Department of Radiology, Radiation Oncology, and Medical Physics, University of Ottawa, Ottawa, ON, Canada

Department of Diagnostic and Interventional Radiology, The Hospital for Sick Children, University of Toronto, Toronto, ON, Canada

P. Maralani
Department of Medical Imaging, University of Toronto, Toronto, ON, Canada

Department of Medical Imaging, Sunnybrook Health Sciences Centre, University of Toronto, Toronto, ON, Canada

H. Mahalingam (ed.), *Temporal Bone Imaging*,
https://doi.org/10.1007/978-981-95-6132-2_37

assessment of the internal auditory canal and labyrinth, including the cochlear nerve and its aperture [2]. CT is vital in examining bony structures, evaluating mastoid pneumatization, determining the course of the facial nerve, identifying ossification associated with labyrinthitis ossificans, and diagnosing dysmorphic syndromes [3].

Presurgical imaging is vital to determine the feasibility and facilitate cochlear implantation. This chapter discusses the stepwise approach to anatomical factors associated with surgical difficulty and increased risk of complications. We also focus on the congenital and acquired anomalies that may preclude cochlear implantation, cause luminal obstruction, and findings that complicate surgical management.

37.2 Anatomical Factors Associated with Surgical Difficulty and Complications

The anatomical factors influencing surgical decision-making include cochlear morphology, status of the mastoid pneumatization, round window accessibility, facial nerve course, and arterial and venous variations [5].

37.2.1 Mastoid and Middle Ear Evaluation

Pneumatization of the temporal bone begins during prenatal development, with the mastoid antrum being the only visible air cell at 24 weeks of gestational age. The pneumatization continues in the postnatal period with an increase in the size and volume of the air cells, which is completed around 10 years of age [6].

The extent of mastoid pneumatization may be classified as poorly aerated, moderately aerated, and well aerated (Fig. 37.1). The tegmen height is the vertical distance between the tegmen and the lateral semicircular canal in the coronal plane (Fig. 37.2). Mastoid pneumatization is a critical prognostic factor in middle ear

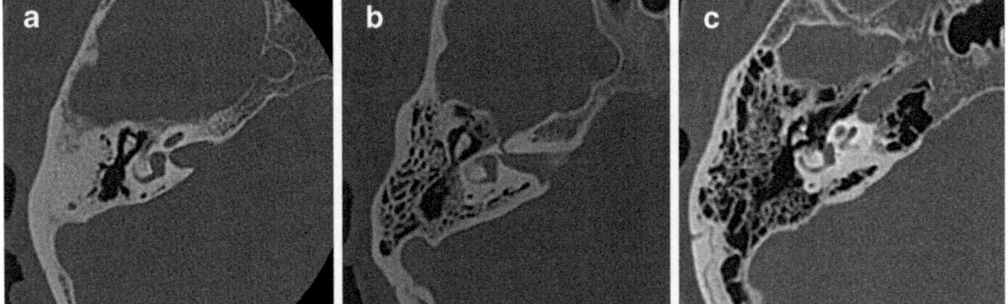

Fig. 37.1 Extent of mastoid pneumatization. Axial HRCT sections of the temporal bone (**a–c**) demonstrate varying extents of mastoid pneumatization, depicting poorly aerated (**a**), moderately aerated (**b**), and well-aerated (**c**) mastoid temporal bone

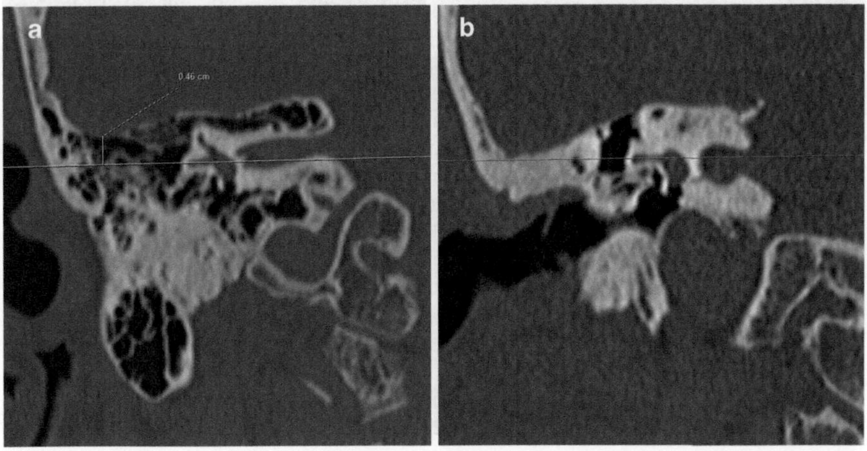

Fig. 37.2 Tegmen height. Coronal HRCT sections of the temporal bone (**a**, **b**) show normal (**a**) and decreased distance (**b**) between the tegmen (floor of the middle cranial fossa) and the horizontal line along the lateral semicircular canal

surgery and cochlear implantation. Reduced mastoid pneumatization and low-lying tegmen (<3.5 mm) are associated with increased surgical difficulty during cortical mastoidectomy with increased risk of dural exposure, meningoencephalocele, CSF leaks, and meningitis [7].

The middle ear is also evaluated for associated pathologies, including chronic otitis media, cholesteatoma, and tympanosclerosis as tympanoplasty or subtotal petrosectomy may be needed for removal of the disease to prevent labyrinthitis and meningitis and avoid cochlear implant explantation (Fig. 37.3).

37.2.2 Cochlear Morphology

The assessment of the cochlear morphology is necessary to determine the optimal cochlear implant length, as deep-inserted electrodes are associated with traumatic insertion, and shallow insertion may result in poor hearing post implantation. The cochlear duct length, defined as scala media length, is measured from the middle of the round window to the helicotrema. The cochlear duct length is calculated using the formula CDL (otic capsule) = 4.16A—3.98 and CDL (lateral wall) = 4.16A—2.7, where A is the distance between the round window to the farthest point on the opposite wall of the cochlea through the center of the cochlea (Fig. 37.4) [8]. The CDL (otic capsule) is relevant for selecting the electrode array length and demonstrates significant variability in cochlear turns, with the mean CDL ranging between 29.8 and 34.6 mm [9, 10]. The diameters of the cochlear turns, cochlear basal turn length, and the mid-modiolar height are assessed to determine the electrode that could be placed beyond one and a half turns of the cochlea (Fig. 37.5).

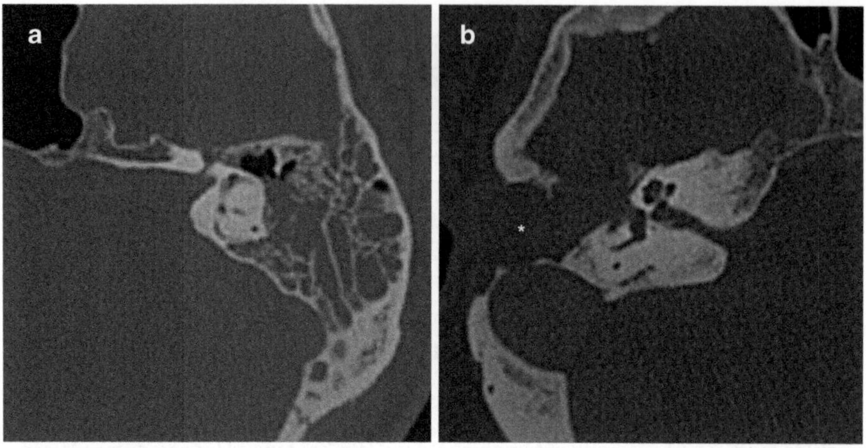

Fig. 37.3 Pathologies affecting the middle ear and mastoid air cells. Axial HRCT section of the left (**a**) temporal bone shows fluid opacification of the left middle ear cavity and mastoid temporal bone (**a**), suggesting mastoid effusion. Axial HRCT section of the right (**b**) mastoid temporal bone shows a soft tissue lesion in the right middle ear cavity and the mastoid temporal bone with osseous erosion and non-visualized ossicles concerning cholesteatoma

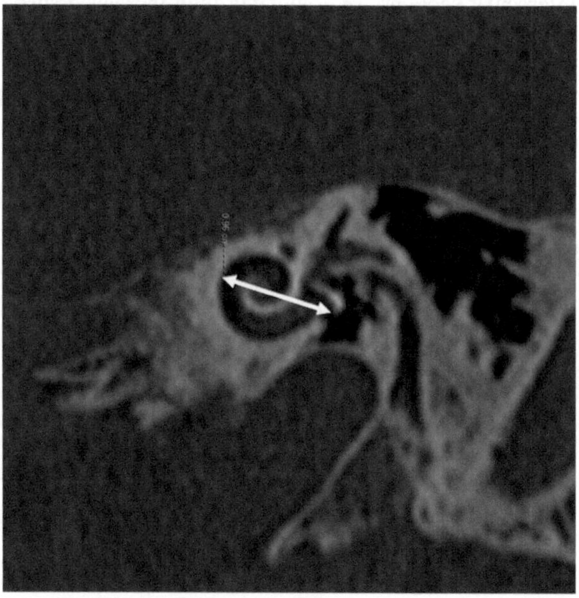

Fig. 37.4 Maximal transverse diameter of cochlea. Oblique coronal HRCT section of the temporal bone demonstrating the cochlear turns with maximal transverse diameter from the round window to the opposite wall through the middle of the cochlea

The basal turn length and the mid-modiolar height are measured in the axial plane. The cochlear basal turn length of less than 7.5 mm and mid-modiolar height of less than 3.42 mm suggest cochlear hypoplasia [11]. The cochlear aperture is the transitional point between the internal auditory canal and the cochlear modiolus, serving as a conduit for entry of the cochlear nerve and the blood vessels. The cochlear aperture is measured in its mid portion at the mid-modiolar level (Fig. 37.6).

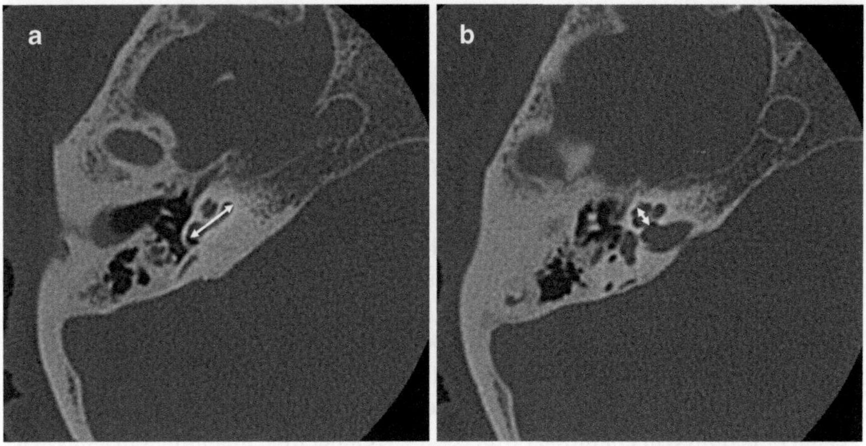

Fig. 37.5 Cochlear basal turn length and mid-modiolar height. Axial HRCT sections of the temporal bone (**a**, **b**) at the level of the round window niche with the cochlear basal turn (**a**) and at the level of modiolus demonstrating mid-modiolar height (**b**). The cochlear basal turn length of less than 7.5 mm and mid-modiolar height of less than 3.42 mm suggest cochlear hypoplasia

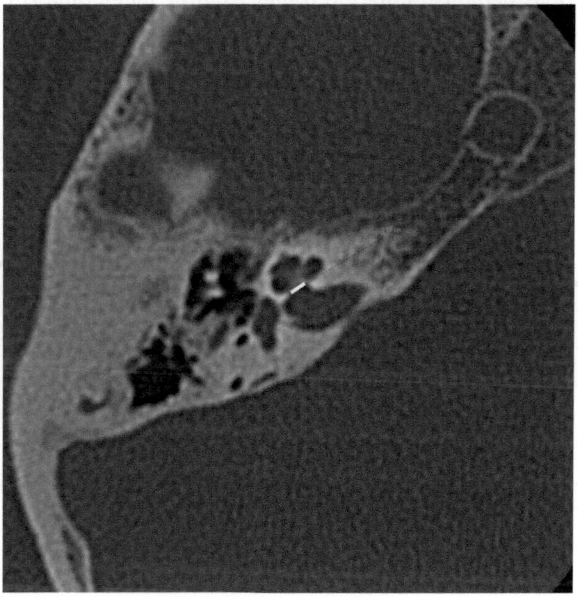

Fig. 37.6 Cochlear aperture. Axial HRCT section of the temporal bone (**a**, **b**) at the cochlear aperture level illustrates the normal cochlear aperture size. The cochlear aperture width of less than 1.4 mm suggests cochlear aperture stenosis

Cochlear aperture stenosis is defined as a width less than 1.4 mm, and aplasia is characterized by bone replacing cochlear aperture [12].

37.2.3 Round Window Accessibility

During cochlear implantation, the parallel trajectory of the electrode to the long axis of the basal turn of the cochlea facilitates scala tympani insertion (Fig. 37.7). The variations of the round window and the long axis of the basal turn are associated with increased surgical difficulty. The round window is assessed for size, orientation, and bony overhang. The diameter of the round window of less than 1.5 mm is suggestive of round window stenosis. Round window stenosis can be either congenital or acquired in conditions with osseous remodeling, including otospongiosis, labyrinthitis ossificans, Paget's disease, and osteogenesis imperfecta [13]. The orientation of the long axis of the basal turn of the cochlea parallel to the posterior wall of the external auditory canal or the axis of the carotid canal is associated with an easier surgical approach. The extent of the round window bony overhang is assessed by the ratio of the full thickness of the bony overhang to the number of image sections demonstrating the round window membrane (Fig. 37.8). An increased bony overhang may need cochleostomy over the preferred posterior tympanotomy approach to access the basal turn of the cochlea during cochlear implantation.

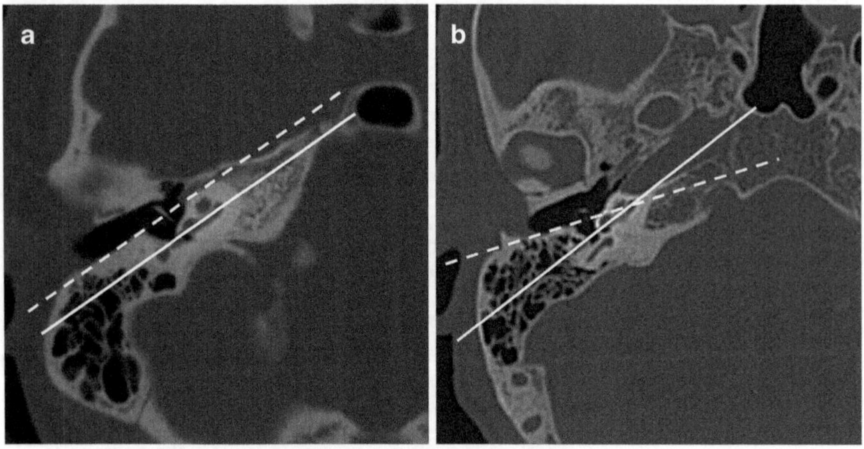

Fig. 37.7 Round window orientation. Axial HRCT sections of the temporal bone (**a**, **b**) at the level of the round window niche show the axes of the basal turn of the cochlea (white line) and posterior wall of the external auditory canal (dashed white line), with parallel orientation (**a**) suggesting likelihood of easier round window accessibility. Intersecting axes (**b**) are associated with surgical difficulty

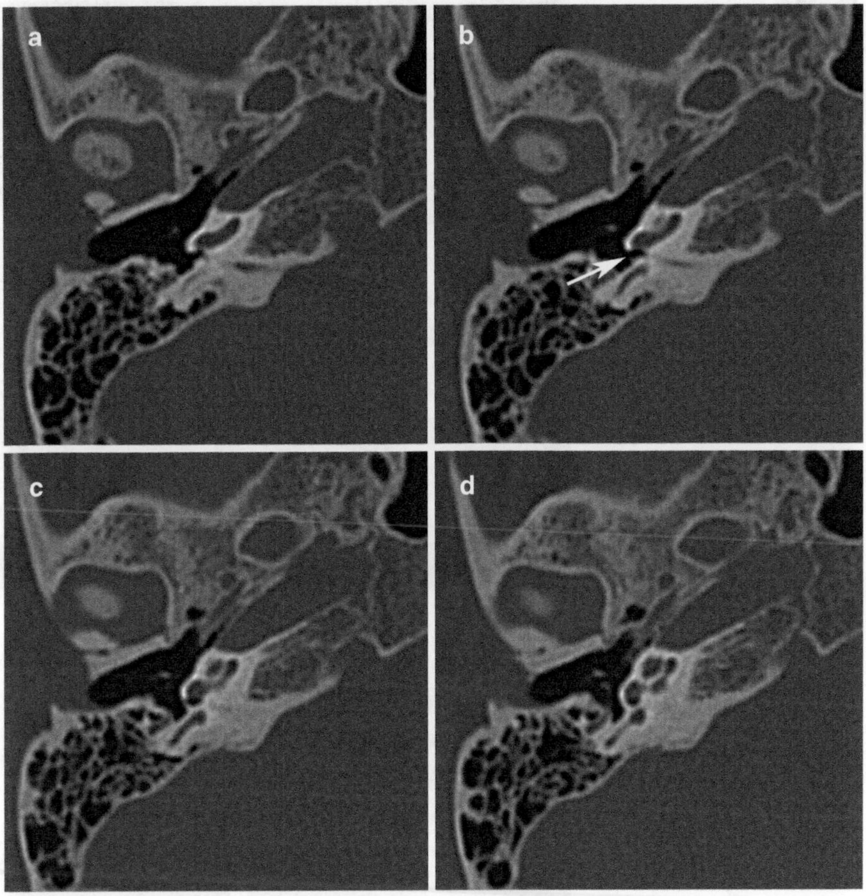

Fig. 37.8 Round window coverage ratio. Axial HRCT sections of the temporal bone (**a**–**d**) demonstrate the round window, and the bony overhang with the round window membrane is seen in one of four sections (arrow in **b**), suggesting a round window coverage ratio of 75%

37.2.4 Facial Nerve and Recess

The mastoid segment of the facial nerve and the chorda tympani nerve form the medial and lateral boundaries of the facial recess. In inner ear malformations, the intra-temporal facial nerve may have an aberrant course with anterior and medial displaced labyrinthine and tympanic facial nerve segments. The mastoid segment of the facial nerve may be anterolaterally displaced with a horizontal course. The facial recess width is the vertical distance between the mastoid segment of the facial nerve and the tympanic annulus at the level of the basal turn of the cochlea and round window (Fig. 37.9). At the same level, the distance between the mastoid cortex and the facial nerve is also assessed in coronal projection. The facial recess width of

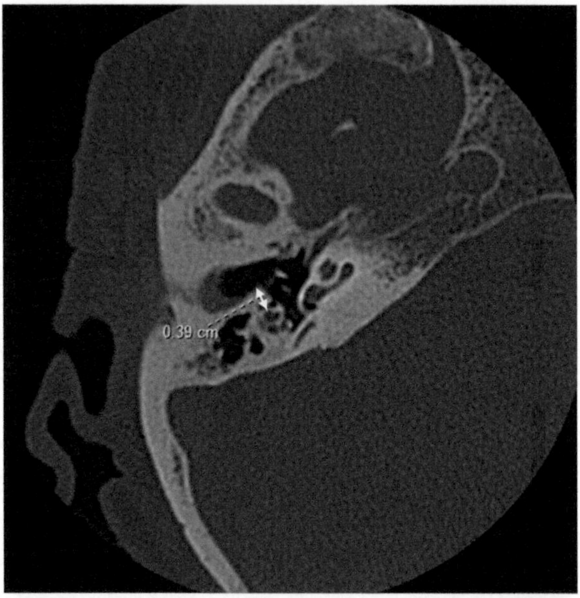

Fig. 37.9 Facial recess width. Axial HRCT section of the temporal bone at the level of the round window niche illustrates the facial recess width, measured as the vertical distance between the posterior tympanic annulus and the mastoid segment of the facial nerve. The facial recess width of less than 3 mm is associated with increased surgical difficulty

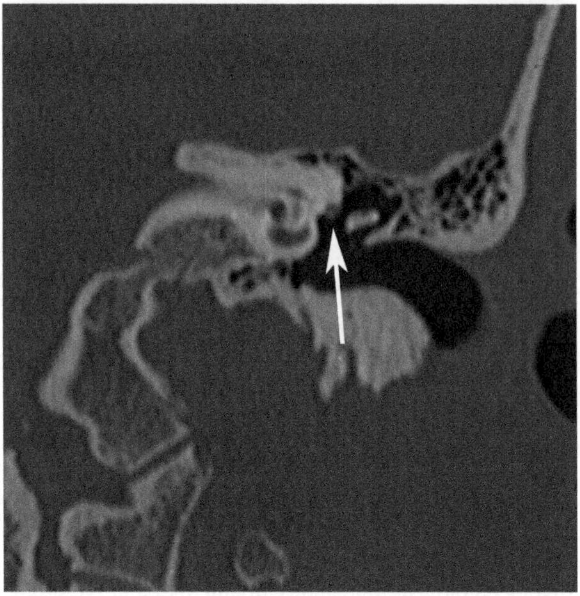

Fig. 37.10 Dehiscent tympanic segment of the facial nerve. Coronal HRCT section of the temporal bone on the left side demonstrates bony dehiscence along the inferior aspect of the tympanic segment of the left facial nerve (arrow)

≥3 mm and the presence of sentinel air cells around the mastoid segment are associated with easier accessibility during posterior tympanotomy.

The facial nerve canal dehiscence most commonly involves the inferior or the lateral wall of the tympanic segment of the facial nerve (Fig. 37.10). Rarely, there is dehiscence of the bone between the superior aspect of the basal turn of the cochlea and the labyrinthine segment of the facial nerve, suggesting cochlear facial dehiscence predisposing to facial nerve twitching, taste disorders, and paralysis post-cochlear implantation (Fig. 37.11) [14].

37.2.5 Arterial and Venous Variations

Vascular variations and anomalies involving the mastoid temporal bone and the middle ear could lead to inadvertent vascular injury and severe hemorrhage, venous thrombosis, ischemia, and rarely venous air embolism. The arterial variants include lateralized internal carotid artery (ICA), aberrant ICA, and persistent stapedial artery. The lateralized ICA is the posterolateral course of the vertical and early horizontal petrous segment and may be associated with focal thinning or dehiscence of the carotid plate and ICA protrusion into the anterior mesotympanum. An aberrant ICA is due to persistent inferior tympanic and caroticotympanic arteries coursing over the cochlear promontory with an absent distal cervical ICA (Fig. 37.12) [15]. The imaging findings associated with the persistent stapedial artery (PSA) include absent hypoplastic foramen spinosum and soft tissue density coursing through the crura of stapes, overlying the cochlear promontory and continuing into or parallel to the tympanic segment of the facial nerve. There are four distinct subtypes of PSA, based on origin from the inferior tympanic artery with a normal or an aberrant ICA, from the caroticotympanic artery, and from the duplicated ICA [15].

Venous abnormalities involving the jugular vein, sigmoid sinus, and mastoid emissary veins include high-riding jugular bulb, jugular bulb dehiscence and

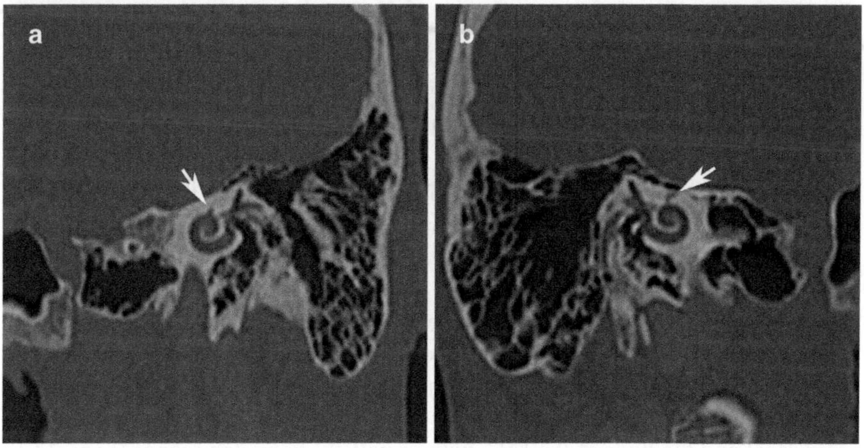

Fig. 37.11 Cochlear facial nerve dehiscence. Oblique coronal HRCT section of the temporal bone on the left side (**a**) demonstrates bony dehiscence (arrow in **a**) between the superior aspect of the cochlea's basal turn and the labyrinthine segment of the facial nerve. In comparison, the normal right side (**b**) with preserved bony separation between the basal turn and the labyrinthine segment of the facial nerve (arrow in **b**)

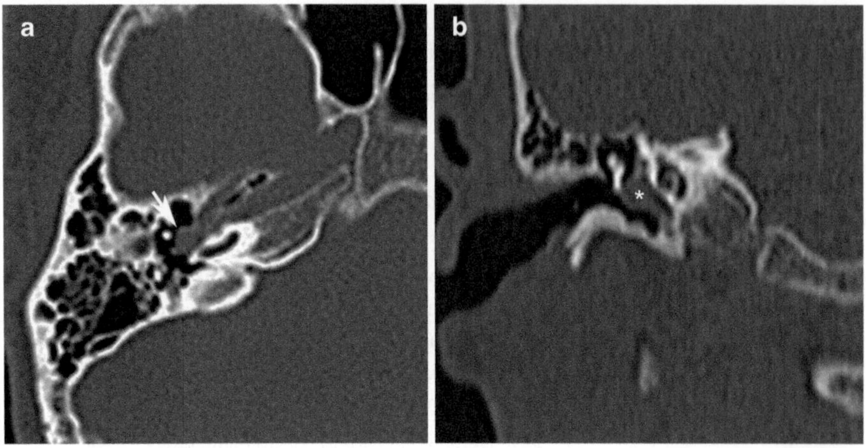

Fig. 37.12 Aberrant right internal carotid artery. Axial (**a**) and coronal (**b**) HRCT sections of the temporal bone show aberrant right internal carotid artery (asterisk in **b**) as a soft tissue density overlying the cochlear promontory (arrow in **a**), continuing as the petrous segment of the internal carotid artery

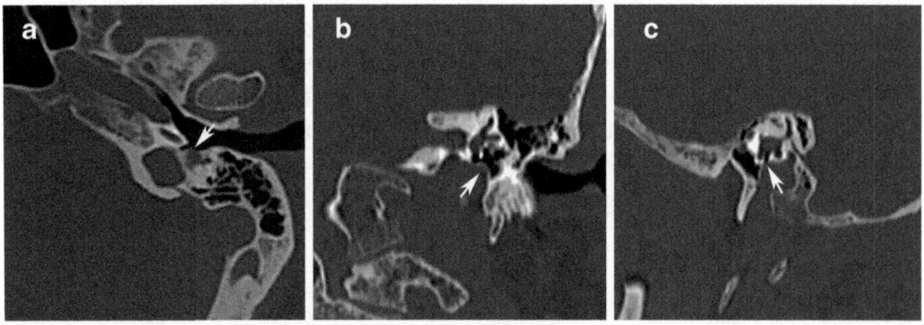

Fig. 37.13 High-riding jugular bulb. Axial (**a**), coronal (**b**), and sagittal (**c**) HRCT sections of the temporal bone show high-riding jugular bulb (arrow) with the jugular dome extending into the mesotympanum, located at the level of the round window niche

diverticulum, anterior and lateral positioned sigmoid sinus, and prominent mastoid emissary vein. Preoperative imaging is crucial for identifying venous variations as they can be asymptomatic. A high-riding jugular bulb is variably defined, with the jugular dome located anywhere from the floor of the IAC to the inferior tympanic annulus to approximately the level of the round window and the basal turn of the cochlea, with a variable reported incidence ranging from 3.5% to 34% depending on the definition used [16]. The high-riding jugular bulb is classified into various subtypes based on the location of the jugular dome in relation to the posterior semicircular canal and the floor of the IAC, with or without bony dehiscence (Figs. 37.13

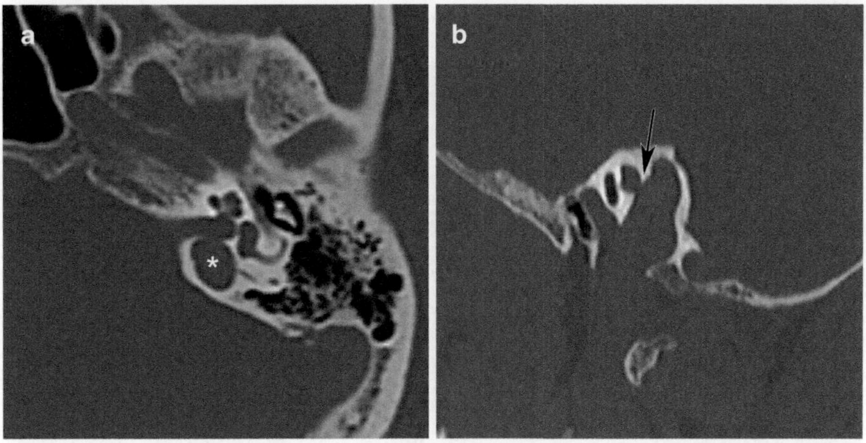

Fig. 37.14 Jugular diverticulum. Axial (**a**) and sagittal (**b**) HRCT section of the temporal bone depicting high-riding jugular bulb with an outpouching in the superior aspect (asterisk in **a**), suggesting jugular diverticulum with dehiscence of the posterior wall of the internal auditory canal (arrow in **b**)

and 37.14) [17]. A jugular diverticulum with a high-riding jugular bulb and bony dehiscence involving the sigmoid plate and superior medial projection from the jugular dome is associated with an increased risk of venous injury during surgery.

The anterior position of the sigmoid sinus is variable and reaches up to the posterior wall of the external auditory canal in up to 1.6% of patients. The anteriorly positioned sigmoid sinus with a distance between the external auditory canal of less than 10 mm may lead to increased predisposition of the sigmoid sinus to injury during mastoid surgery [18]. The lateralized sigmoid sinus is classified based on the anterolateral extent in relation to the common crus of the posterior semicircular canal, the tympanic segment of the facial nerve, and the malleoincudal axis (Fig. 37.15) [5, 19]. The emissary veins are valveless veins connecting the intracranial and the extracranial venous circulation. The mastoid emissary veins are seen in up to 63–92% of HRCT studies (Fig. 37.16). Enlarged mastoid emissary veins larger than 3 mm may be associated with complicated receiver-stimulator placement, and inadvertent injury could lead to venous infarction and incessant hemorrhage.

Presurgical imaging should also identify bone thinning or dehiscence between the cochlea and the internal auditory canal, carotid canal, jugular bulb, and eustachian tube. Additionally, it should highlight the presence of Hyrtl's fissure, which extends from the posterior fossa to the inferior aspect of the round window, to alert the operating surgeon about the potential risk of electrode misplacement (Fig. 37.17).

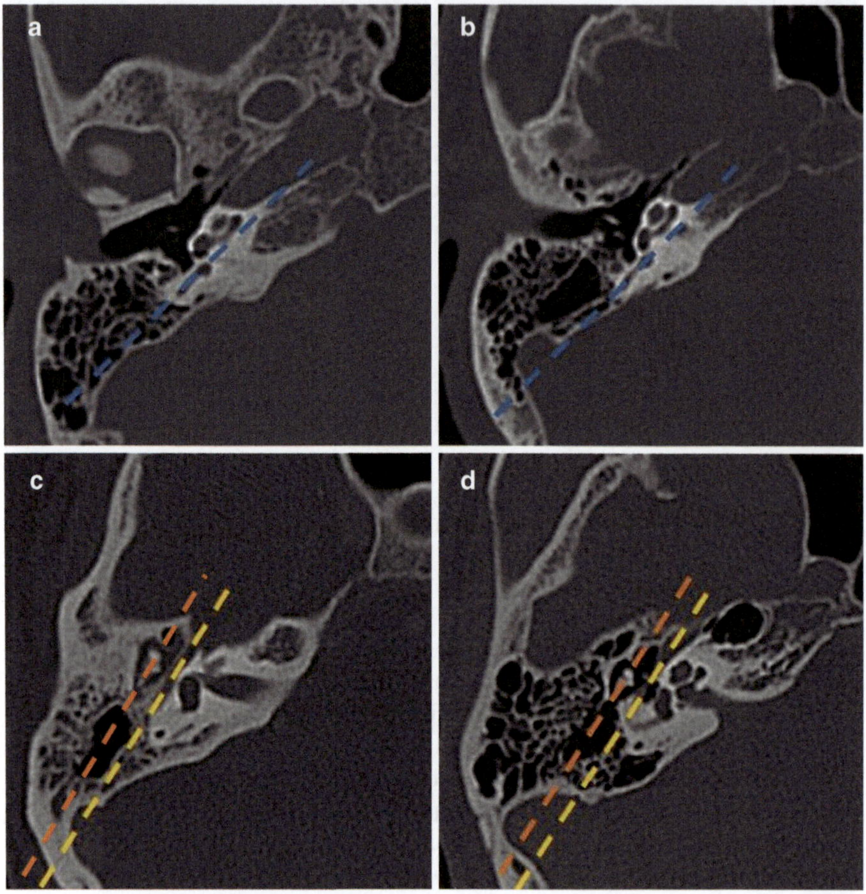

Fig. 37.15 Lateralization of the sigmoid sinus. Axial HRCT sections of the temporal bone (**a**-**d**) demonstrate types of sigmoid sinus based on the extension beyond the axis of the posterior SCC (blue line in **a** and **b**), the tympanic segment of the facial nerve (yellow line in **c** and **d**), and the malleal-incudal axis (orange line in **c** and **d**): type 1, located medial to the long axis of the posterior SCC (**a**); type 2, located between the long axis of the posterior SCC and the tympanic segment of the facial nerve (**b**); type 3, located between the long axis of the tympanic segment of the facial nerve and the malleal-incudal axis (**c**); and type 4, located beyond the malleal-incudal axis (**d**)

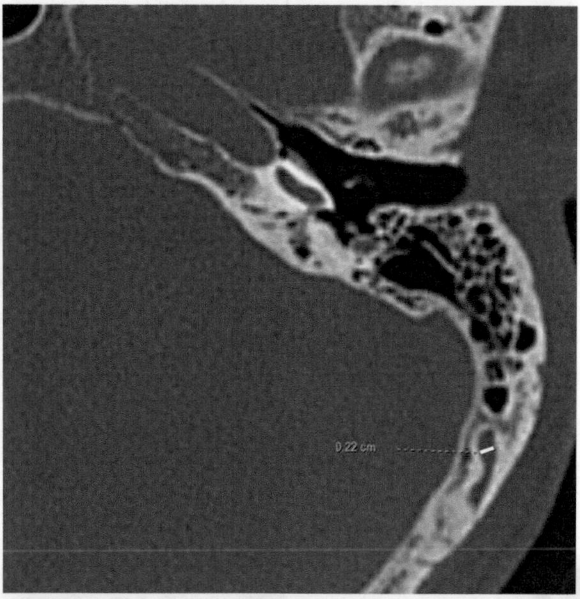

Fig. 37.16 Mastoid emissary vein. Axial HRCT section of the temporal bone shows the normal size of the left mastoid emissary vein

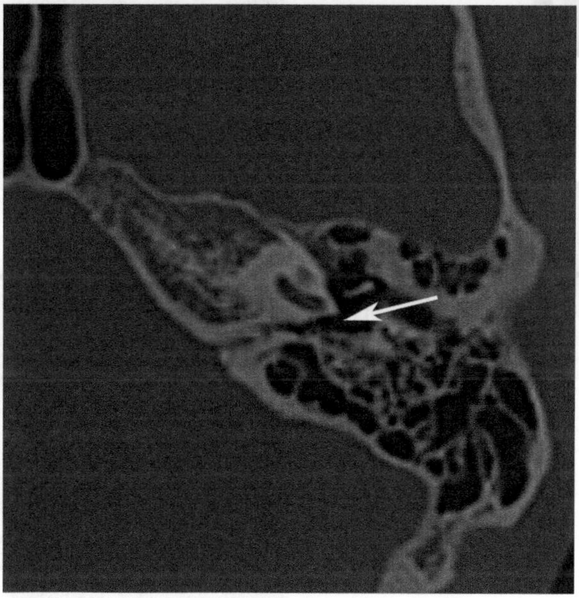

Fig. 37.17 Hyrtl's fissure. Axial HRCT section of the temporal bone shows a tympanomeningeal (Hyrtl's) fissure on the left side inferior to the round window (arrow)

37.3 Presurgical Assessment of Inner Ear Malformations

The presurgical assessment is crucial to assess the inner ear malformations (IEMs) that preclude cochlear implantation, characterized by the absence of the cochlea and the cochlear nerve, as well as lack of communication between the otocyst and the brainstem, including complete labyrinthine aplasia, rudimentary otocyst, cochlear aplasia, and cochlear nerve aplasia (Figs. 37.18 and 37.19) [7, 12]. Auditory brainstem implantation may be considered for hearing rehabilitation in these patients.

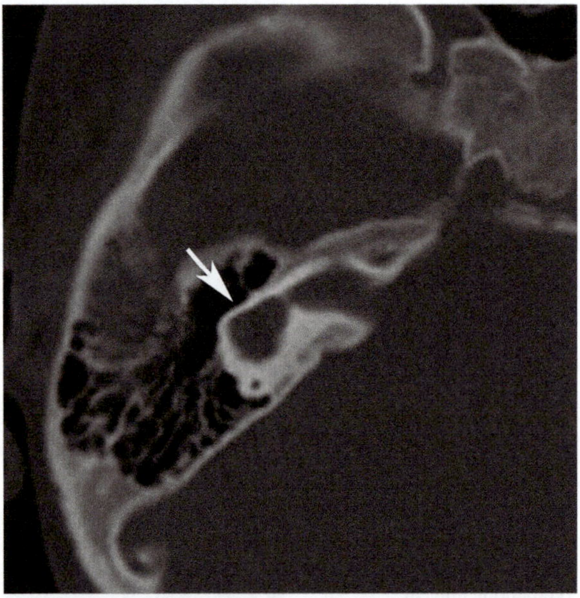

Fig. 37.18 Cochlear aplasia with dilated vestibule. Axial HRCT section of the temporal bone shows the absence of cochlea and dysplastic vestibule (arrow) posterior to the lateral end of the internal auditory canal

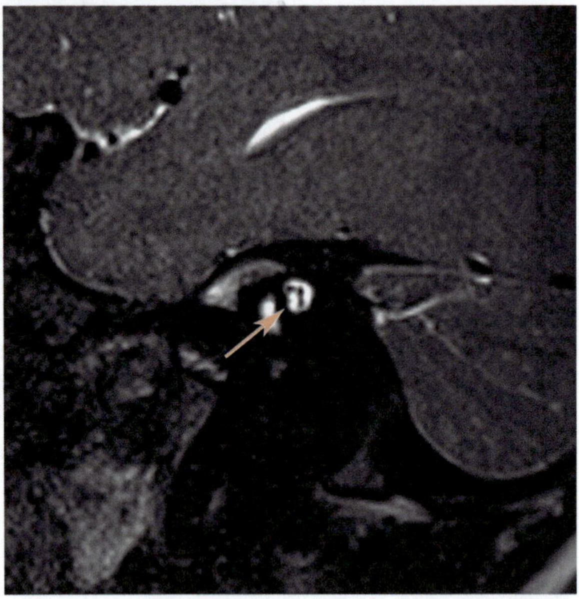

Fig. 37.19 Cochlear nerve aplasia. Sagittal oblique T2-weighted image through the internal auditory canal demonstrates the absence of the cochlear nerve in the anteroinferior aspect of the internal auditory canal (arrow)

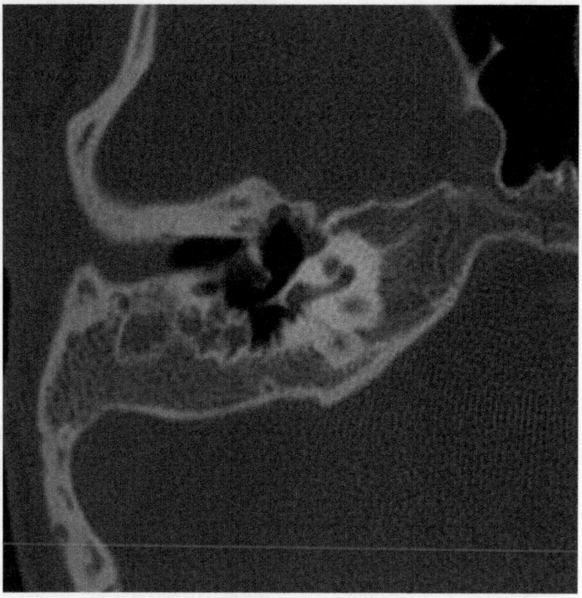

Fig. 37.20 Cochlear hypoplasia with unwound cochlea. Axial HRCT section of the temporal bone shows hypoplasia of the middle and apical turns of the cochlea with increased separation in the lateral aspect suggesting cochlear hypoplasia

The choice of the cochlear implant electrode depends on the malformed cochlea in cases of IEMs. U-shaped electrodes are placed along the inner wall near the IAC fundus in common cavity malformations to maximize cochlear neuroepithelial stimulation [20], while a short electrode array is used in cases of cochlear hypoplasia (Fig. 37.20) [12]. The incidence of postoperative facial nerve stimulation has been reported to be more than 50% in patients with common cavity malformation, especially with abnormal course of the facial nerve and a combined cochleovestibular structure.

In patients with vestibulocochlear nerve abnormalities, the choice for hearing rehabilitation depends on the presence of an intact cochlear nerve that may be assessed by cochlear promontory stimulation. Auditory brainstem implantation may be necessary in cases with non-visualized vestibulocochlear and cochlear nerves for acceptable language development [12].

Focused attention on the enlarged vestibular aqueduct, absent modiolus, and the corkscrew appearance of the cochlea is necessary due to the potential risk of CSF leaks and gushers in patients with common cavity malformation, cochlear hypoplasia, and incomplete partition types II and III [12, 21–23]. CSF gusher occurs in only 3% of patients with normal inner ear anatomy, compared to 29% of patients with IP II and an enlarged vestibular aqueduct, and 38% of patients with cochlear hypoplasia [24, 25].

Other potential complications include the risk of perilymphatic fistula and meningitis in a few inner ear malformations with defective footplate of stapes, including common cavity malformation, cochlear hypoplasia type II, and incomplete partition types I, II, and III (Figs. 37.21, 37.22, and 37.23).

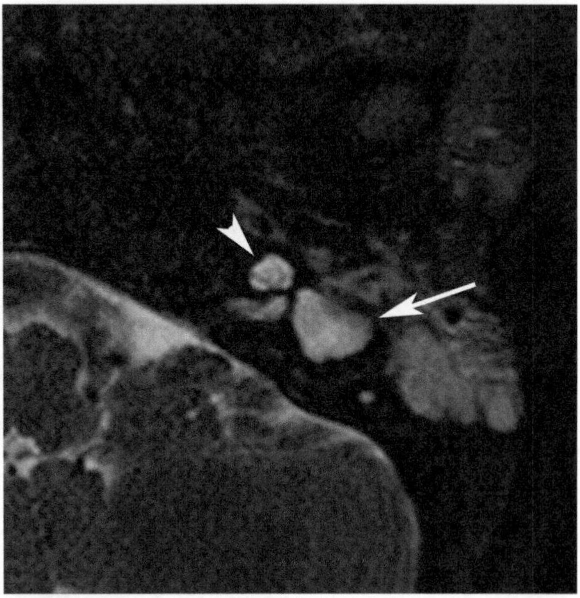

Fig. 37.21 Incomplete partition type 1. Axial heavily T2-weighted image through the left inner ear shows a cystic enlarged cochlea (arrowhead) without modiolus and interscalar septum and separated from a dilated vestibule (arrow) posterior to the IAC and demonstrates a typical figure-of-8 appearance

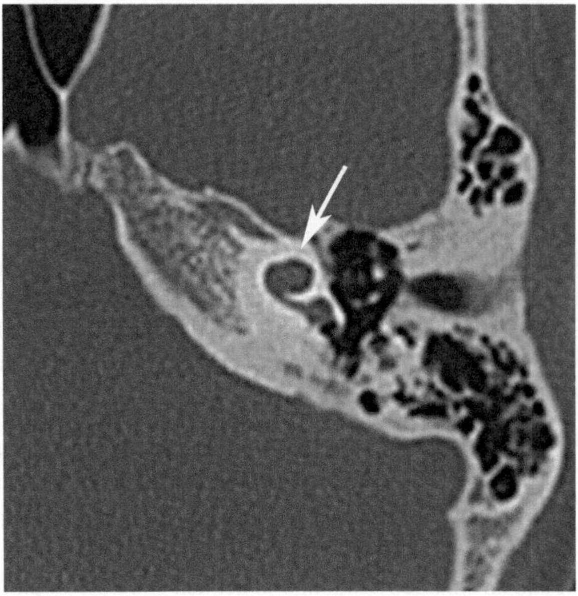

Fig. 37.22 Incomplete partition type 2. Axial HRCT section of the temporal bone shows cystic fusion of the apical and middle turns (arrowheads) along with absent modiolus and interscalar septum in the apex

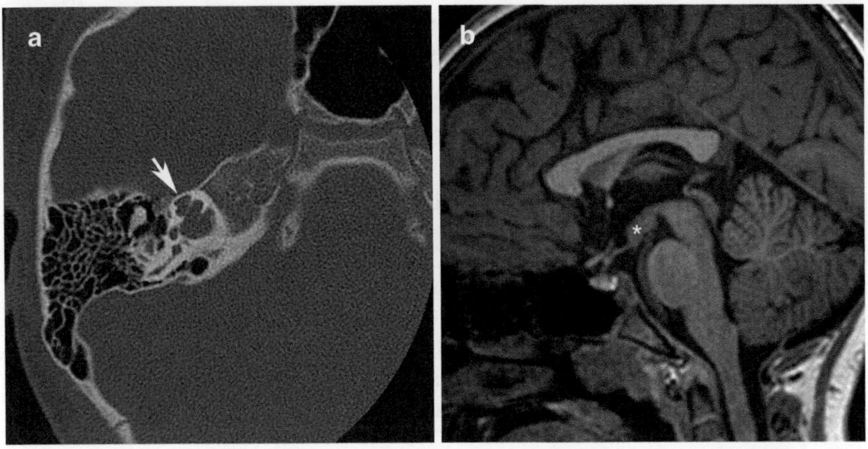

Fig. 37.23 Incomplete partition type 3 with hypothalamic hamartoma. Axial HRCT of the temporal bone (**a**) shows cochlear aperture widening with absent modiolus and corkscrew appearance of the cochlea (arrow in **a**). Sagittal T1-weighted image (**b**) shows increased lobulated thickening involving the hypothalamus (asterisk) suggesting hypothalamic hamartoma

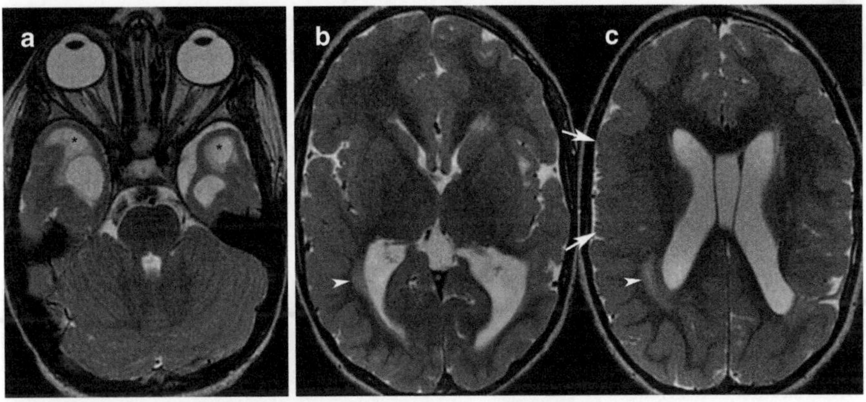

Fig. 37.24 Congenital CMV infection. Axial T2-weighted images of the brain (**a-c**) showing anterior temporal lobe cysts (asterisk in **a**), posterior periventricular white matter hyperintensity (arrowhead in **b**), and abnormal gyration in both frontal lobes (arrows in **c**)

37.3.1 Brain Parenchymal Assessment

The presurgical assessment of the brain is necessary to evaluate for the presence of foci of white matter signal abnormality, anterior temporal lobe cysts, and/or polymicrogyria in congenital cytomegalovirus infections due to their potential impact on auditory outcome after cochlear implantation (Fig. 37.24). A thorough assessment is essential to identify related hypothalamic abnormalities in incomplete partition type III (Fig. 37.23) and posterior fossa malformations in patients with congenital muscular dystrophy, LAMA1 mutations, and pontine tegmental cap dysplasia. Additionally, it is essential to assess imaging findings that may indicate associated metabolic disorders [7, 26–28].

37.4 Presurgical Assessment of Acquired Sensorineural Hearing Loss

The acquired causes of sensorineural hearing loss, affecting the cochlear patency, otic capsule, round window, and the internal auditory canal include labyrinthitis ossificans, otospongiosis, round window stenosis, and tumors involving the internal auditory canal and cerebellopontine angle cistern.

37.4.1 Labyrinthitis Ossificans

The inner ear inflammation due to otogenic and tympanic infections, trauma, metabolic disorders, labyrinthine hemorrhage, and autoimmune disorders may result in luminal obstruction due to fibrosis and neo-ossification of the cochlea. The most common etiology encountered in pediatric cochlear implant candidates includes meningitis, resulting in varying degrees of neo-ossification in up to 70% of patients [29]. The cochlear basal turn neo-ossification may be seen in up to 15% of adults and between 28% and 35% of pediatric patients with hearing loss (Fig. 37.25) [30, 31].

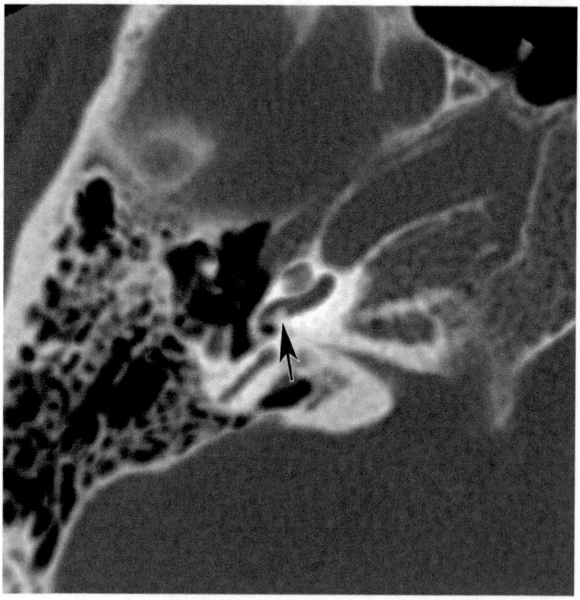

Fig. 37.25 Labyrinthitis ossificans with neo-ossification in the basal turn of the cochlea. Axial HRCT section of the right temporal bone demonstrates isolated focal ossification in the lateral aspect of the scala tympani in the basal turn of the cochlea (arrow)

There are three stages of labyrinthitis, including the initial acute inflammatory stage, followed by the fibrotic stage, usually between 2 weeks and 2 months after primary insult and eventual labyrinthitis ossificans progressing to calcification and luminal obliteration (Figs. 37.26, 37.27, and 37.28). The proximal scala tympani in the basal turn of the cochlea adjacent to the cochlear aqueduct opening and the round window are usually involved in meningogenic and tympanogenic labyrinthitis [32]. The involvement of the middle and apical turns is uncommon, with relative sparing of the scala vestibuli. Complete ossification of the cochlea with luminal obliteration may occur, more commonly in children than adults [33].

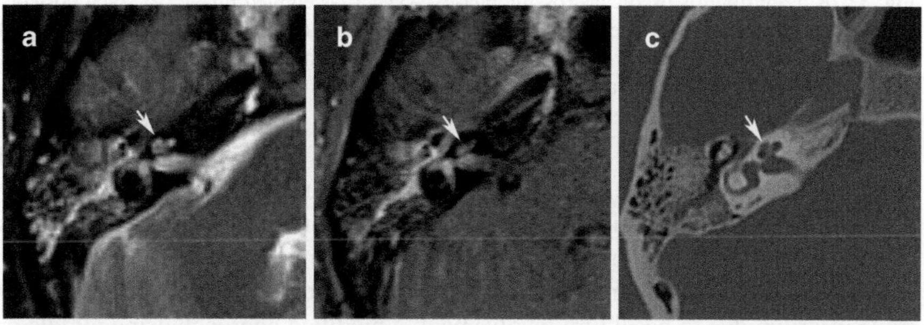

Fig. 37.26 Labyrinthitis ossificans (inflammatory phase). Axial T2-weighted image (**a**), axial postcontrast T1-weighted image (**b**), and axial CT of the temporal bone (**c**) demonstrate slightly decreased fluid signal intensity in the inner ear structures (arrow in **a**) with enhancement in the cochlea, vestibule, and semicircular canals (arrow in **b**) and lack of ossification (arrow in **c**)

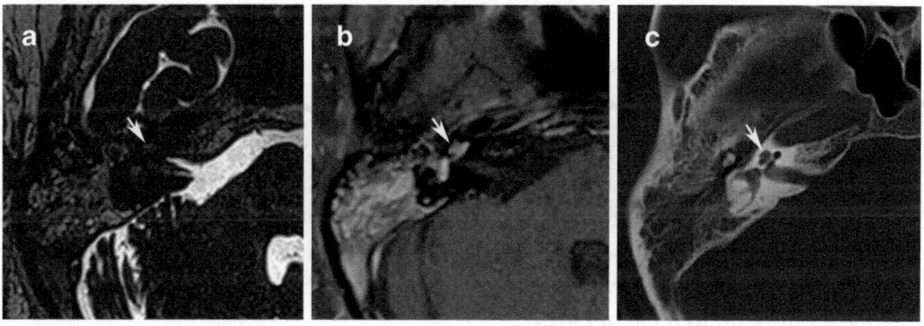

Fig. 37.27 Labyrinthitis ossificans (fibrotic phase). Axial heavily T2-weighted image (**a**), axial postcontrast T1-weighted image (**b**), and axial CT of the temporal bone (**c**) demonstrate loss of fluid signal intensity in the inner ear structures (arrow in **a**) with enhancement in the cochlea, vestibule, and semicircular canals (arrow in **b**) and lack of ossification (arrow in **c**)

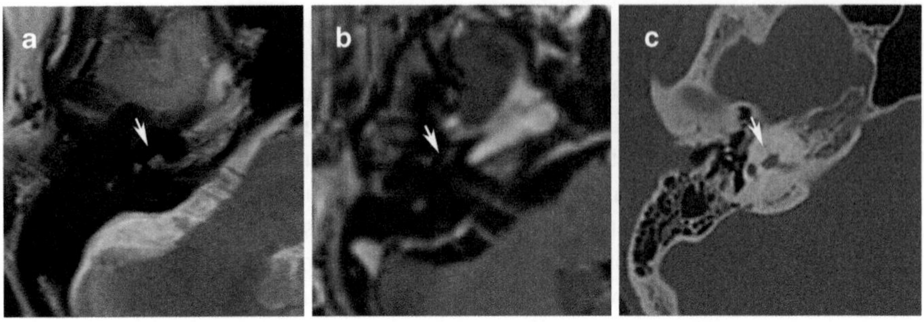

Fig. 37.28 Labyrinthitis ossificans (ossific phase). Axial T2-weighted image (**a**), axial postcontrast T1-weighted image (**b**), and axial CT of the temporal bone (**c**) demonstrate loss of fluid signal intensity in the inner ear structures (arrow in **a**) with lack of enhancement (arrow in **b**) and ossification in the apical, middle, and basal turns of the cochlea (arrow in **c**)

Cochlear ossification is associated with severe loss of cochlear hair cells and a reduction in the spiral ganglion cell population [34]. Labyrinthitis ossificans is usually partial with asymmetric luminal obstruction, and the presurgical evaluation is crucial in assessing the severity of cochlear involvement, delineating the scalar chambers, side selection, and prognostication [35]. In cases with complicated electrode insertion due to basal turn involvement, a modified approach using middle or apical cochleostomy and a circum-modiolar drill-out procedure may be required for cochlear implantation [36]. Scala vestibuli insertion may be performed for isolated obliteration of the scala tympani. Extensive cochlear obliteration in advanced labyrinthitis ossificans precludes cochlear implantation.

37.4.2 Otospongiosis

Otospongiosis is an autosomal dominant osteodystrophy characterized by abnormal bony remodeling with initial osteoclastic resorption, otic capsule demineralization, and irregular woven spongiotic vascular bone formation that is eventually replaced by dense abnormal sclerotic bone [37]. It usually presents in the second to fourth decade of life with conductive, sensorineural, or mixed hearing loss and bilateral involvement in up to 85% of cases.

Fenestral otosclerosis typically involves the fissula ante fenestram, along with possible involvement of the cochlear promontory, round window niche, and the tympanic segment of the facial nerve. The retrofenestral form, a continuum of fenestral otosclerosis, is associated with the involvement of the cochlear capsule, which may extend to the vestibule, semicircular canals, and internal auditory canal. On HRCT, the fenestral form appears as focal lucency involving the fissula ante fenestram that progresses into retrofenestral form, with lucency surrounding the cochlea (double-ring sign), vestibule, semicircular canals, and the internal auditory canal [38]. The dense, heaped-up otospongiotic plaques may lead to round and oval window stenosis (Fig. 37.29). Rarely, there is membranous labyrinth ossification that is usually limited to the basal turn of the cochlea [39].

An early cochlear implantation would facilitate electrode placement using a round window insertion technique. Otospongiotic plaques causing the round window obliteration are usually associated with surgical difficulty, suboptimal insertion, and misplaced electrodes and may need a cochleostomy and bony drilling [7].

Obliteration of the basal turn of the cochlea is a relative contraindication to cochlear implantation [38]. Otospongiosis is associated with an increased risk of postoperative facial nerve stimulation due to bone demineralization between the superior aspect of the basal turn of the cochlea and the labyrinthine segment of the facial nerve (Fig. 37.30). In the postsurgical period, the cochleostomy approach is associated with significant fibrosis and neo-osteogenesis in the basal turn of the cochlea, causing obliteration of scala tympani and extending into the scala media and scala vestibuli in some cases compared to minimal neo-osteogenesis with the round window insertion [40].

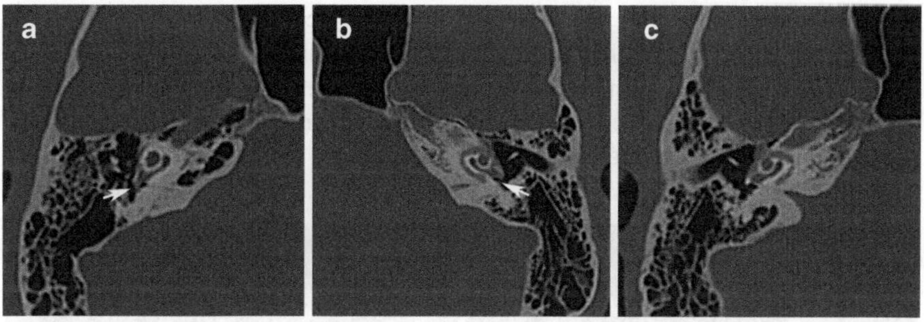

Fig. 37.29 Otospongiosis with round window stenosis. Axial HRCT sections of the temporal bone (**a–c**) demonstrating pericochlear lucency with heaped-up non-ossified plaques causing the round window stenosis (arrow in **a** and **b**). The normal appearance of the round window in another case of otospongiosis is shown in **c**

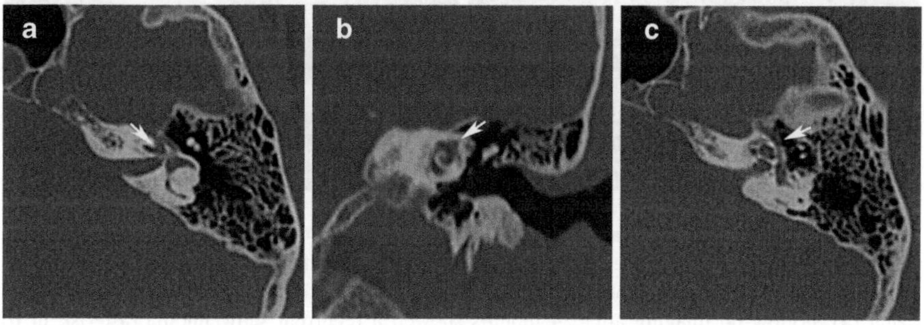

Fig. 37.30 Otospongiosis with facial nerve dehiscence. Axial and coronal (**a**, **b**) HRCT sections of the temporal bone demonstrate lucency with loss of bony separation between the basal turn of the cochlea and the labyrinthine segment of the facial nerve. Axial HRCT section of the temporal bone (**c**) showing pericochlear lucency reaching up to the tympanic segment of the facial nerve

37.4.3 Vestibular Schwannoma

Sensorineural hearing loss in vestibular schwannoma is multifactorial and postulated to be due to mechanical compression and cochlear nerve damage secondary to tumor growth and cellular damage from tumor-secreted factors, including tumor necrosis factor-alpha and extracellular vesicles [41]. Stereotactic neurosurgery may result in tissue damage from vascular injury with postulated stria vascularis injury leading to posttreatment hearing loss [42]. Hearing loss following vestibular schwannoma resection may be due to injury to the cochlear nerve, otic capsule of the membranous labyrinth, and vascular insult [43].

Cochlear implantation is associated with favorable outcomes in sporadic and neurofibromatosis 2-related vestibular schwannomas in patients with long-term tumor stability, small tumor size, and preserved cerebrospinal fluid between the lateral margin of the tumor and the fundus of the internal auditory canal [44, 45]. Large tumors, multifocal involvement, and involvement of the neurovascular structures may result in less favorable outcomes in neurofibromatosis 2 [46].

Cochlear implantation is performed along with tumor resection or as an early second surgery due to the potential risk of postsurgical labyrinthine fibrosis and eventual cochlear obliteration from labyrinthitis ossificans occurring after about 16 months (median duration; interquartile range 12–18.9 months) (Fig. 37.31) [47]. The presence of an intact cochlear nerve is assessed intraoperatively by electrical promontory stimulation or electrically evoked auditory brainstem response.

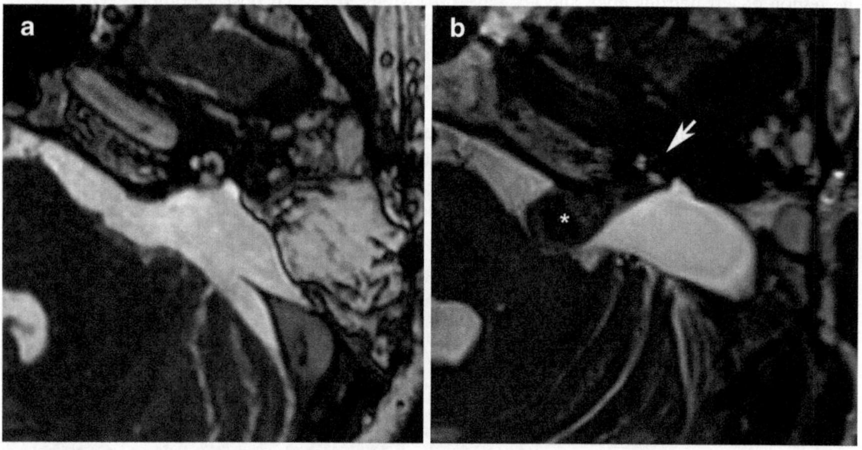

Fig. 37.31 Labyrinthitis ossificans after translabyrinthine resection of schwannoma. Axial heavily T2-weighted images through the posterior fossa (**a**, **b**) demonstrate postsurgical changes related to left translabyrinthine resection of schwannoma involving the posterior wall of the internal auditory canal (**a**). Follow-up imaging after 24 months showed a recurrent schwannoma (asterisk in **b**) along with loss of fluid signal intensity in the apical and middle turns of the cochlea suggesting labyrinthitis ossificans

37.5 Conclusion

Presurgical assessment using CT and MRI is crucial for assessing anatomical factors and congenital or acquired sensorineural hearing loss. These imaging modalities provide critical information to the operating surgeon regarding factors influencing the surgical technique, implant selection, and electrode type. In addition, the radiologist needs to highlight key findings associated with surgical challenges to help prevent potential complications.

References

1. Deafness and hearing loss [Internet]. [cited 2024 Nov 27]. Available from: https://www.who.int/news-room/fact-sheets/detail/deafness-and-hearing-loss.
2. Benson JC, Carlson ML, Lane JI. MRI of the internal auditory canal, labyrinth, and middle ear: how we do it. Radiology. 2020;297:252–65.
3. Chin O, Dharsono F, Kuthubutheen J, Thompson A. Is CT necessary for imaging paediatric congenital sensorineural hearing loss? Cochlear Implants Int. 2020;21:75–82.
4. Mackeith S, Joy R, Robinson P, Hajioff D. Pre-operative imaging for cochlear implantation: magnetic resonance imaging, computed tomography, or both? Cochlear Implants Int. 2012;13:133–6.
5. Malhotra V, Kumar S, Menon GS, Hejjaji Krishnamurthy A, Medikeri S, Dutt SN. Morphometric analysis of temporal bone radiology for cochlear implant candidacy. Indian J Otolaryngol Head Neck Surg. 2024;76:702–11.
6. Aladeyelu OS, Olaniyi KS, Olojede SO, Mbatha W-BE, Sibiya AL, Rennie CO. Temporal bone pneumatization: a scoping review on the growth and size of mastoid air cell system with age. PLoS One. 2022;17:e0269360.
7. Hiremath SB, Biswas A, Mndebele G, Schramm D, Ertl-Wagner BB, Blaser SI, et al. Cochlear implantation: systematic approach to preoperative radiologic evaluation. Radiographics. 2023;43:e220102.
8. Alexiades G, Dhanasingh A, Jolly C. Method to estimate the complete and two-turn cochlear duct length. Otol Neurotol. 2015;36:904–7.
9. Dhanasingh A. Cochlear duct length along the outer wall vs organ of corti: which one is relevant for the electrode array length selection and frequency mapping using Greenwood function? World J Otorhinolaryngol Head Neck Surg. 2019;5:117–21.
10. Spiegel JL, Polterauer D, Hempel J-M, Canis M, Spiro JE, Müller J. Variation of the cochlear anatomy and cochlea duct length: analysis with a new tablet-based software. Eur Arch Otorrinolaringol. 2022;279:1851–61.
11. Pamuk G, Pamuk AE, Akgöz A, Bajin MD, Özgen B, Sennaroğlu L. Radiological measurement of cochlear dimensions in cochlear hypoplasia and its effect on cochlear implant selection. J Laryngol Otol. 2021;135:501–7.
12. Sennaroğlu L, Bajin MD. Classification and current management of inner ear malformations. Balkan Med J. 2017;34:397–411.
13. Marsot-Dupuch K, Meyer B. Cochlear implant assessment: imaging issues. Eur J Radiol. 2001;40:119–32.
14. Bunne M, Myhrum M, Iftikhar M, Rasmussen K, Falkenberg-Jensen B. Cochlear-facial dehiscence – the most common cause of facial nerve stimulation from a cochlear implant? A case–control study. Cochlear Implants Int [Internet]. 2024 [cited 2024 Dec 25]. Available from: https://www.tandfonline.com/doi/abs/10.1080/14670100.2024.2316452.

15. Sullivan AM, Curtin HD, Moonis G. Arterial anomalies of the middle ear: a pictorial review with clinical-embryologic and imaging correlation. Neuroimaging Clin N Am. 2019;29:93–102.
16. Clarke R, Booth T. CT and MR imaging of the pediatric temporal bone: normal variants and pitfalls. Curr Radiol Rep. 2017;5:34.
17. Manjila S, Bazil T, Kay M, Udayasankar UK, Semaan M. Jugular bulb and skull base pathologies: proposal for a novel classification system for jugular bulb positions and microsurgical implications. Neurosurg Focus. 2018;45:E5.
18. Atmaca S, Elmali M, Kucuk H. High and dehiscent jugular bulb: clear and present danger during middle ear surgery. Surg Radiol Anat. 2014;36:369–74.
19. Mandour M, Tomoum M, El Zayat S, Hamad H, Amer M. Surgeon oriented preoperative radiologic evaluation in cochlear implantation – our experience with a proposed checklist. Int Arch Otorhinolaryngol. 2019;23:137–41.
20. Bae SH, Choi J, Choi JY. Cochlear implants for patients with common cavity deformities and the impact of electrode positioning. Clin Exp Otorhinolaryngol. 2022;15:77–83.
21. Casselman JW, Offeciers EF, De Foer B, Govaerts P, Kuhweide R, Somers T. CT and MR imaging of congenital abnormalities of the inner ear and internal auditory canal. Eur J Radiol. 2001;40:94–104.
22. Ginat DT. Imaging findings in syndromes with temporal bone abnormalities. Neuroimaging Clin N Am. 2019;29:117–28.
23. O'Brien WT, D'Arco F, Onofrj V, Koch BL. Nonsyndromic congenital causes of sensorineural hearing loss in children: an illustrative review. AJR Am J Roentgenol. 2021;216:1048–55.
24. Kamogashira T, Akamatsu Y, Kashio A, Ogata E, Karino S, Kakigi A, et al. Development of auditory skills after cochlear implantation in children with inner ear malformations. Acta Otolaryngol. 2016;136:78–82.
25. Vashist S, Singh S. CSF Gusher in Cochlear Implant Surgery-does it affect surgical outcomes? Eur Ann Otorhinolaryngol Head Neck Dis. 2016;133(Suppl 1):S21–4.
26. Trinh T-T, Blasco H, Maillot F, Bakhos D. Hearing loss in inherited metabolic disorders: a systematic review. Metabolism. 2021;122:154841.
27. Alarcón A, de Vries LS, Parodi A, Arnáez J, Cabañas F, Steggerda SJ, et al. Neuroimaging in infants with congenital cytomegalovirus infection and its correlation with outcome: emphasis on white matter abnormalities. Arch Dis Child Fetal Neonatal Ed. 2024;109:151–8.
28. D'Arco F, Youssef A, Ioannidou E, Bisdas S, Pinelli L, Caro-Dominguez P, et al. Temporal bone and intracranial abnormalities in syndromic causes of hearing loss: an updated guide. Eur J Radiol. 2020;123:108803.
29. Seidman DA, Chute PM, Parisier S. Temporal bone imaging for cochlear implantation. Laryngoscope. 1994;104:562–5.
30. Balkany T, Gantz B, Nadol JB. Multichannel cochlear implants in partially ossified cochleas. Ann Otol Rhinol Laryngol Suppl. 1988;135:3–7.
31. Harnsberger HR, Dart DJ, Parkin JL, Smoker WR, Osborn AG. Cochlear implant candidates: assessment with CT and MR imaging. Radiology. 1987;164:53–7.
32. Green JD, Marion MS, Hinojosa R. Labyrinthitis ossificans: histopathologic consideration for cochlear implantation. Otolaryngol Head Neck Surg. 1991;104:320–6.
33. Ketten DR. The role of temporal bone imaging in cochlear implants. Curr Opin Otolaryngol Head Neck Surg. 1994;2:401–8.
34. Otte J, Schunknecht HF, Kerr AG. Ganglion cell populations in normal and pathological human cochleae. Implications for cochlear implantation. Laryngoscope. 1978;88:1231–46.
35. Isaacson B, Booth T, Kutz JW, Lee KH, Roland PS. Labyrinthitis ossificans: how accurate is MRI in predicting cochlear obstruction? Otolaryngol Head Neck Surg. 2009;140:692–6.
36. Balkany T, Gantz BJ, Steenerson RL, Cohen NL. Systematic approach to electrode insertion in the ossified cochlea. Otolaryngol Head Neck Surg. 1996;114:4–11.
37. Davis GL. Pathology of otosclerosis: a review. Am J Otolaryngol. 1987;8:273–81.
38. Purohit B, Hermans R, Op de Beeck K. Imaging in otosclerosis: a pictorial review. Insights Imaging. 2014;5:245–52.

39. Rotteveel LJC, Proops DW, Ramsden RT, Saeed SR, van Olphen AF, Mylanus EAM. Cochlear implantation in 53 patients with otosclerosis: demographics, computed tomographic scanning, surgery, and complications. Otol Neurotol. 2004;25:943–52.
40. Hodge SE, Ishiyama G, Lopez IA, Ishiyama A. Histopathologic analysis of temporal bones with otosclerosis following cochlear implantation. Otol Neurotol. 2021;42:1492.
41. Early S, Rinnooy Kan CE, Eggink M, Frijns JHM, Stankovic KM. Progression of contralateral hearing loss in patients with sporadic vestibular schwannoma. Front Neurol [Internet]. 2020 [cited 2024 Dec 4];11. Available from: https://www.frontiersin.org/journals/neurology/articles/10.3389/fneur.2020.00796/full.
42. Wackym PA, Runge-Samuelson CL, Nash JJ, Poetker DM, Albano K, Bovi J, et al. Gamma knife surgery of vestibular schwannomas: volumetric dosimetry correlations to hearing loss suggest stria vascularis devascularization as the mechanism of early hearing loss. Otol Neurotol. 2010;31:1480–7.
43. Babbage MJ, Feldman MB, O'Beirne GA, MacFarlane MR, Bird PA. Patterns of hearing loss following retrosigmoid excision of unilateral vestibular schwannoma. J Neurol Surg B Skull Base. 2013;74:166–75.
44. Carlson ML, Vivas EX, McCracken DJ, Sweeney AD, Neff BA, Shepard NT, et al. Congress of neurological surgeons systematic review and evidence-based guidelines on hearing preservation outcomes in patients with sporadic vestibular schwannomas. Neurosurgery. 2018;82:E35.
45. Tadokoro K, Bartindale MR, El-Kouri N, Moore D, Britt C, Kircher M. Cochlear implantation in vestibular schwannoma: a systematic literature review. J Neurol Surg B Skull Base. 2021;82:643–51.
46. Hallak D, Macielak RJ, Zhang L, Ren Y. Cochlear implantation and vestibular schwannoma management. Curr Otorhinolaryngol Rep. 2024;12:66–75.
47. Feng Y, Lane JI, Lohse CM, Carlson ML. Pattern of cochlear obliteration after vestibular Schwannoma resection according to surgical approach. Laryngoscope. 2020;130:474–81.

Chapter 38
Postoperative Imaging in Temporal Bone

Shivaprakash B. Hiremath, Neetika Gupta, Paula Alcaide Leon, Pradeep Krishnan, and Elka Miller

38.1 Introduction

The combination of preexisting abnormalities and a wide variety of complex surgical techniques leads to distortion of the regional anatomy of the temporal bone, middle, and posterior cranial fossa. Understanding surgical techniques and imaging findings is necessary to distinguish between the expected postoperative changes, recurrent disease, and complications and to inform the surgeon about critical findings.

The most common surgical techniques involving the temporal bone can be classified as procedures for middle ear drainage and equalizing the tympanic pressure (myringotomy and tympanostomy tubes), functional reconstruction of the conductive apparatus (tympanoplasty, ossicular reconstruction, including stapedotomy and stapedectomy), eradication of the middle ear disease and cholesteatoma (mastoidectomy), hearing rehabilitation in severe sensorineural hearing loss (cochlear and auditory brain implantation), and access for surgical management of the internal auditory canal, middle, and posterior cranial fossa pathology (middle cranial fossa, retrosigmoid, and translabyrinthine approach).

S. B. Hiremath (✉) · P. Alcaide Leon
Division of Neuroradiology, Joint Department of Medical Imaging, Toronto Western Hospital, University Health Network, University of Toronto, Toronto, ON, Canada

N. Gupta
Department of Medical Imaging, Children's Hospital of Eastern Ontario, Department of Radiology, Radiation Oncology, and Medical Physics, University of Ottawa, Ottawa, ON, Canada

P. Krishnan · E. Miller
Department of Diagnostic and Interventional Radiology, The Hospital for Sick Children, University of Toronto, Toronto, ON, Canada

H. Mahalingam (ed.), *Temporal Bone Imaging*,
https://doi.org/10.1007/978-981-95-6132-2_38

Radiographs are commonly used for intraoperative imaging, while postoperative evaluation is typically performed with CT and MRI. CT is the primary imaging modality used to assess the continuity of the prosthesis, as well as the aeration and opacification of the mastoid cavity. MRI is better for monitoring recurrent cholesteatoma and further characterize mastoid opacification. This chapter discusses the neuro-otologic surgical techniques involving the temporal bone, highlighting the postsurgical findings, recurrent disease, and postoperative complications described in Table 38.1.

Table 38.1 Surgical techniques in the temporal bone and postoperative complications

Surgical technique	Complications
Tympanostomy tubes	Tympanostomy tube obstruction Persistent middle ear and mastoid opacification Granulation tissue and cholesteatoma formation Accidental displacement and partial extrusion
Tympanoplasty and ossicular chain reconstruction	Ossicular chain dislocation and graft necrosis Prosthetic malpositioning, fixation, and dislocation Labyrinthitis and perilymphatic fistula
Mastoidectomy	Inflammatory mucosa and granulation tissue Fibrosis and cholesterol granuloma Residual and recurrent cholesteatoma
Middle cranial fossa approach	Residual and recurrent tumor Labyrinthine inflammation, vascular injury, and fenestration
Retrosigmoid approach	Residual and recurrent tumor Labyrinthine inflammation, vascular injury, and fenestration Cerebellar infarction and hemorrhage Fat graft necrosis and transverse and sigmoid sinus thrombosis Cerebrospinal fluid leaks
Translabyrinthine approach	Residual and recurrent tumor Fat graft necrosis and labyrinthitis ossificans
Transcutaneous bone conduction devices	Bleeding and extra-axial hemorrhage Sigmoid sinus injury and thrombosis CSF leaks, meningitis, and cerebritis Failure of osseointegration, idiopathic resorption, and rarely bone overgrowth
Cochlear implantation	Early: Pinching, tip and basal fold-over, and malpositioning Delayed: Recurrent otitis media, cholesteatoma, and labyrinthitis Fibrosis and delayed nerve injury

38.2 Myringotomy and Tympanostomy Tubes

Tympanostomy tubes are small cylindrical tubes inserted into the tympanic membrane to treat middle ear effusion often associated with recurrent acute or chronic otitis media due to eustachian tube dysfunction [1]. Tympanostomy tubes facilitate middle ear fluid drainage, equalize intratympanic pressure, and improve hearing by reducing middle ear effusion. They are made of various materials, including plastics and metals, and are evident on CT (Fig. 38.1). Depending on the size, shape, and material, they are spontaneously expelled, generally by 3–24 months.

It is essential to recognize the imaging appearance of tympanostomy tubes to avoid potential misdiagnosis as a foreign body or ossicular dislocation. On clinical examination, fluid opacification and malpositioning hinder tube identification. CT is usually performed to evaluate possible complications, including tube obstruction, persistent opacification of the middle ear and mastoid, granulation tissue and cholesteatoma formation, accidental displacement into the eustachian tube, and partial extrusion into the middle ear (Fig. 38.2). The presence of tympanostomy tubes beyond 2 years is concerning for retained tympanostomy tubes [2].

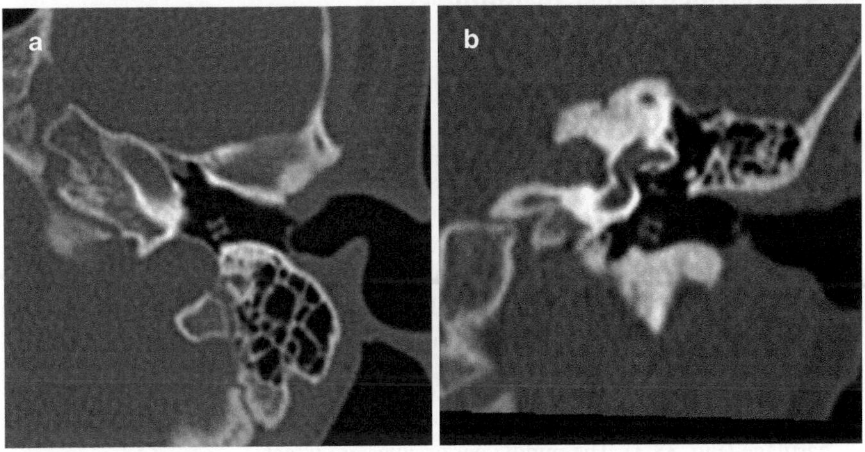

Fig. 38.1 Tympanostomy tubes. Axial (**a**) and coronal CT (**b**) shows a Teflon grommet tube across the tympanic membrane

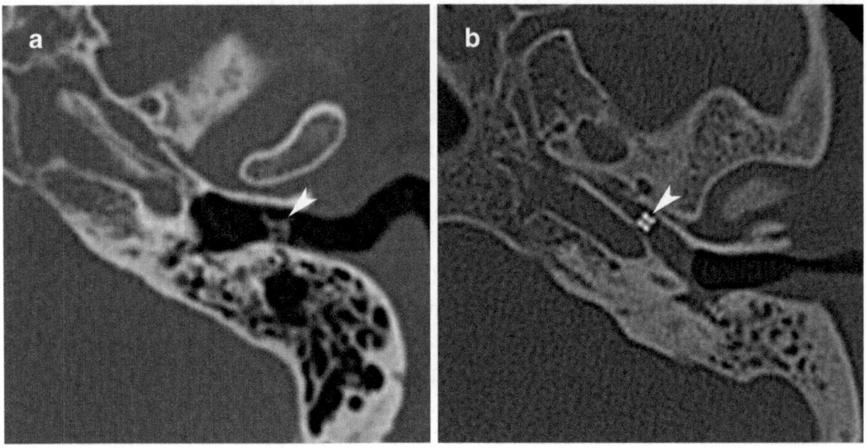

Fig. 38.2 Extrusion and displaced tympanostomy tubes. Axial CT of the left temporal bone (**a**) shows partial extrusion of the Teflon grommet tube (arrowhead) in the external auditory canal. Axial CT of the temporal bone (**b**) shows the metal grommet (arrowhead) displacement into the eustachian tube

38.3 Reconstructive Techniques

38.3.1 Tympanoplasty

Tympanoplasty involves surgically eradicating middle ear disease and restoring the middle ear conductive mechanism. The surgical repair includes varying combinations based on the extent of impairment and potential for functional recovery, involving tympanic membrane repair/reconstruction, inspection and removal of the middle ear disease (cholesteatoma, fibrotic scars, and adhesions), and repair of the involved ossicles. Tympanoplasty procedures are most commonly classified using the Wullstein classification into five distinct types [3].

Type 1 tympanoplasty (myringoplasty) refers to the repair of the perforated tympanic membrane using various grafts, commonly temporalis fascia and auricular cartilage (Fig. 38.3). The middle ear ossicles are intact.

Type 2 tympanoplasty is performed for malleus erosion and involves tympanic graft placement over the residual malleus and incus.

Type 3 tympanoplasty, or myringostapediopexy, refers to placing the tympanic membrane over the head of the stapes after removal of the eroded malleus and incus (Fig. 38.4).

Type 4 tympanoplasty refers to attaching the tympanic membrane to the stapes footplate in cases with extensive erosion of the malleus and incus and involvement of the head, anterior and posterior crus of the stapes, and mobile footplate.

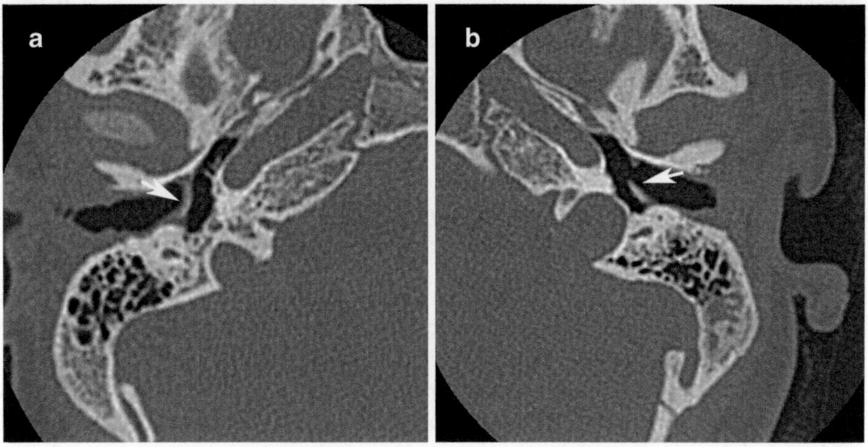

Fig. 38.3 Complicated type 1 tympanoplasty. Axial CT of the temporal bone (**a**, **b**) shows a calcified and thickened tympanic membrane on both sides with a perforation on the left side (arrow in **a** and **b**)

Fig. 38.4 Type 3 tympanoplasty. Axial CT of the temporal bone shows a medialized tympanic membrane placed directly over the head of the stapes (arrow)

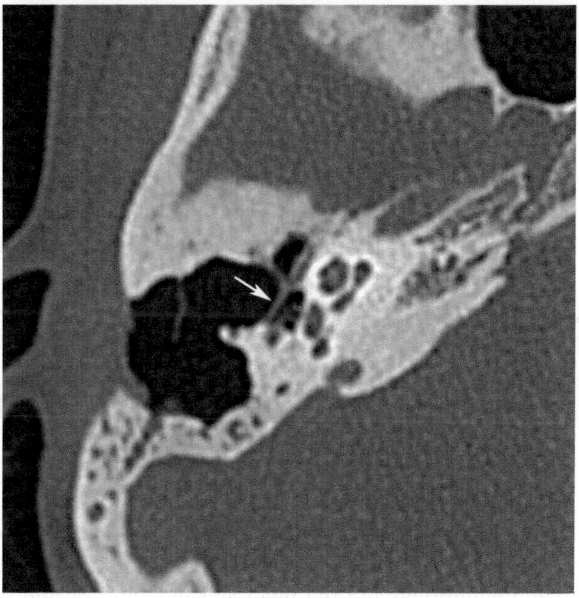

Type 5 tympanoplasty, or fenestration operation, refers to the tympanic membrane attachment to fenestration in the lateral semicircular canal in cases with ossicular chain erosion and stapes footplate fixation.

Types 1 and 3 are most commonly performed, and type 5 tympanoplasty is obsolete. The transcanal and postauricular approaches are used to assess the middle ear.

The CT findings with the transcanal approach include soft tissue thickening, flattening, and defects in the vault of the external auditory canal. Awareness of postoperative findings is essential to avoid misdiagnosing cholesteatoma or malignancy-related osseous erosion.

38.3.2 Ossicular Chain Reconstruction

Ossicular chain reconstruction comprises graft or prosthesis placement between the tympanic membrane and the inner ear to restore the continuity of the conductive mechanism. The common indications include congenital abnormalities of the middle ear, ossicular discontinuity, ossicular erosion due to chronic otitis media and cholesteatoma, and otosclerosis. Ossicular chain reconstruction can be performed with materials such as ossicles, bone, cartilage, and synthetic prostheses (stainless steel, gold, teflon, hydroxyapatite, and titanium) [4]. The choice of the material depends on its properties, indication, extent of disease, and operator experience. The most commonly used prosthetic material includes hydroxyapatite and titanium [5].

38.3.2.1 Incus Interposition Graft

Incus interposition graft is performed in cases with erosion of the lenticular process of the incus. The diseased incus is removed after being carefully disarticulating from the malleus. The remaining incus, including the body and short process, is then reshaped by drilling a notch to receive the manubrium and the stapes head [6, 7]. CT demonstrates preserved continuity with altered morphology of the ossicular chain.

38.3.2.2 Partial and Total Ossicular Replacement Prosthesis

Partial or total ossicular replacement prostheses (PORP and TORP) are used in cases with extensive ossicular discontinuity or lateral fixation of the ossicular chain [8–10]. In cases with an intact head and anterior and posterior crura of the stapes, a PORP is used to restore the conductive mechanism between the tympanic membrane and the head and the anterior and posterior crura of the stapes (Fig. 38.5). A TORP is used when the stapes is either absent or impaired to connect the tympanic membrane to the footplate of the stapes or the oval window (Fig. 38.6a).

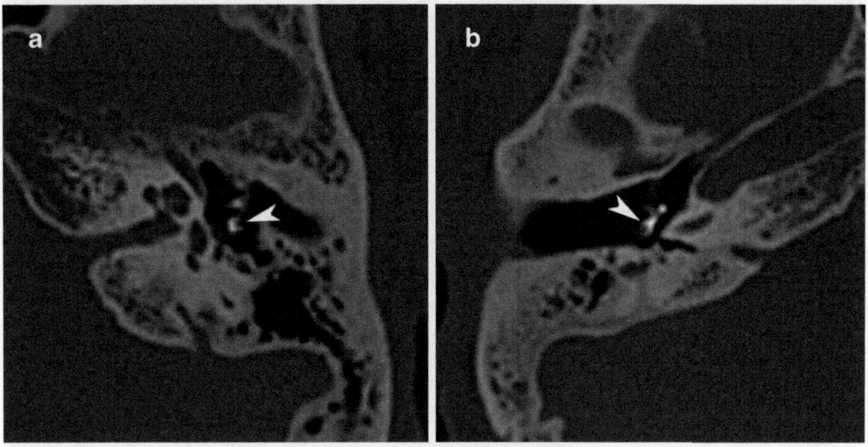

Fig. 38.5 Partial ossicular replacement ossicular prosthesis. Axial CT of the temporal bone (**a**) shows a partial ossicular replacement prosthesis between the tympanic membrane and the head of the stapes. Axial CT of the temporal bone (**b**) shows a partial ossicular replacement prosthesis between the malleus handle and the head of the stapes

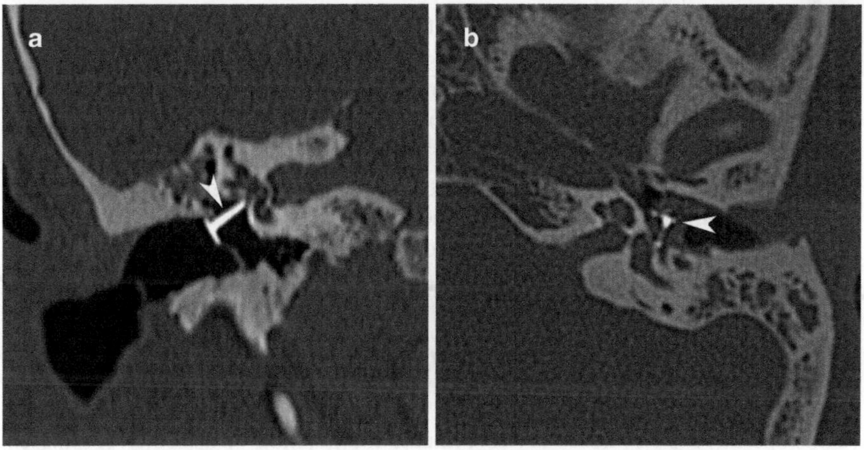

Fig. 38.6 Total ossicular replacement prosthesis. Coronal CT of the temporal bone (**a**) shows a T-shaped prosthesis between the tympanic membrane and the oval window. Axial CT of the temporal bone (**b**) shows soft tissue opacification of the mesotympanum and a displaced total ossicular replacement prosthesis with the tip directed toward the sinus tympani

38.3.2.3 Stapes Surgery

Stapes surgery is commonly performed in patients with otosclerosis, resulting in stapes footplate fixation due to spongiotic and sclerotic plaques to restore the conductive mechanism. The surgical management in such patients involves stapedotomy or stapedectomy with partial or total ossicular replacement prostheses [11, 12].

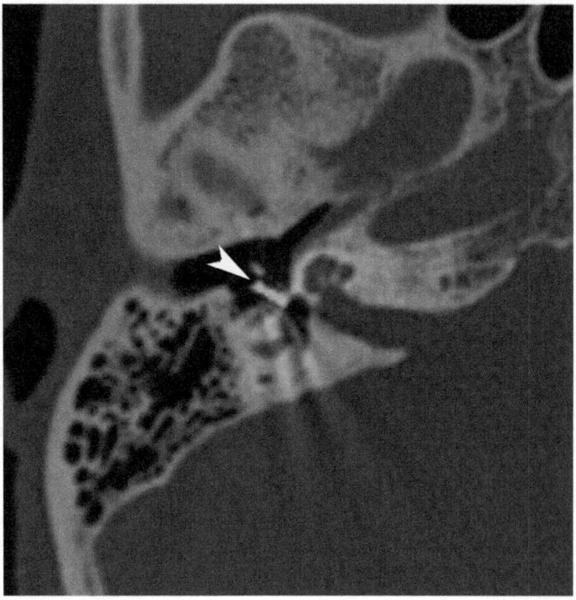

Fig. 38.7 Stapes prosthesis. Axial CT of the temporal bone shows a metallic piston and bucket handle prosthesis articulating with the oval window

In stapedotomy, a small hole is drilled in the footplate with the insertion of a stapes prosthesis, usually between the long process of incus, or infrequently, the lenticular process and the oval window. Stapedectomy involves removing the stapes superstructure and footplate to facilitate the prosthesis insertion into the oval window (Fig. 38.7).

The anatomical factors influencing surgical planning in patients undergoing ossicular chain reconstruction include the status of the oval window, facial nerve dehiscence/prolapse, and persistent stapedial artery [13].

38.3.3 Complications of Ossicular Chain Reconstruction

A postoperative CT is necessary to evaluate the position of ossicular prostheses, assess the underlying disease progression, and identify the factors that may contribute to new or recurrent hearing loss and an abnormal audiogram. Complications involving the ossicular chain reconstruction include ossicular chain dislocation and graft necrosis, prosthetic malpositioning, and prosthetic extrusion [14]. Nonspecific opacification of the middle ear may be due to granulation tissue, fluid, or recurrent cholesteatoma, resulting in reduced mobility or dislocation of the prosthesis (Fig. 38.6b). Ossicular erosion involving incus due to necrosis or resorption may result in disarticulation of the prosthesis (Fig 38.8) [15].

The medial end of the stapes prosthesis can extend 0.25 mm into the vestibule in asymptomatic cases (Fig. 38.9). In cases with vestibular symptoms, the vestibular penetration may be considered abnormal when it exceeds 50% of the vestibule

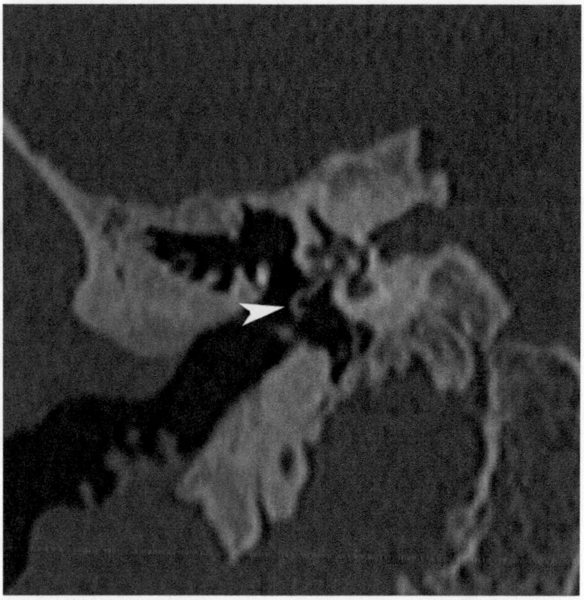

Fig. 38.8 Dislocated loop prosthesis. Coronal CT of the temporal bone shows an empty loop of the stapes prosthesis, suggesting disarticulation of the prosthesis

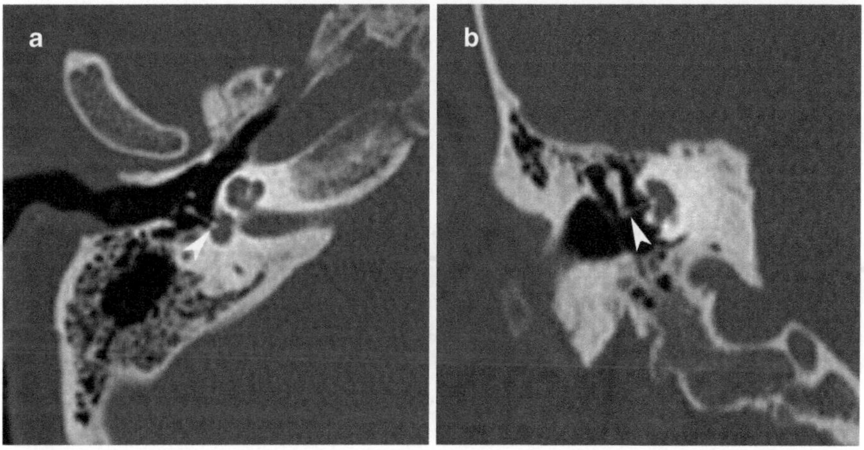

Fig. 38.9 Intravestibular protrusion of the stapes prosthesis. Axial (**a**) and coronal (**b**) CT of the temporal bone shows subtle acceptable protrusion of the stapes prosthesis into the vestibule

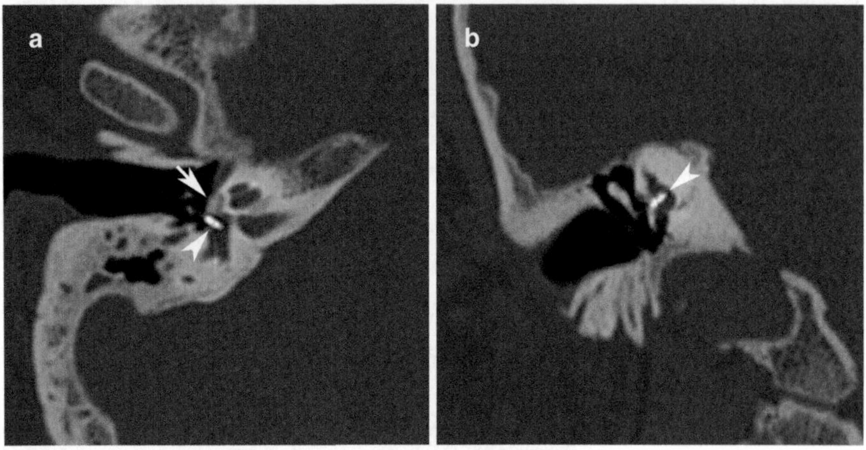

Fig. 38.10 Vestibular penetration of the stapes prosthesis. Axial (**a**) and coronal (**b**) CT of the temporal bone shows the penetration of the prosthesis into the medial aspect of the vestibule (arrowhead in **a** and **b**). Focal hypodensity in the fissula ante fenestram (arrow in **a**) suggests otosclerosis

(Fig. 38.10) [16]. Stapes prosthesis fixation, malposition, and dislocation may occur in the presence of obliterative otosclerosis and granulation tissue [17]. Other complications include labyrinthitis and perilymphatic fistula [18].

38.4 Mastoidectomy

Mastoidectomy is a surgical procedure for treating chronic middle ear infections and their complications. It provides surgical access to the facial nerve, inner ear, floor of the middle cranial fossa, and internal auditory canal. The extent of the resection depends on the involvement and may include the removal of the mastoid air cells, middle ear cavity, and ossicles.

Cortical mastoidectomy includes resection of the mastoid cortex and lateral air cells while preserving the Koerner septum [8]. It is used to treat acute or chronic mastoiditis and subperiosteal abscess, typically without extending to the mastoid antrum and epitympanum (Fig. 38.11) [19].

Canal wall-up (CWU) mastoidectomy involves resection of the mastoid cortex and air cells, including removal of the Koerner septum extending into the mastoid antrum and epitympanum (Fig. 38.12) [20]. The facial recess approach includes resection of the facial recess (between the chorda tympani nerve and the mastoid segment of the facial nerve), facilitating access to the round window and the cochlear promontory. The CWU mastoidectomy is also performed in cochlear implantation and endolymphatic sac surgery.

Canal wall-down (CWD) mastoidectomy includes resection of the posterior wall of the external auditory canal and the scutum. The surgical cavity, which involves the mastoid antrum, middle ear, and mastoid air cells, communicates with the

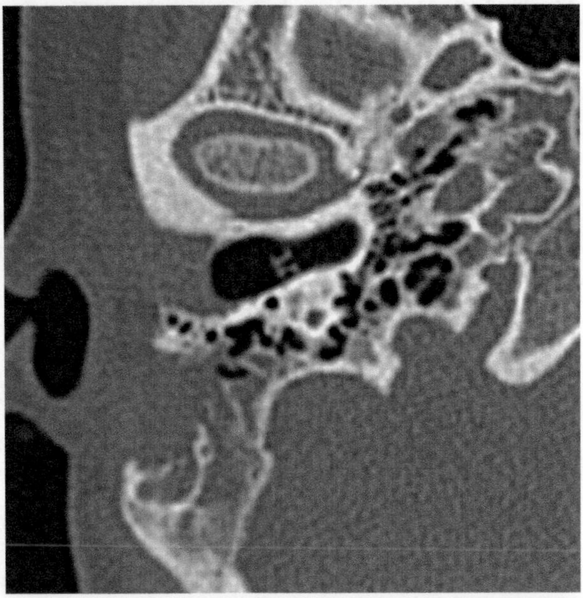

Fig. 38.11 Cortical mastoidectomy. Axial CT of the temporal bone shows resection of the lateral cortex of the mastoid temporal bone, sparing the Koerner septum and not extending into the antrum and middle ear (not shown). A partially extruded Teflon tympanostomy tube is seen in the external auditory canal

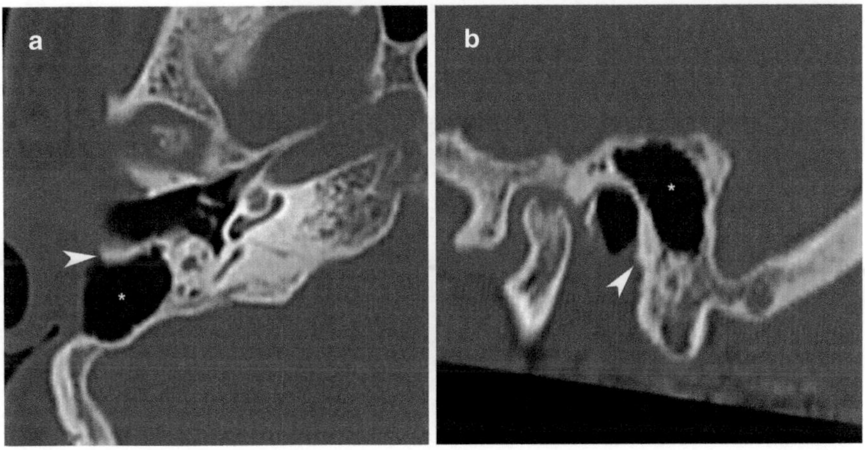

Fig. 38.12 Canal wall-up mastoidectomy. Axial (**a**) and sagittal (**b**) CT of the temporal bone shows an aerated mastoid cavity (asterisk in **a** and **b**) with the preserved posterior wall of the external auditory canal (arrowhead in **a** and **b**)

external environment through the defect in the external auditory canal (Fig. 38.13). The extensive approach enables visualization and periodic cleaning of the surgical cavity in the postoperative period. The CWD mastoidectomy can be further divided into modified radical mastoidectomy, including tympanostomy and/or ossicular chain reconstruction, and radical mastoidectomy with removal of the ossicles and preservation of stapes with no attempt for tympanic membrane or ossicular chain

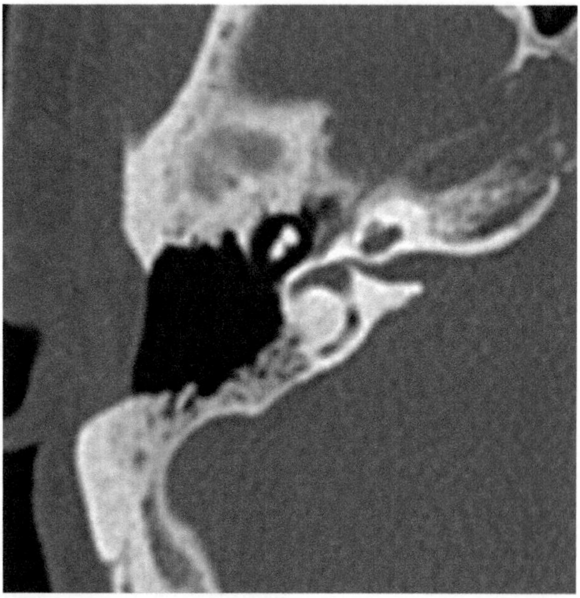

Fig. 38.13 Canal wall-down mastoidectomy. Axial CT of the temporal bone shows resection cavity and mastoid temporal bone involving the Koerner septum and extending into the mastoid antrum along with resection of the posterosuperior wall of the external auditory canal (not shown)

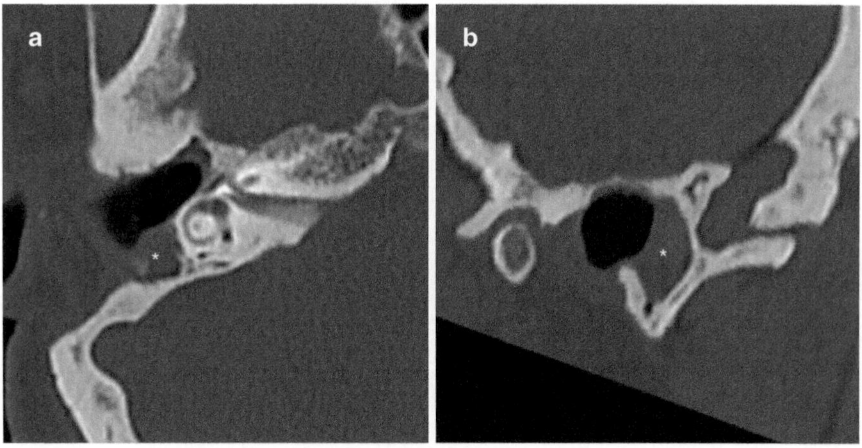

Fig. 38.14 Obliteration of the CWD mastoidectomy cavity. Axial (**a**) and sagittal (**b**) CT of the temporal bone shows nonspecific soft tissue opacification of the mastoidectomy cavity due to obliteration in the postoperative period

reconstruction. Radical mastoidectomy is reserved for tumor resection and surgical management of extensive middle ear disease [19, 20].

The obliteration of the mastoid cavity can be performed using fat, cartilage, muscle flaps, bone, or hydroxyapatite to reduce the complications associated with CWD mastoidectomy (Fig. 38.14).

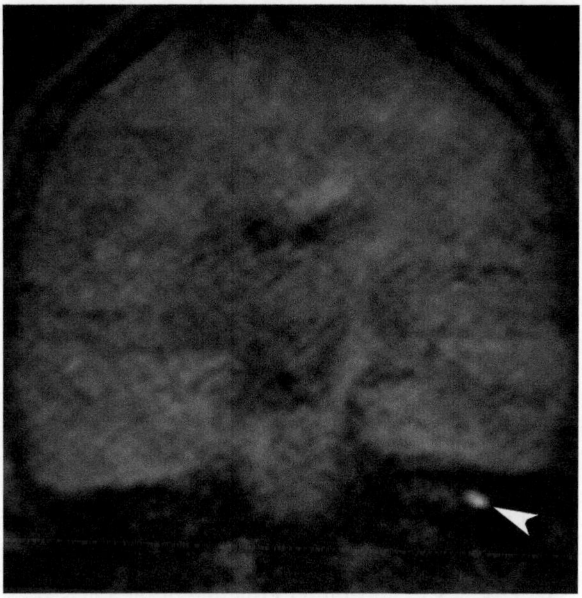

Fig. 38.15 Recurrent cholesteatoma. Coronal non-EPI diffusion of the temporal bone shows a small focal restricted diffusion in the left mastoidectomy cavity, suggesting recurrent cholesteatoma

38.4.1 Complications

The presence of a lobulated or irregular soft tissue attenuation lesion within the mastoid cavity, along with bone erosion, raises suspicion for residual or recurrent cholesteatoma. In about 20% of cases, there is a nonspecific soft tissue mass within the mastoid cavity lacking definite features on CT, which may represent inflammatory mucosa, granulation tissue, fibrosis, cholesterol granuloma, or cholesteatoma [21]. On MRI, non-EPI diffusion enables the detection of up to 3 mm cholesteatoma, distinguishing it from the inflammatory and scar tissue (Fig. 38.15) [22, 23]. The delayed postcontrast T1-weighted imaging about 30 min after contrast administration may also aid in differentiating nonspecific soft tissue mass as cholesteatoma lacks enhancement compared to other soft tissue lesions [5].

38.5 Approaches to the IAC and CP Angle

The surgical access to the internal auditory canal and the cerebellopontine angle includes the middle cranial fossa, retrosigmoid, and translabyrinthine approaches. The middle cranial fossa and retrosigmoid approaches are associated with limited access along with the possibility of preserved hearing. The translabyrinthine approach provides optimal access to the internal auditory canal and cerebellopontine angle cistern, invariably leading to postsurgical hearing loss. The presurgical evaluation assesses factors associated with limiting surgical access to IAC (high-riding jugular bulb and jugular diverticulum), CSF leak (pneumatization of the posterior wall of the IAC), and technical difficulty during cortical mastoidectomy and suboccipital craniotomy (sigmoid sinus variations) [24, 25].

38.5.1 Middle Cranial Fossa Approach

The middle cranial fossa approach is usually performed for small schwannomas (<1.5 cm) restricted to the internal auditory canal, superior semicircular canal dehiscence repair, temporal lobe encephaloceles involving the floor of the middle cranial fossa, and access to lesions affecting the labyrinthine and tympanic segments of the facial nerve (Figs. 38.16 and 38.17) [26, 27]. A temporal craniotomy is performed initially, followed by elevation of the temporal lobe from the middle cranial fossa to expose the tegmen and the internal auditory canal. The surgical defect in the floor of the cranial fossa is reconstructed using fascia, muscle and bone grafts, hydroxyapatite, and titanium mesh.

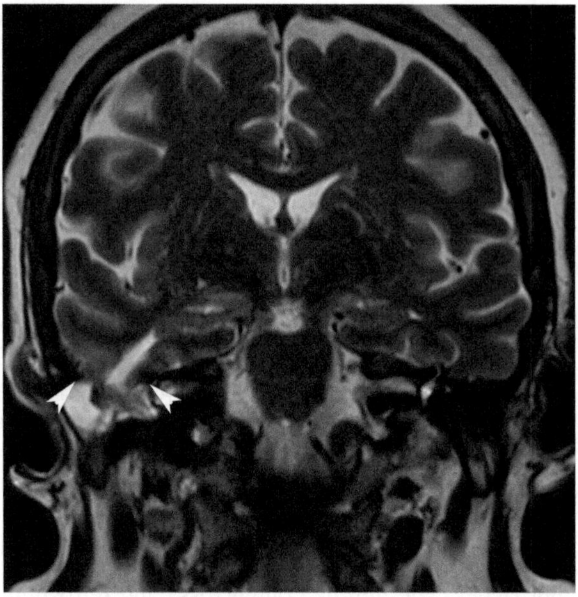

Fig. 38.16 Right temporal encephalocele. Coronal T2-weighted MR image shows a large defect in the tegmen with gliosis and herniation of the inferior temporal gyrus in keeping with temporal encephalocele

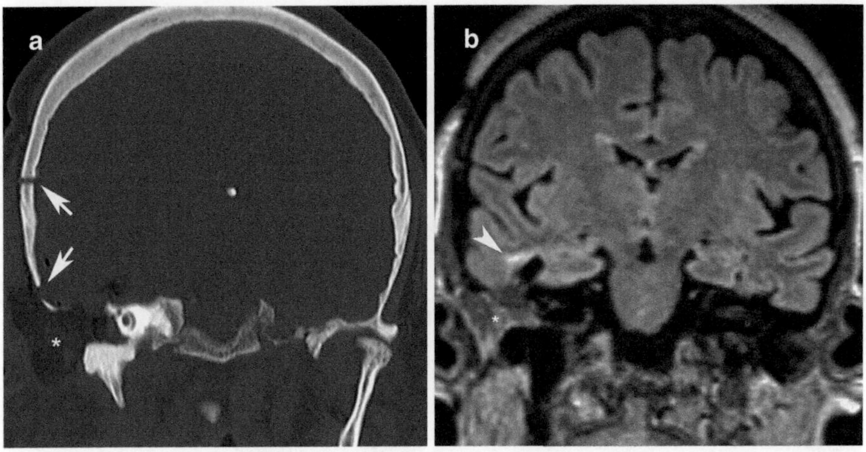

Fig. 38.17 Middle cranial fossa approach and mastoidectomy. Coronal CT (**a**) and FLAIR (**b**) images of the right temporal bone show postsurgical changes from right temporal craniotomy for placement of the temporalis fascia graft (arrowhead in **a**) with a mastoidectomy defect filled with fat graft (asterisk in **a** and **b**) for encephalocele repair

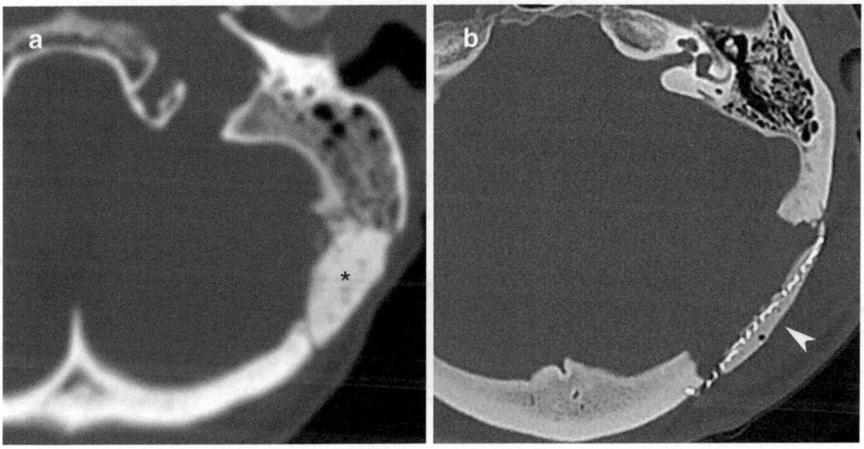

Fig. 38.18 Retrosigmoid approach. Axial CT of the temporal bone (**a**) shows left retrosigmoid mastoidectomy (asterisk) with opacification of the left mastoid air cells. Axial CT of the temporal bone (**b**) shows left retrosigmoid mastoidectomy with mesh tympanoplasty (arrowhead in **b**)

38.5.2 Retrosigmoid Approach

The retrosigmoid approach includes suboccipital craniotomy posterior to the sigmoid sinus, retraction of the anterior aspect of the cerebellum, and resection of the posterior wall of the internal auditory canal to provide access to the canalicular segment of the facial and vestibulocochlear nerves (Fig. 38.18) [27, 28]. The retrosigmoid approach is typically performed to resect the vestibular schwannomas, CP angle meningiomas, and epidermoid cysts.

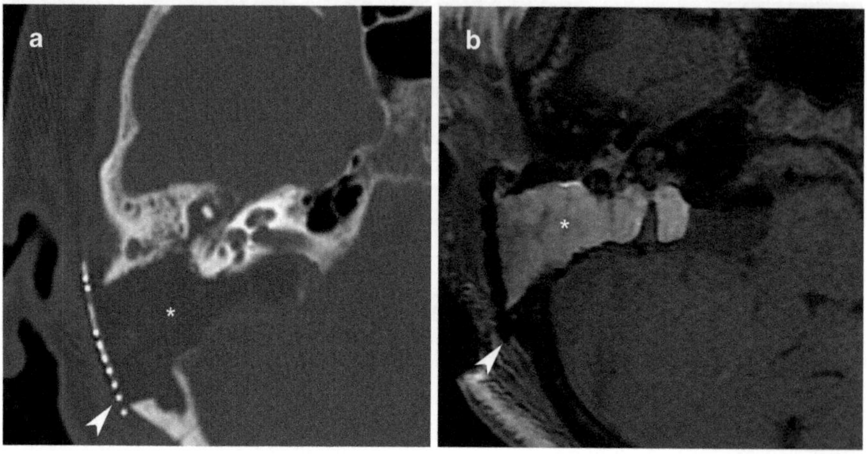

Fig. 38.19 Translabyrinthine approach. Axial CT (**a**) and axial T1-weighted MRI (**b**) images show right translabyrinthine mastoidectomy with mesh tympanoplasty (arrowhead in **a** and **b**) and fat graft (asterisk in **a** and **b**) obliterating the surgical cavity

38.5.3 Translabyrinthine Approach

The translabyrinthine approach includes CWU mastoidectomy anterior to the sigmoid sinus, followed by resection of the semicircular canals and the posterior wall of the internal auditory canal to access the facial and vestibulocochlear nerves (Fig. 38.19) [21, 27, 28]. The translabyrinthine approach is performed for intralabyrinthine and translabyrinthine schwannomas in cases with hearing loss. The surgical cavity is obliterated using fat, bone powder, fascia, or fibrin glue to prevent CSF leak.

38.5.4 Postsurgical Imaging and Complications

Magnetic resonance imaging using fat-suppressed postcontrast T1-weighted images enables differentiation between the fat graft and possible residual/recurrent tumor. The typical findings in the immediate postsurgical period include thin linear enhancement along the IAC margins and labyrinthine enhancement, typically after the translabyrinthine approach [13, 20, 28]. However, labyrinthine enhancement after the middle cranial fossa and retrosigmoid approach is usually due to inflammation, vascular injury, or labyrinthine fenestration. The presence of nodular or mass-like enhancement and increased enhancement within the resection cavity on follow-up concerns residual or recurrent tumors.

The surgical complications include the temporal lobe and cerebellar injury due to the retraction, intracranial hemorrhage, and infarction due to vascular injury, fat graft necrosis, and transverse sinus or jugular vein thrombosis (Figs. 38.20, 38.21, and 38.22) [13, 20, 28]. The retrosigmoid approach is potentially associated with the risk of CSF leak, and the translabyrinthine approach invariably leads to labyrinthitis ossificans (Fig. 38.23) [13, 20, 28].

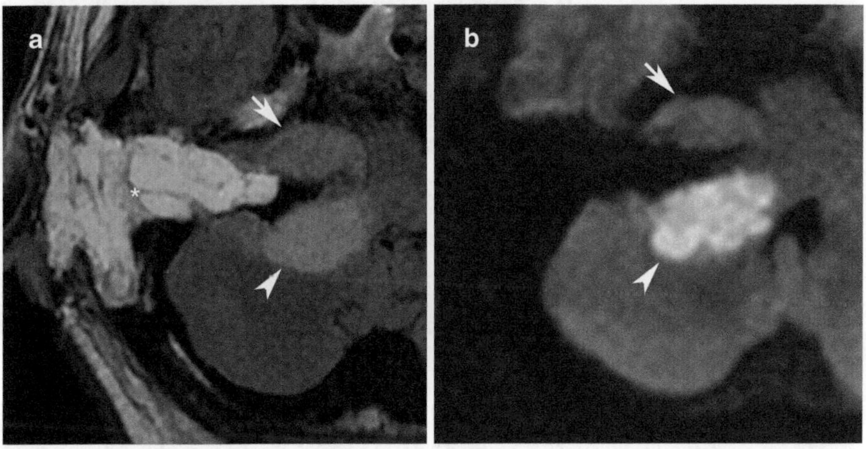

Fig. 38.20 Cerebellar infarction. Axial T2 FLAIR (**a**) and diffusion-weighted images (**b**) show right translabyrinthine mastoidectomy with fat graft. A residual tumor is seen in the right CP angle cistern (arrow in **a** and **b**) and right AICA territory infarction (arrowhead in **a** and **b**)

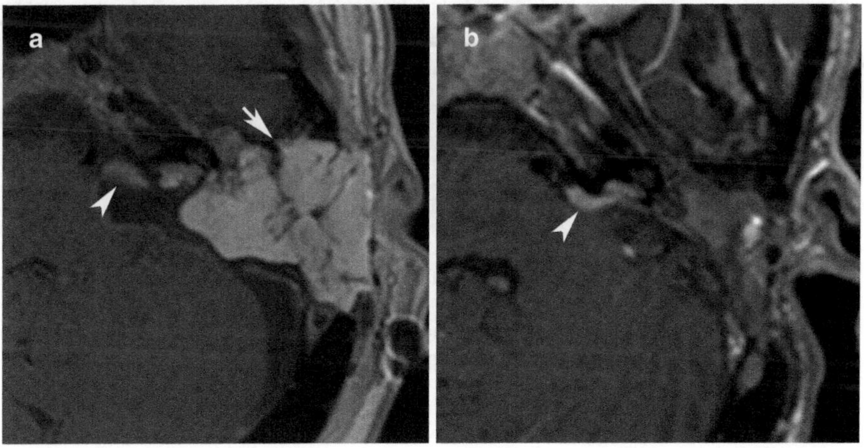

Fig. 38.21 Fat graft necrosis. Axial postcontrast T1-weighted images (**a**, **b**) show a residual tumor (arrowhead in **a** and **b**) and fat graft obliterating the translabyrinthine mastoidectomy cavity (arrow in **a**), with significantly decreased fat on follow up study within the resection cavity, suggesting fat graft necrosis

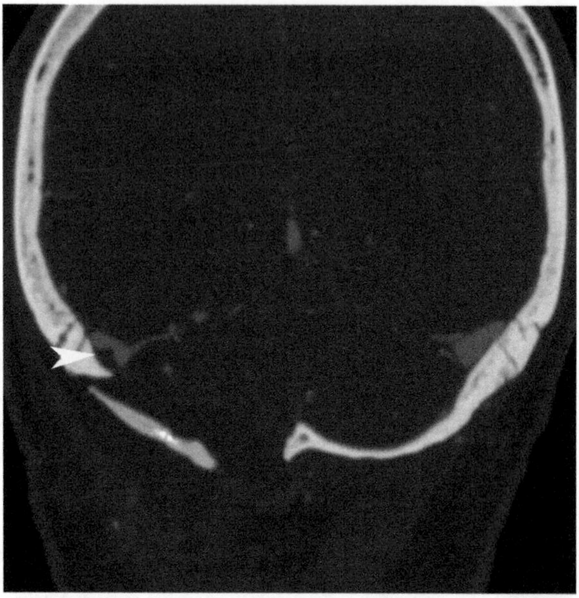

Fig. 38.22 Sigmoid sinus thrombosis. Coronal postcontrast CT image after the right retrosigmoid approach demonstrates an eccentric nonocclusive filling defect in the lateral aspect of the right sigmoid sinus

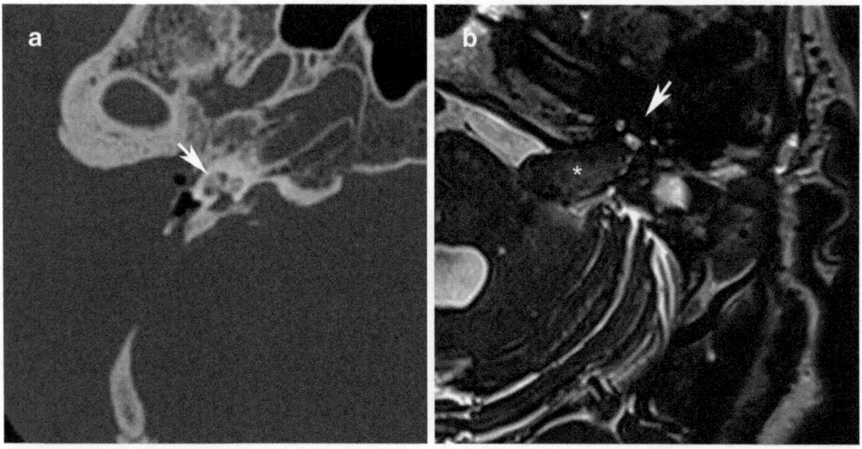

Fig. 38.23 Labyrinthitis ossificans. Axial CT of the temporal bone (**a**) shows hyperdensity in the apical and middle turns of the cochlea after translabyrinthine mastoidectomy. Axial heavily T2-weighted image of the temporal bone (**b**) shows a residual tumor in the left CP angle cistern (asterisk) along with T2 hypointensity (arrow) and loss of normal in the apical and middle turns of the cochlea, suggesting labyrinthitis ossificans

38.6 Transcutaneous Bone Conduction Implants (TBCI)

The transcutaneous bone conduction implants are classified as passive, i.e., bone-anchored hearing aid (BAHA) and active transcutaneous bone conduction implants (Bonebridge and Osia devices) [29, 30]. The passive transcutaneous devices consist of an external processor, the abutment, and the fixture (Fig. 38.24). The detachable external processor transmits the sound to the inner ear through the bone via the socket and the titanium screw fixture that is firmly anchored to the bone by osseointegration. Bonebridge BCI 601 and 602 use bone conduction transducers communicating via electromagnetic induction (Fig. 38.25), and the Osia ear is based on a piezoelectric transducer using a digital radiofrequency link, benefiting high-frequency hearing. Passive transcutaneous devices are associated with inferior audiological outcomes due to the scalp and soft tissue attenuation of the sound, along with an overall increased complication rate of 24.4-26.6 % compared to 11.8 % for active transcutaneous bone conduction implants .

The indications for transcutaneous bone conduction implants include congenital, infectious, and inflammatory causes associated with severe unilateral or bilateral conductive or mixed hearing loss and single-sided sensorineural deafness with functioning cochlea. Presurgical planning is necessary to evaluate the temporal bone thickness, proximity to the dura and sigmoid sinus, skin and soft tissue thickness, and prior mastoid surgeries. The preferred implant insertion site and calvarial thickness necessary for optimal bone drilling vary depending on the choice of transcutaneous bone conduction implants, as described in Table 38.2.

Postsurgical complications may include violation of the dura or sigmoid sinus during bone drilling, leading to bleeding; venous sinus thrombosis; extra-axial hemorrhage; CSF leaks; infectious complications such as soft tissue abscess, meningitis, and cerebritis; and reduced hearing outcome (Fig. 38.26). The delayed

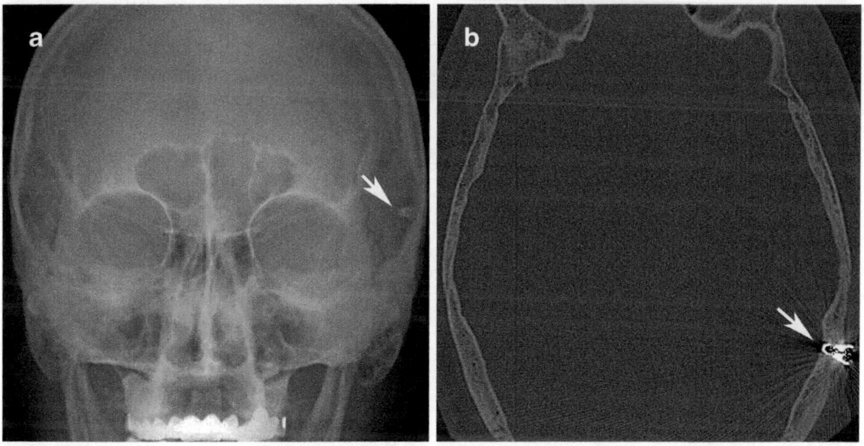

Fig. 38.24 Bone-anchored hearing aid. Frontal radiograph of the skull (**a**) and axial CT of the temporal bone (**b**) demonstrate an implant in the left temporoparietal region

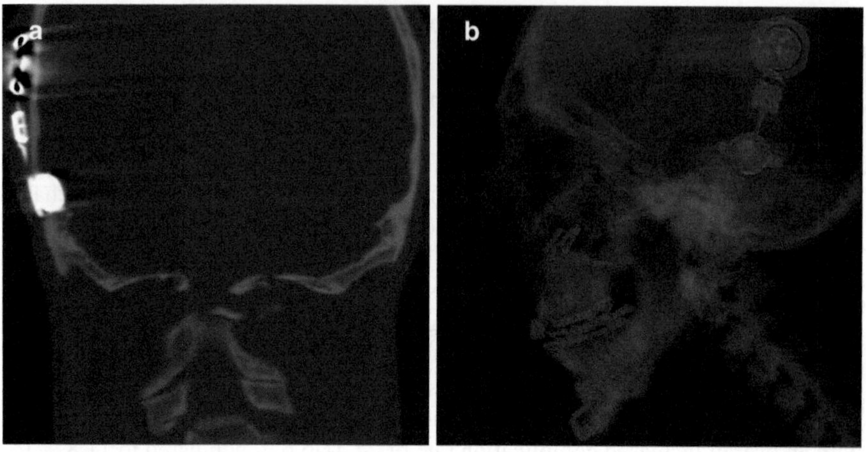

Fig. 38.25 Bonebridge active TBCI. Coronal CT of the temporal bone (**a**) and reconstructed image of prostheses overlying the calvarium (**b**) demonstrating Bonebridge bone conduction implant

Table 38.2 Calvarial thickness and device placement in transcutaneous bone conduction implants

Device	Calvarial thickness	Preferred site
Bone-anchored hearing aid	3–3.5 mm	Posterior to the temporoparietal suture—5–5.5 cm behind the external auditory canal
Bonebridge BCI 601	8.7 mm	Sinodural angle or retrosigmoid placement
Bonebridge BCI 602	4.5 mm	Sinodural angle or retrosigmoid placement
Osia device	3–4 mm	Based on cortical thickness, anatomical complexity, and position of the dura

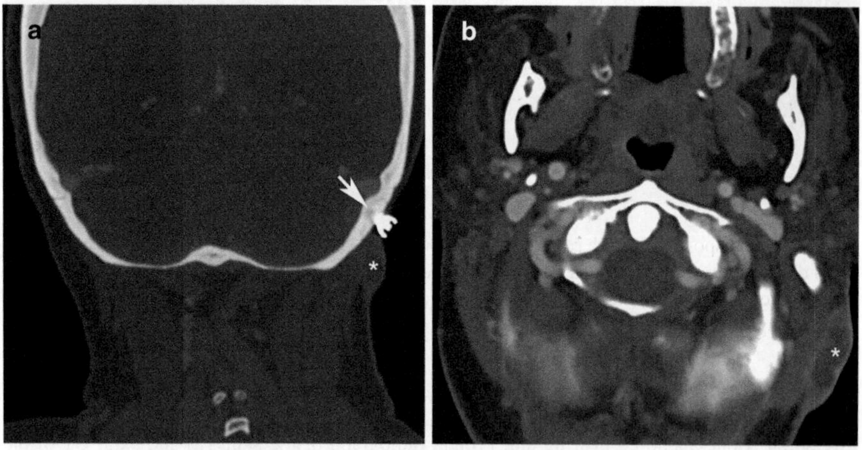

Fig. 38.26 Retromastoid abscess. Coronal (**a**) and axial (**b**) CT images of the temporal bone show a BAHA implant (arrow in a) with rim-enhancing subcutaneous collection in the left retromastoid region (asterisk in **a**, **b**)

complications include failure of osseointegration, idiopathic bone resorption, and rarely bone overgrowth.

38.7 Cochlear Implantation

A cochlear implant is an electronic device that directly stimulates the spiral ganglion cells of the cochlear nerve, bypassing the damaged hair cells in the organ of Corti. The external components process the sound waves into an electrical signal, including the microphone and battery, speech processor, external magnet, and transmitter antenna, and send the impulses to the receiver transmitter. The internal components include an internal magnet, antenna coil, receiver transmitter, electrode lead, and array (Fig. 38.27). The reference electrode calibrates the electrode array and functions as a grounding electrode. It is within the receiver transmitter or as a separate electrode beneath the temporalis muscle [31].

The first step in cochlear implant surgery involves a canal wall-up mastoidectomy, followed by posterior tympanotomy and a facial recess approach to provide access to the middle ear. Preferably, the round window access to the cochlea is considered over round window cochleostomy to preserve any residual hearing as it allows for easier insertion into the scala tympani, minimizes damage to the hair cells and osseous spiral lamina, and prevents displacement of bony fragments into the cochlea. A subperiosteal pocket is created in the outer table of the mastoid temporal bone for the receiver-stimulator component [31].

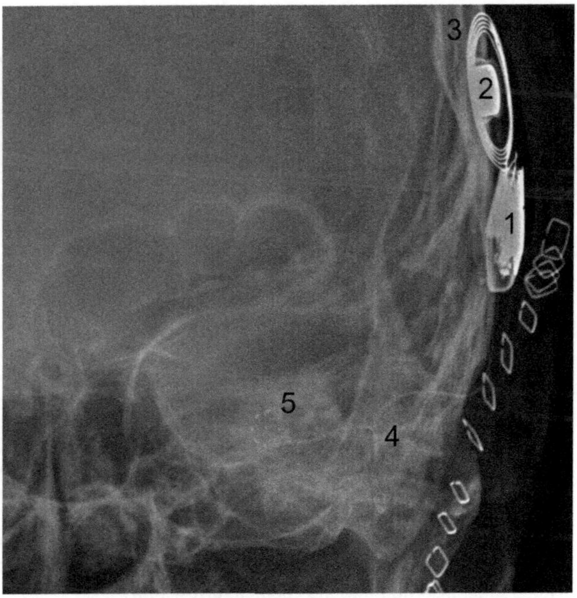

Fig. 38.27 Cochlear implant. Modified Stenvers view of the temporal bone shows a left cochlear implant with a receiver transmitter (1), magnet (2), antenna coil (3), intramastoid course of the electrode lead (4), and intracochlear electrode array (5)

The modified endomeatal and suprameatal approaches can be utilized in cases with a small mastoid cavity, anomalous facial nerve course, and decreased facial recess width. In cases with excessive bone covering of the round window, drilling the bone to expose the round window membrane may be necessary. A middle or apical cochleostomy may be considered when the otospongiotic plaques and calcification involve the round window. In cases with suspected mastoiditis, cholesteatoma, and an increased risk of CSF leak, a subtotal petrosectomy may be needed for wider resection and access.

Postoperative imaging ensures proper placement of the implanted electrode for improved programming accuracy, frequency allocation, and deactivation of extra cochlear electrodes (Fig. 38.28). The location of the first electrode is usually within 3 mm from the round window opening (Fig. 38.29). The immediate postsurgical complications include scala vestibuli insertion, scalar translocation, and over-insertion (more than 3 mm beyond the round window) (Fig. 38.30). An under-inserted electrode array may be seen in patients with otosclerosis, labyrinthitis ossificans, and neurofibromatosis type II. An earlier revision surgery should be performed for under-inserted electrodes before healing and scar formation.

Electrode-related complications include pinching, tip and basal fold-over, and malpositioning in the tympanic cavity, internal auditory canal, vestibule, and semicircular canals, and rarely into the carotid canal and eustachian tube [32]. Late complications encountered after the immediate postsurgical period include electrode migration due to loss of support, movement, and tension, recurrent otitis media, cholesteatoma and labyrinthitis, fibrosis, and delayed nerve injury [32].

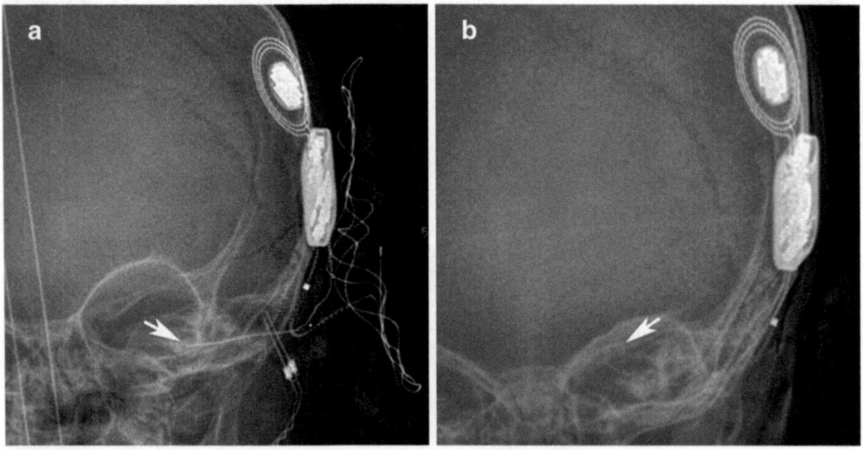

Fig. 38.28 Intraoperative fluoroscopy for cochlear implantation. Modified Stenvers view of the left temporal bone (**a**, **b**) shows the medial end of the electrode array in the middle ear (arrow in **a**) with gradual insertion into the cochlea (arrow in **b**)

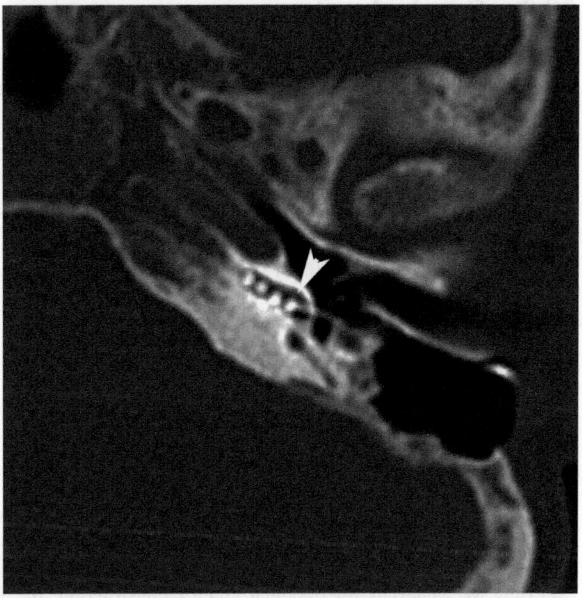

Fig. 38.29 Normal electrode position. Axial CT of the left temporal bone shows the optimal position of the first electrode in the basal turn of the cochlea medial to the round window (arrowhead)

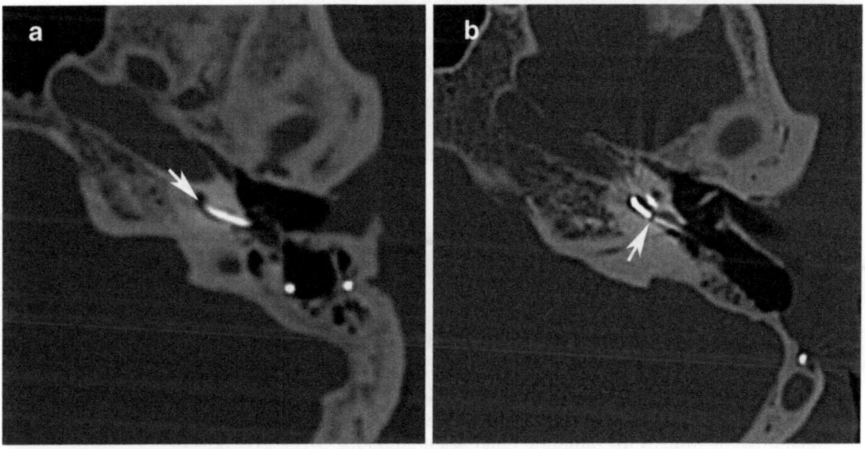

Fig. 38.30 Cochlear implant over-insertion. Axial CT of the left temporal bone (**a**, **b**) shows a lack of an electrode in the inferior aspect of the basal turn of the cochlea beyond 3 mm from the round window

38.8 Conclusion

An adequate understanding of the neurotological surgical techniques and expected imaging findings is essential to diagnose recurrent disease and postsurgical complications. CT is optimal for assessing the position and continuity of the reconstructed ossicular chain and opacification of the mastoidectomy cavity. MRI is necessary to identify recurrent cholesteatoma and follow-up after schwannoma resection to assess residual or recurrent tumors.

References

1. Rosenfeld RM, Tunkel DE, Schwartz SR, Anne S, Bishop CE, Chelius DC, et al. Clinical practice guideline: tympanostomy tubes in children (update). Otolaryngol Head Neck Surg. 2022;166:S1–55.
2. Michel M, Nahas G, Preciado D. Retained tympanostomy tubes: who, what, when, why, and how to treat? Ear Nose Throat J. 2020;145561320950490:014556132095049.
3. Wullstein H. Theory and practice of tympanoplasty. Laryngoscope. 1956;66:1076–93.
4. Yung M. Materials for ossicular chain reconstruction. In: Hildmann H, Sudhoff H, editors. Middle ear surgery [Internet]. Berlin, Heidelberg: Springer; 2006 [cited 2024 Oct 1]. p. 55–61. Available from: https://doi.org/10.1007/978-3-540-47671-9_12.
5. Williams MT, Ayache D. Imaging of the post-operative middle ear. Eur Radiol. 2004;14:482–95.
6. Swartz JD, Lansman AK, Berger AS, Wolfson RJ, Bell G, Popky GL, et al. Stapes prosthesis: evaluation with CT. Radiology. 1986;158:179–82.
7. Wehrs RE. Incus interposition and ossiculoplasty with hydroxyapatite prostheses. Otolaryngol Clin N Am. 1994;27:677–88.
8. Mukherji SK, Mancuso AA, Kotzur IM, Slattery WH, Swartz JD, Tart RP, et al. CT of the temporal bone: findings after mastoidectomy, ossicular reconstruction, and cochlear implantation. AJR Am J Roentgenol. 1994;163:1467–71.
9. Goldenberg RA. Ossiculoplasty with composite prostheses. PORP and TORP. Otolaryngol Clin N Am. 1994;27:727–45.
10. Kartush JM. Ossicular chain reconstruction. Capitulum to malleus. Otolaryngol Clin N Am. 1994;27:689–715.
11. Shea JJ. Forty years of stapes surgery. Am J Otol. 1998;19:52–5.
12. Bailey HA, Pappas JJ, Graham SS. Small fenestra stapedectomy technique: reducing risk and improving hearing. Otolaryngol Head Neck Surg. 1983;91:516–20.
13. Tames HLVC, Padula M, Sarpi MO, Gomes RLE, Toyama C, Murakoshi RW, et al. Post-operative imaging of the temporal bone. Radiographics. 2021;41:858–75.
14. Stone JA, Mukherji SK, Jewett BS, Carrasco VN, Castillo M. CT evaluation of prosthetic ossicular reconstruction procedures: what the otologist needs to know. Radiographics. 2000;20:593–605.
15. Langman AW, Lindeman RC. Revision stapedectomy. Laryngoscope. 1993;103:954–8.
16. Rangheard AS, Marsot-Dupuch K, Mark AS, Meyer B, Tubiana JM. Post-operative complications in otospongiosis: usefulness of MR imaging. AJNR Am J Neuroradiol. 2001;22:1171–8.
17. Seicshnaydre MA, Sismanis A, Hughes GB. Update of reparative granuloma: survey of the American Otological Society and the American Neurotology Society. Am J Otol. 1994;15:155–60.
18. Bordure P, Legent F, Calais C, Loheac D, Beauvillain C. Pneumolabyrinth and perilymphatic fistula after stapedectomy. Ann Otolaryngol Chir Cervico-Fac. 1990;107:359–62.

19. Bennett M, Warren F, Haynes D. Indications and technique in mastoidectomy. Otolaryngol Clin N Am. 2006;39:1095–113.
20. Penta M, Pinho MC, Isaacson B, Kutz JW, Perez CL. Postsurgical temporal bone: a pictorial essay of commonly encountered neuro-otologic surgical approaches and post-operative imaging appearance. Neurographics. 2016;6:138–50.
21. Juliano AF, Ginat DT, Moonis G. Imaging review of the temporal bone: part II. Traumatic, post-operative, and noninflammatory nonneoplastic conditions. Radiology. 2015;276:655–72.
22. De Foer B, Vercruysse J-P, Bernaerts A, Deckers F, Pouillon M, Somers T, et al. Detection of post-operative residual cholesteatoma with non-echo-planar diffusion-weighted magnetic resonance imaging. Otol Neurotol. 2008;29:513–7.
23. Schwartz KM, Lane JI, Bolster BD, Neff BA. The utility of diffusion-weighted imaging for cholesteatoma evaluation. AJNR Am J Neuroradiol. 2011;32:430–6.
24. Jackler RK, Pitts LH. Selection of surgical approach to acoustic neuroma. 1992. Neurosurg Clin N Am. 2008;19:217–38. vi
25. Lin EP, Crane BT. The management and imaging of vestibular schwannomas. AJNR Am J Neuroradiol. 2017;38:2034–43.
26. Jackler RK. Chapter 66. Neurotologic skull base surgery. In: Lalwani AK, editor. Current diagnosis & treatment in otolaryngology—head & neck surgery [Internet]. 3rd ed. New York: The McGraw-Hill Companies; 2012 [cited 2024 Oct 1]. Available from: accesssurgery.mhmedical.com/content.aspx?aid=55773108.
27. Silk PS, Lane JI, Driscoll CL. Surgical approaches to vestibular schwannomas: what the radiologist needs to know. Radiographics. 2009;29:1955–70.
28. Ginat DT, Martuza RL. Postoperative imaging of vestibular schwannomas. Neurosurg Focus. 2012;33:E18.
29. Willenborg K, Lenarz T, Busch S. Surgical and audiological outcomes with a new transcutaneous bone conduction device with reduced transducer thickness in children. Eur Arch Otorrinolaringol. 2023;280:4381–9.
30. Gaffney PJ, Ahmad JG, Gong SW, Kaul VF. Implantable devices in otolaryngology: pediatric application of active bone conduction devices. Curr Otorhinolaryngol Rep. 2024;12:82–9.
31. Hiremath SB, Biswas A, Mndebele G, Schramm D, Ertl-Wagner BB, Blaser SI, et al. Cochlear implantation: systematic approach to preoperative radiologic evaluation. Radiographics. 2023;43:e220102.
32. Widmann G, Dejaco D, Luger A, Schmutzhard J. Pre- and post-operative imaging of cochlear implants: a pictorial review. Insights Imaging. 2020;11:1–20.

Further Reading

Bhatt PR, Alyono JC, Fischbein NJ, Penta M. Imaging of the postoperative temporal bone. Neuroimaging Clin N Am. 2022;32(1):175–92.

Ginat DT, Martuza RL. Postoperative imaging of vestibular schwannomas. Neurosurg Focus. 2012;33(3):E18.

Stone JA, Mukherji SK, Jewett BS, Carrasco VN, Castillo M. CT evaluation of prosthetic ossicular reconstruction procedures: what the otologist needs to know. Radiographics. 2000;20(3):593–605.

Tames HLVC, Padula M, Sarpi MO, Gomes RLE, Toyama C, Murakoshi RW, Olivetti BC, Gebrim EMMS. Post-operative imaging of the temporal bone. Radiographics. 2021;41(3):858–75.

Widmann G, Dejaco D, Luger A, Schmutzhard J. Pre- and post-operative imaging of cochlear implants: a pictorial review. Insights Imaging. 2020;11(1):93.

GPSR Compliance

The European Union's (EU) General Product Safety Regulation (GPSR) is a set of rules that requires consumer products to be safe and our obligations to ensure this.

If you have any concerns about our products, you can contact us on ProductSafety@springernature.com

In case Publisher is established outside the EU, the EU authorized representative is:

Springer Nature Customer Service Center GmbH
Europaplatz 3
69115 Heidelberg, Germany

Batch number: 10732090

Printed by Printforce, the Netherlands